Principles and Applications of Nanotherapeutics

This book covers a vast range of information regarding nanotherapeutics, including knowledge based on fundamentals, history and progress, applications, practical aspects and examples, and prospects of nanotherapeutics. It includes the fundamentals of nanotherapeutics, including mechanisms and theories behind the phenomena, summarizing various approaches of nanotherapeutics in the field of medicine. By considering the emerging pandemics and other issues regarding public health, the timely need for novel solutions is also described.

Features:

- Provides a comprehensive knowledge on fundamentals, applications, current situations, and ongoing research in nanotherapeutics.
- Highlights the practical aspects and prospects to enhance the use of nanotherapeutics in the health field.
- Illustrates the significance of using nanotherapeutics in futuristic life.
- Discusses sustainable resolutions to issues in public health.
- Explores the latest implementations and merits of the fields supported by pertinent examples.

This book is aimed at undergraduate, graduate students, and researchers in drug delivery, gene and cancer therapy, biomedical engineering, and nanotechnology.

Emerging Materials and Technologies

Series Editor: Boris I. Kharissov

The *Emerging Materials and Technologies* series is devoted to highlighting publications centered on emerging advanced materials and novel technologies. Attention is paid to those newly discovered or applied materials with potential to solve pressing societal problems and improve quality of life, corresponding to environmental protection, medicine, communications, energy, transportation, advanced manufacturing, and related areas.

The series takes into account that, under present strong demands for energy, material, and cost savings, as well as heavy contamination problems and worldwide pandemic conditions, the area of emerging materials and related scalable technologies is a highly interdisciplinary field, with the need for researchers, professionals, and academics across the spectrum of engineering and technological disciplines. The main objective of this book series is to attract more attention to these materials and technologies and invite conversation among the international R&D community.

Impedance Spectroscopy and its Application in Biological Detection
Edited by Geeta Bhatt, Manoj Bhatt and Shantanu Bhattacharya

Nanofillers for Sustainable Applications
Edited by N.M Nurazzi, E. Bayraktar, M.N.F. Norrrahim, H.A. Aisyah, N. Abdullah, and M.R.M. Asyraf

Chemistry of Dehydrogenation Reactions and its Applications
Edited by Syed Shahabuddin, Rama Gaur and Nandini Mukherjee

Biosorbents
Diversity, Bioprocessing, and Applications
Edited by Pramod Kumar Mahish, Dakeshwar Kumar Verma and Shailesh Kumar Jadhav

Principles and Applications of Nanotherapeutics
Imalka Munaweera and Piumika Yapa

For more information about this series, please visit: www.routledge.com/ Emerging-Materials-and-Technologies/book-series/CRCEMT

Principles and Applications of Nanotherapeutics

Imalka Munaweera and Piumika Yapa

CRC Press
Taylor & Francis Group
Boca Raton London New York

CRC Press is an imprint of the
Taylor & Francis Group, an **informa** business

Designed cover image: © Shutterstock

First edition published 2024
by CRC Press
2385 NW Executive Center Drive, Suite 320, Boca Raton FL 33431

and by CRC Press
4 Park Square, Milton Park, Abingdon, Oxon, OX14 4RN

CRC Press is an imprint of Taylor & Francis Group, LLC

ISBN: 978-1-032-53875-4 (hbk)
ISBN: 978-1-032-58034-0 (pbk)
ISBN: 978-1-003-44220-2 (ebk)

DOI: 10.1201/9781003442202

Typeset in Times
by Apex CoVantage, LLC

Contents

Preface

Nanotechnology is an emerging field of technology in the twenty-first century that allows for a variety of solutions to challenges in numerous fields. It manipulates the characteristics of materials within a unique range that give rise to the special features of nanoparticles resulting in an ability of super performance. In the field of medicine, nanotherapeutics is a revolutionary idea that refers to the use of nanomaterials as medicinal remedies for a variety of diseases and circumstances that are associated with diseases, such as diagnostics and monitoring aids.

This book will disseminate knowledge based on the fundamentals, history and progress, applications, practical aspects and examples, and prospects of the field of nanotherapeutics. The goal of doing so is to delve more deeply into the field of nanotherapeutics.

New research on nanotherapeutics will be accelerated as a result of the findings of various research projects, as well as the benefits and drawbacks of specific applications, implementations, and rates of success. Additionally, this will open up new horizons for unresolved issues in the realm of public health. This book will present information that is up to date for relevant parties that are engaging in this notion in order to make it a reality. As a result of this, this book is suitable for use not only as a textbook for undergraduate and graduate students, but also as a reference book for researchers working in the pharmaceutical industry, biotechnology, nanotechnology, biomaterials, medicine, and bioengineering, among other fields.

My expectation is that the material presented in this book will be sufficient to provide an understanding of nanotherapeutics and their applications in a variety of fields, including diagnostic agents, monitoring therapies, drug discovery and development, drug delivery, gene therapy, cancer therapy, surgery, orthopedics, non-communicable diseases, infectious diseases, global sanitary issues, and so on. The references at the end of each chapter will allow readers to dive further into specific topics and see specific examples.

Dr. Imalka Munaweera

About the Authors

Dr. Imalka Munaweera is Senior Lecturer in the Department of Chemistry at the University of Sri Jayewardenepura in Sri Lanka. She has over 15+ years of research experience in the field of nanotechnology and its applications, and more than ten years of teaching experience in nanotechnology, application of nanotechnology, inorganic chemistry, polymer chemistry, and instrumental analysis. She obtained her Ph.D. in Chemistry from the University of Texas at Dallas, Richardson, TX, United States in 2015. She has served as Assistant Professor of Chemistry at Prairie View A&M University, Prairie View, TX, United States, and was a postdoctoral researcher at the University of Texas Southwestern Medical Center, Dallas, TX, United States. Her research interests are nanotechnology for drug delivery/pharmaceutical applications, agricultural applications, and water purification applications. She also pursues research toward development of nanomaterials from natural resources for various industrial applications. She has authored many publications in indexed journals and is also an inventor of US-granted patents (licensed and commercialized), international patents, and Sri Lankan-granted patents related to nanoscience and nanotechnology-based research. Furthermore, she is a recipient of many awards related to nanoscience and nanotechnology research. She is a winner of the 2021 OWSD-Elsevier foundation award for early-career women scientists in the developing world for her research contribution to the nanotechnology-related projects.

Ms. Piumika Yapa is a graduate research assistant. She obtained her Bachelor's degree in Pharmacy and Pharmaceutical Sciences from the University of Sri Jayewardenepura, Sri Lanka. Currently, she is working toward a sustainable future through nanotechnology-based findings. Her research interests include nanotechnology, nanomedicine, nanopharmaceuticals, material sciences, and microbiology. She is engaged in generating new research ideas and devising feasible solutions to broadly relevant problems.

Introduction

As a result of recent developments in the realm of nanotechnology, the study of nano-therapeutics has become an extremely popular subject among researchers and pharmaceutical industry professionals. When compared to more conventional approaches to medical care, nanotherapeutics have been shown to be superior in terms of performance. Several benefits entice people to focus on finding answers to public health issues. However, there is only a limited amount of information available regarding nanotherapeutics and the developments in the field. Because of this, additional advancements and developments in this sector have become more difficult, and as a result, there may be a dearth of innovations in this subject as a direct consequence of this.

Nanotherapeutics traced back to the ancient eras when colloidal gold was used as a medicine. Since then, nanotherapeutics has achieved many breakthroughs, and today, it is a goal of many scientists in the fight against new pandemic threats. Therefore, this information may help to spread the knowledge based on nanotherapeutics among the population who is interested in this field without barriers in access to the relevant information.

This book provides a broad overview of information pertaining to nanotherapeutics, including knowledge based on fundamentals, history and progress, applications, practical elements and examples, and the prospects of nanotherapeutics. Fundamentals of nanotherapeutics will explain the mechanisms and theories behind the phenomena. Moreover, future prospects of nanotherapeutics enable the research interests of young scientists toward nanotherapeutics and accelerate drug entities to resolve public health concerns that have become a serious threat globally.

The book offers comprehensive coverage of the most essential topics:

1. Provides a comprehensive knowledge on fundamentals, applications, current situation and ongoing research, latest implementations and merits of nanotherapeutics to gain manufacturing advantages, medical benefits, environmental effects and economic issues, and risk assessment on humans.
2. Highlights the practical aspects and prospects in order to enhance the use of nanotherapeutics in health field.
3. Discusses in detail the significance of using nanotherapeutics in futuristic life with appropriate examples.
4. Provides novel research ideas through the information to scientists in order to find sustainable resolutions to issues in public health matters.
5. Fulfills the timely need of an up-to-date book that covers emerging trends and all aspects of nanotherapeutics, including fundamentals, applications, implementations, practical examples (Failures and success), and future prospects.

DOI: 10.1201/9781003442202-1

In summary, the proposed book gives comprehensive and up-to-date information on nanotherapeutics that will help to win hurdles in this field and that knowledge will lead to new chapters in medical and health fields regarding the sustainable and economic solutions for latest health concerns.

1 Introduction to Nanotherapeutics

1.1 DEFINITION OF NANOTHERAPEUTICS

Nanotechnology has influenced healthcare tactics in the modern era and is expected to have a significant impact on the provision of better healthcare services. Nanotherapeutics have developed into a gold mine in the world of pharmaceuticals and medicine that is also owed to a number of achievements at the intersection of nanotechnology and medicine. Nanotherapeutics, which operate at the level of individual molecules or molecular complexes at the "nano" scale of around 100 nm or less, offer new avenues in various medical diagnosis, monitoring, and treatments (Ventola, 2012). The use of engineered nanostructures and nanodevices to "monitor, repair, construct, and govern biological systems at the molecular levels of humans" represents what is meant by the term "nanotherapeutics" (Prasad et al., 2018). The use of nanoscale technology and applications in healthcare industry can be referred to as nanotherapeutics. It is basically utilized for better understanding of the fundamental disease mechanisms in addition to disease diagnosis, prevention, and treatments (Freitas, 2005).

The size of nanotherapeutics, which resembles biological macromolecules and makes them suitable for both *in vitro* and *in vivo* applications, is its most intriguing aspect. Nanotherapeutics is the discovery, modification, and manipulation of atomic or molecular structures of objects with a size of 1–100 nm (Bharali and Mousa, 2010). The development of multifunctional nanotherapeutics holds great promise for filling several gaps in the current therapeutic field. The discipline of nanotherapeutics is integrating the use of several biological tools and nanobiosensors, as well as a broad spectrum of techniques related to the nanotechnology. Researchers can benefit from these phenomena because quantum effects at the nanoscale affect biological, chemical, physical, optical, and mechanical aspects (Wagner et al., 2006).

The driven forces of nanotherapeutics are biological macromolecules, their structures or chemical substances, that have a xenobiotic nature. As a result of combining nanotechnology with various biological materials, a number of diagnostic tools, analytical tools, monitoring tools, therapeutic agents, physiotherapy applications, and drug delivery agents have been developed. As a result, there is enormous potential for studying and developing nanotherapeutics. The nanotechnology-related drug or therapy acts more precisely and efficiently than traditional medication procedures, with fewer side effects. As a result, nanotherapeutics offers distinct opportunities to improve the safety and efficacy of traditional therapeutic methods (Freitas, 2005).

According to a recent analysis by Grand View Research, sales of nanotherapeutics has surged up to $16 in 2018. Furthermore, the analysis indicates that the nanomedicine sector, which is expected to reach $ 350.8 billion by 2025, will have a significant impact on the global economy (*Nanomedicine Market Analysis by Products, (Therapeutics, Regenerative Medicine, Diagnostics), by Application, (Clinical Oncology, Infectious diseases), By Nanomolecule (Gold, Silver, Iron Oxide, Alumina), & Segment Forecasts, 2013–2025*, 2017).

The healthcare industry is currently working to increase productivity, increase access, and provide higher-quality care at a lower cost. In treating chronic and dangerous diseases such as cancer, diabetes, Parkinson's, Alzheimer's, HIV/AIDS, and various cardiac problems, healthcare practitioners have faced numerous challenges. Infectious diseases pose an additional challenge because the standard antimicrobial medications used to treat them may cause unfavorable side effects and multiple drug resistance (Freitas, 2005).

Target specificity is one of the most significant barriers to achieving therapeutic effectiveness. Nanotherapeutics has amassed substantial evidence as a rational and encouraging tool for the controlled and selective delivery of medicine. Nanotherapeutics plays a crucial role in addressing a variety of challenges in the field of health, because nanotechnology-based formulations improve pharmacokinetic characteristics, bioavailability, and drug targeting in numerous diseases. Nanotherapeutics, which use molecular recognition of human biological systems, have practical applications in drug discovery, diagnostics, monitoring therapy, drug delivery, surgery, orthopedics, and gene delivery, as well as the prevention and treatment of various diseases (Farokhzad and Langer, 2006). Figure 1.1 illustrates the major biological barriers that nanoparticles (NPs) could overcome and therapeutic applications that benefit from NP-based nanotherapeutics (Mitchell et al., 2021).

With the aforementioned merits, explaining the prospects of nanotherapeutics can be focused on the synthesis and application of innovative nanomaterials and nanostructures, biomimetic nanostructures that mimic biological systems to create synthetic goods, nanosensors and nanodevices for diagnosing diseases and pathogens (such as PCR-coupled fluidic devices in micro- or nanostructures), as well as diagnostic tools for finding new therapeutic targets, receptors, and ligands for imaging, screening, therapy, and diagnostics (e.g., for cancers, cardiac abnormalities, neurogenerative diseases, etc.), nanotherapeutics for regenerative medicine and tissue engineering systems and equipment for screening and combinatorial medication delivery, and nanotheranostics for the development of multipurpose biological nanostructured materials, therapies that are physically targeted and stimuli-sensitive nanodevices, systems and nanofluidic tools that are more efficiently capable of transporting fluids to the delivery site (more effective site-specific targeting of nanotherapeutics decreases systemic adverse effects and improves patient compliance). Next-generation nanotherapeutics include nanodevices and implants with sensors on the same chip for closed-looped drug delivery, nanobots, molecular motors, or minimally invasive surgical tools that can travel throughout the body to eliminate tumors or viruses or even carry out gene therapy (Bawa and Bawa, 2005).

1.2   HISTORY OF THE USE OF NANOTHERAPEUTICS

Nanomaterials have a wide range of applications, which is nothing new. As early as 2500 BC, natural asbestos was used to strengthen a ceramic blend for ornamentals.

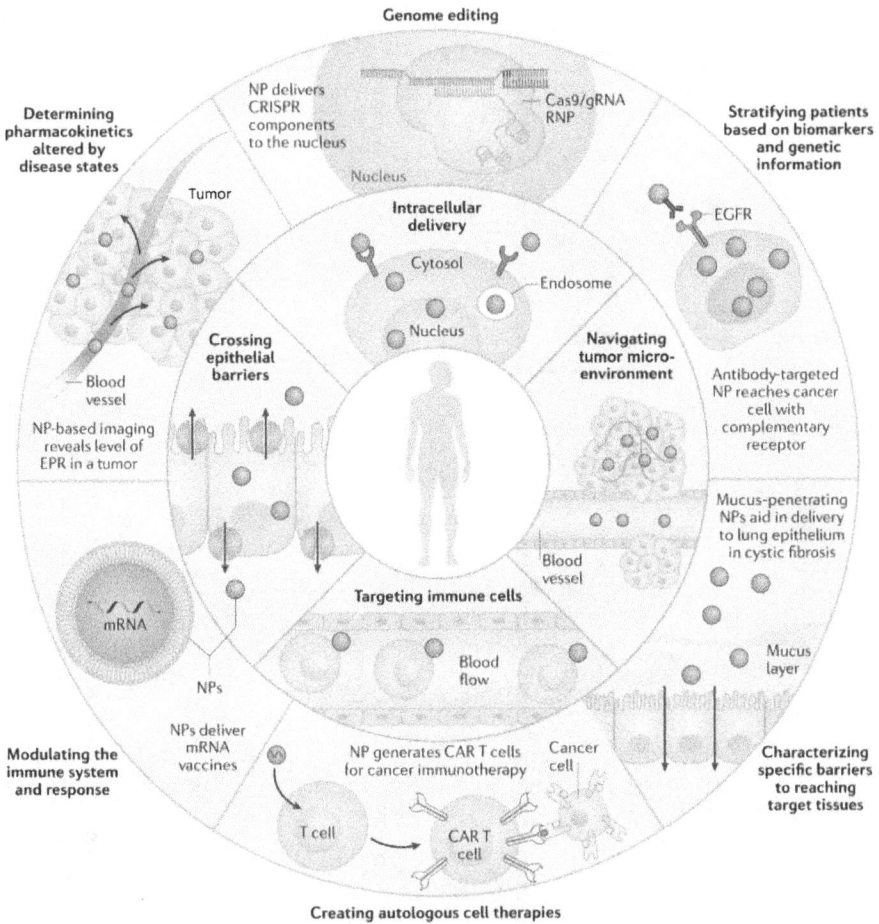

FIGURE 1.1 Overview highlighting some of the biological barriers that nanoparticles (NPs) can overcome (inner ring) and precision medicine applications that may benefit from NPs (outer ring). Next-generation NP designs that improve delivery have the potential to enhance the performance of precision medicines and, thus, accelerate their clinical translation. CAR, chimeric antigen receptor; EGFR, epidermal growth factor receptor; EPR, enhanced permeation and retention; gRNA, guide RNA; RNP, ribonucleoprotein.

Source: Reproduced with permission from Mitchell et al., 2021.

When illuminated from within, the legendary Lycurgus cup, designed by the Romans in the fourth century AD, displayed many colors both during the day and at night. This was the first concrete evidence of the production and consumption of gold colloids. Mesopotamians introduced ceramics with silver and copper glazes in the ninth century AD (Reibold et al., 2006).

The word "nanotechnology" was not coined until exactly ten years after Feynman's famous remark that "there is plenty of room at the bottom" in 1959 thrust

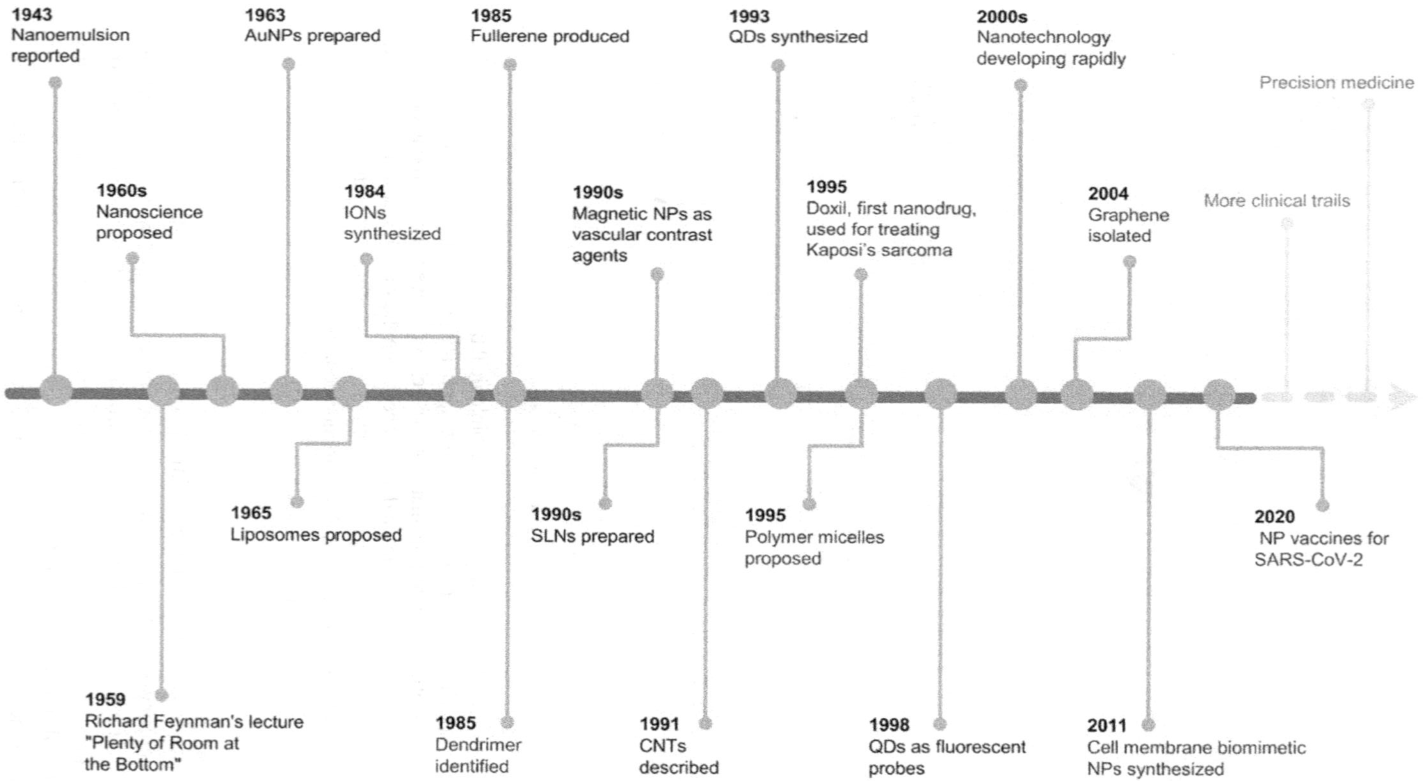

FIGURE 1.2 Timeline of the discovery and research history of nanoparticles. Key discoveries are highlighted. Research on nanoparticles began in the 1960s. Over the last two decades, an increasing number of scientists have devoted themselves to the study of nanoparticles, yielding impressive results in the biomedical field. AuNPs, gold nanoparticles; IONs, iron oxide nanoparticles; NPs, nanoparticles; SLNs, solid lipid nanoparticles; CNTs, carbon nanotubes; QDs, quantum dots.

Source: Reproduced with permission from Xu, Li, and Liu, 2022.

nanotechnology back into the spotlight of the current scientific community (Feynman, 1960). The use of nanoparticles in biomedicine has grown significantly over time, and the addition of inorganic and polymeric materials has strengthened their function in drug transport and prolonged drug release (Yamamoto et al., 2014). Important milestones in the development of nanotherapeutics, from their discovery or invention to various uses, are shown in Figure 1.2 from nineteenth century to the present.

It is acceptable to assert Prof. Peter P. Speiser's labs at the ETH in Zurich, Switzerland, where everything originated. In 1965, when his research first began, he focused on intensive emulsification to convert emulsions from micrometer-sized droplets to ultrafine nanodroplets. He also worked on chemically altering surfactants and micelles before polymerizing these systems. Furthermore, Gerd Birrenbach, who was a Ph.D. student, has conducted his research work on development of sera and vaccinations with prolonged activity by their inclusion in nanosized structures. Birrenbach submitted his thesis based on polymerized micelles, possible inclusion complexes (nanocapsules), and their usage as adjuvants after nearly four years of in-depth research (Birrenbach, 1973). This was the first time the term "nanocapsules" was used and medicinal polymeric nanoparticles were invented. Almost until his retirement in 1998, Professor Speiser worked hard on his nanoparticle research, culminating more than 25 years of productive work in the field (Kreuter, 2007). The work of Professor Speiser sparked other initiatives in the study of nanoparticulate systems in general. The pharmaceutical industry enthusiastically adopted his ideas at the start of the 1980s, and research centers were established to take those ideas from the laboratory benchtop to the real world.

A few years later, it became clear that nanotherapeutics are challenging and will take longer than anticipated to reach the market. It took a lot of fundamental academic research to prove that these systems were clinically effective. Nevertheless, liposomes were introduced to consumers with the first goods in the 1990s. Therefore, it is important to note that all the newly synthesized nanotherapeutics cannot be undergone clinical use unless there is strong evidence of effectiveness and safety concerns.

However, the number of pharmaceutical items is still lower than analysts predicted. In this case, the cost of technological advancements must be borne. Following the initial excitement for nanotherapeutics in the 1980s, more realistic assessments resulted in significant disillusionment. Around the turn of the millennium, nanotherapeutics offered a solution for the development of pharmaceuticals with better efficacy or patient convenience. With problematic novel compounds like extremely weakly soluble medicines, conventional formulation strategies frequently missed the mark. Naturally, the success of nanotechnology in many other spheres of daily life also acted as a trigger for its comeback. In the year 2000, a novel nanoformulation was introduced to the market with the production of medicinal nanocrystals (product Emend). The innovative product Tricor became one of the most popular pharmaceutical nanoproducts, with annual US sales of more than $1 billion. Tricor can thus be exemplified as a succeeded commercially available nanoformulation and it has been applied as a tool for management of the productive life cycle (Müller and Keck, 2010).

Nanotherapeutics have long been used in various research fields, but their use in medicine is new. Nanotherapeutics are particularly suited for interactions at that scale of cellular organelles because of their minuscule sizes, which relate with the submicrometer elements of the biological world. Nanomaterials exhibit a wide range of unique physicochemical characteristics that set them apart from the analogous bulk materials. Their outstanding performance for numerous biological applications, including as drug delivery, gene delivery, screening, tissue engineering, biomicroelectromechanical systems (bioMEMS), nanobots, biosensors, microfluidics, and diagnostic tools, is mostly dictated by their size-related features. Nanomaterial-based delivery of drugs has become the predominant therapeutic use of nanotechnology due to the great possibility it represents. Nanotherapeutics help to improve medication absorption characteristics after administration, circulation time and biodistribution, solubility, intracellular delivery, metabolism, excretion, and bridging biological membranes in addition to increasing targeted drug delivery and control drug release. Traditionally, nanotherapeutics have only been employed for medication delivery purposes; nevertheless, novel nanoscale frameworks have been created that also have a diagnostic purpose. Researchers are increasingly focused on multifunctional nanotherapeutics, which combine therapeutic, targeting, and monitoring capabilities for cutting-edge drug delivery systems (Krukemeyer et al., 2015).

1.3 DIVERSITY OF NANOTHERAPEUTICS

Nanotherapeutics can be used in the medical field as treatments to cure, prevention, and diagnostic and monitoring purposes of various diseases. Nanotherapeutics use as mono type of nanoparticles itself to gain the respective action or nanoparticles in combination as bi, tri, quadra or multiparticle systems. These nanoparticles are typically used to treat diseases, as diagnostic agents, and for preventive care. As a result, these nanoparticles function as nanotherapeutics. Besides consuming nanoparticles as nanotherapeutics, there are emerging nanotherapeutic agents which have improved with many technologies. They have been developed with the assistance of biosensing, robotic, imaging, and miniaturized nanofluidic, photothermal, and photodynamic technologies. These technologies, in conjunction with nanotechnology and medicine, have opened up new avenues for the advancement of the medical field by providing the opportunity to break through bottlenecks and overcome medical field obstacles. Nonetheless, these technological combinations result in a wide range of nanotherapeutics.

1.3.1 Nanotherapeutics as Delivery Agents

Nanotherapeutics are emerging delivery agents for drugs, genes, proteins, and peptides, among other things. Nanotherapeutics have piqued the interest of researchers due to their ability to overcome issues related to drug absorption, distribution, poor solubility with body fluids, metabolism, bioavailability, excretion, and elimination.

Nanotechnology used in drug delivery has the potential to completely transform how various diseases, such as cancer, infections, diabetes, neurological diseases, blood diseases, and orthopedic abnormalities, are treated. These strategies should ideally improve medication absorption, therapeutic concentration, and stability in order to allow more precise drug targeting. Other characteristics of nanotherapeutics-based drug delivery systems include reproducibility and long-term release of the medication within the target tissue. The creation of nano-platforms with certain shape, size, and surface characteristics that are essential for biological interactions and the therapeutic effects that follow results from the rational design of nanotherapeutics. Nanotechnology-based formulations have distinct physical and chemical properties that are responsible for a wide range of applications in the treatment of various disorders (Bhaskar et al., 2010).

Nanoformulations, as recently reported, are critical to the healthcare industry. While some nano-therapeutic products on the market are intended for oral administration, the vast majority are available for parenteral administration. A large number of preclinical and clinical trials are expected to result in the development of emerging nanotherapeutics for non-parenteral distribution platforms such as pulmonary, ophthalmic, nasal, vaginal, and cutaneous. For drug delivery systems, the decision of the distribution route and the related obstacles to be overcome is of special significance (European Commission/ETP). Over time, a number of formulations based on nanoparticles, such as polymeric nanotherapeutics, nanobubbles, nanogels, nanosponges, dendrimers, nanocapsules, liposomes, nanoemulsions, and nanostructured lipid-based carriers, were designed to improve the drug delivery mechanisms (Joseph et al., 2023). Figure 1.3 illustrates the intracellular application of NPs designed using different material composition based on the classes and functionality of NPs, shape, size, and targeting ligands leading to high maneuverability and target-specific delivery of drugs.

Proteins and peptides have numerous biological actions in practically every discipline of medicine, and they have shown significant promise for treating a variety of diseases when used as proteins and peptide delivery agents in nanotherapeutics (Chen and Guan, 2011). Additionally, these have a role in the diagnosis of a number of metabolic, cardiovascular, neurological (Alzheimer's, Parkinson's), and other illnesses, such as diabetes and cancer (Kaspar and Reichert, 2013). Proteins and peptides are delivered more efficiently and with controlled release when they are delivered using dendrimers and nanoparticles. Furthermore, they have high localization specificity, as evidenced by the unique localization signal generated on peptides (Minamihata et al., 2020). The design of effective, nontoxic, easily manipulated vehicles that can enclose and transport new genetic material into particular cell types is essential for the success of gene therapy. Because nanoparticles have a high surface area-to-volume ratio, it is relatively easy to add different functional groups to their surfaces. Some tumor cells can be found and bound using these functional groups. More significantly, aggregation is hampered by the lower size of nanoparticles (Wang, Langer and Farokhzad, 2012). The selection of the right substance is crucial for the delivery of genes. These substances release to the target after conjugating with genes or medications. Lipid-based, metal-based, and polymer-based nanoparticles are the three groups into which nanoparticles for gene therapy are divided (Herrero and Medarde, 2015). For gene therapy to be successful, the nucleic acid needs to be encased and shielded by a delivery formulation. The hope for successful gene therapy is increased by the nanotherapeutics. Significant research has been conducted in the last ten years to develop nonviral delivery vehicles for gene therapy, particularly in the treatment of cancer (Ngoc et al., 2015).

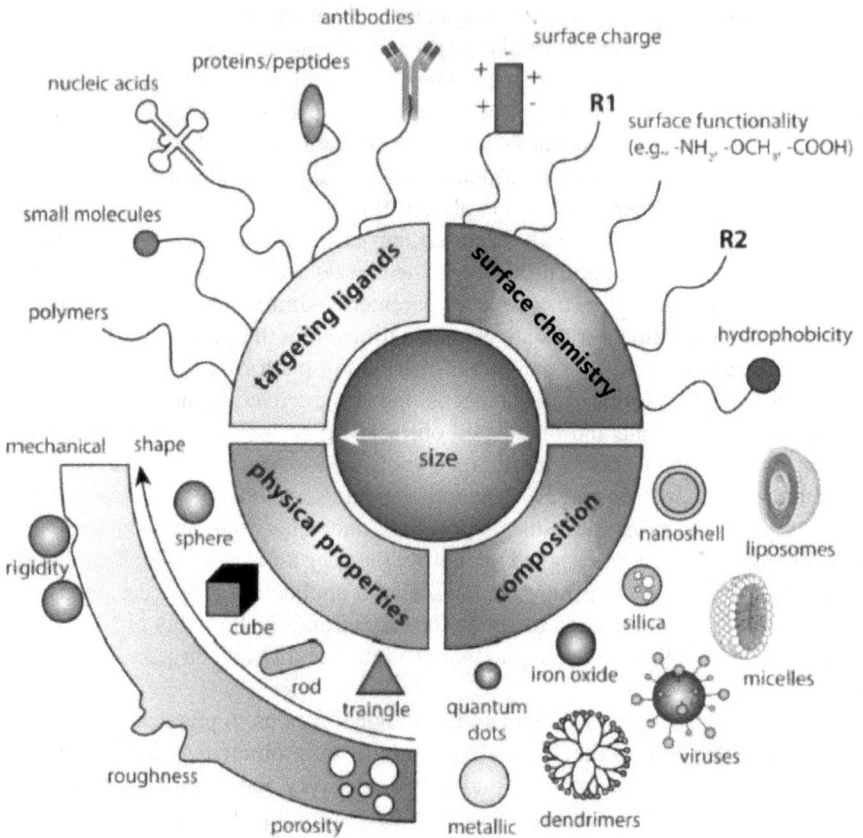

FIGURE 1.3 Intracellular application of NPs designed using different material composition based on the classes and functionality of NPs, shape, size, and targeting ligands leading to high maneuverability and target-specific delivery of drugs.

Source: Reproduced with permission from Shah et al., 2021.

Treatment of metastatic cancer is required for cancer gene therapy to be successful. The wild-type p53 functions as a tumor suppressor and is crucial to understanding the biology of cancer. It has been shown that wt p53 has been transduced into malignant cells via a virus-mediated gene delivery method. The low quantity of transduced cells and the diagnosis of infected cells, however, hampered the efficacy (Misra et al., 2014). Charge reversal polymers like polyethylenimine (PEI), polylysine (PLL), and nanogels may be used for gene delivery in cancer treatment therapy based on nanotechnology. Additionally, they transport substantial molecules like deoxyribose nucleic acid (DNA) straight into the nucleus, greatly enhancing their cellular absorption. Such cationic polymers have been shown to have nuclear localization features by Zhang et al. in 2014 (Zhang et al., 2014). Recently, a number of charge-reversal carriers for drug delivery and effective cancer therapy were created. Nonviral (physical and chemical approaches)-based gene delivery techniques have been evaluated to combat immunogenic issues. For better outcomes and prognosis, medication combinations can be used in the delivery platform (Mujokoro et al., 2016).

1.3.2 NANOTHERAPEUTICS AS AGENTS IN THERAPEUTIC DRUG MONITORING

The primary goal of therapeutic drug monitoring (TDM), an intervention technique, is to determine the appropriate dosage for difficult-to-administer medications in order to improve patient's responses and reduce harmful drug reactions. Nanoelectromechanical systems were created as a way to apply nanotherapeutics to TDM that have crucial structural components smaller than 100 nm. Their impact is being examined for the active release of medications and sustaining their level in the patient's body. With the aid of iron nanoparticles and gold nanoshells, the use of this technique could be crucial in the treatment of cancer. This has been shown to be quite helpful in people with insulin-dependent diabetic mellitus (IDDM) (Roorda, 2001). Nanoelectromechanical systems allow for the maintenance of drug levels in the body while preventing drug toxicity or overdose (Cimalla et al., 2007).

1.3.3 NANOTHERAPEUTICS AS IMPLANTS

Since a few years ago, there has been a persistent necessity for alternative and reformative medications to treat organ damage or failure. Nanotherapeutics-based implantations have been used to manage pathological diseases and regulate the release of therapeutic medications. Drug modifications have been carried out at the nanogram to microgram scale. Recently, titanium implants using nanotechnology have been developed for controlled release of various antibacterial nanoparticles like ZnO (Wang et al., 2021). The titanium tube demonstrated improved binding capacity of osteoblast and was utilized to deliver hormones and medications simultaneously for rapid bone healing (Gulati et al., 2023). The idea of nano-engineered implants could be used for epidermal, dental brain, cochineal, and cardiovascular engineering in addition to bones. Figure 1.4 shows various nanoimplants that are recently developed.

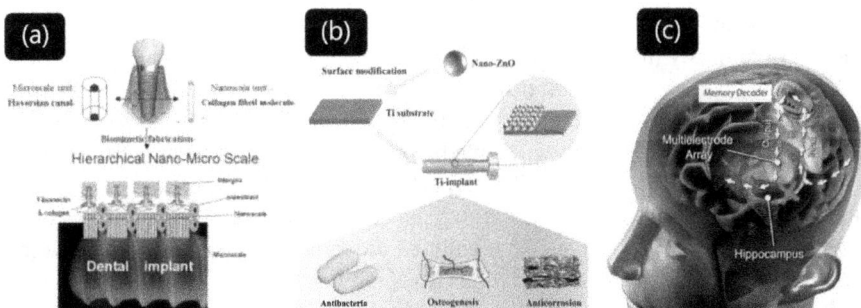

FIGURE 1.4 (a) Dental implant with nanoscale dimensions. (b) Titanium nanoimplants for osteogenesis, as antimicrobials and as anticorrosive agents. (c) Brain implants in nanoscale.

Source: (a) Reproduced with permission from Wang et al., 2013. (b) Reproduced with permission from Wang et al., 2021. (c) Reproduced with permission from Kumar, 2020.

1.3.4 NANOTHERAPEUTICS FOR PHOTODYNAMIC THERAPY

To eradicate skin cancer, photosensitive dyes are used in photodynamic therapy (PDT), also known as nontoxic pigment therapy (Figure 1.5). Nontoxic medicines such as photosensitizers (PS) and eosin pigment are combined with light and various nanomaterials to treat tumor cells. Additionally, PDT has been utilized as a nontoxic medicine with visible red light, which extends new advancements of clinical study in gene therapy (Correia et al., 2021). Nanotherapeutics-based PDT is typically used to treat skin ailments like sunburn, acne, and other infections of the skin. These nanoparticles are injected on a specific skin area or bloodstream and triggered with exposure to external light, based on which portion of the body is impacted. To restore the tissue architecture, these particles absorb a specific wavelength of light. When these particles reach the excited state, they react with oxygen, which eventually leads to the creation of stronger free radicals (Correia et al., 2021).

Additionally, PDT destroys the blood arteries that typically supply blood to malignant tissue. Graphene oxide (GO) combined with PDT was employed as a cancer treatment in a study conducted, as described by Tian et al. (2013). Moreover, they demonstrated successful applications of mild light-triggered PDT and GO (Tian et al., 2013). Due to its lower toxicity and its less adverse effects than other long-term complementary therapies, this treatment is rising to fame. Therapies like these have a special ability because they are less invasive than surgical operations. Typically, it is regarded as more cost-effective and target-specific than standard neoplastic therapies. Targeting particular affected tissues, organs, and cancer cells, gold nanoparticles have demonstrated some specialized therapeutic approaches (Yao, Epstein and Akey, 2006).

The basis of photodynamic cancer therapy is the potential cytotoxic laser-generated atomic oxygen that kills cancer cells. Typically, cancer cells consume a greater amount of special photosensitive dye than healthy cells. The atomic oxygen that is generated inside the cancer cells is the reason behind this phenomenon. From this point forward, only the cancer cells may be eliminated by laser radiation in the photodynamic cancer therapy. However, the residual dye molecules, which may stay in the body up to certain weeks or longer, migrate to the skin tissues and eyes, where they induce irritation and sensitivity and make the patient more susceptible to sunlight. A hydrophobic form of compound was encapsulated inside a porous nanoparticle in order to prevent this undesirable impact of the dye. For an example, some dyes are encapsulated in organically modified silica (Ormosil) nanoparticles. The dye was then found to have remained inside the Ormosil nanoparticle rather than spreading to other areas in the body (Xu et al., 2021). On the contrary extreme, the capacity to produce oxygen is unaltered, and oxygen can be readily expelled through pores with a diameter of around 1 nm in these Ormosil nanoparticles. Furthermore, patients undergoing this therapy could ingest fluids containing nanorobots that are programmed to target viruses and cancer cells while also rebuilding the molecular machinery and internal structures of the cells. This tactic diminishes the consequences of the residual dye molecules that are mentioned before. Moreover, in one technique, healthy cells might be surgically inserted to speed up the processes once cancer cells were discovered and destroyed. A whole branch of nanosurgery may also be developed in the future to support photodynamic therapy (Hong, Choi and Shim, 2016).

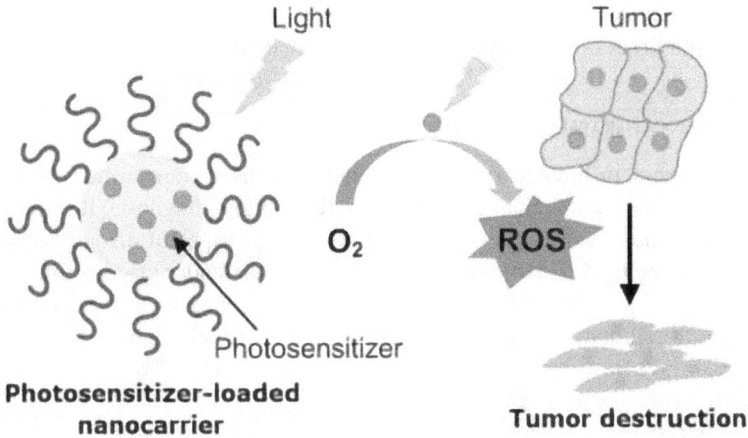

FIGURE 1.5 Photodynamic therapy for tumor destruction.

Source: Reproduced with permission from Hong, Choi, and Shim, 2016.

1.3.5 NANOTHERAPEUTICS-BASED NUTRACEUTICALS

Nanotherapeutics could make it easier to add nutrients and increase their bioavailability, allowing animals to grow more quickly. The nanoparticles can stabilize bioactive substances, increasing their cellular uptake. Because of their small size, they move quickly through the digestive tract and make it easier for nutrients to be delivered. Phenolic molecules are essential micronutrients in our diet that inhibit the progression of neuro- and degenerative diseases. They are rapidly degraded by environmental triggers and have poor bioavailability. These phenolics function well as a delivery mechanism when enclosed in nanoparticles. The nanocarriers are therefore the most useful for delivering and protecting phenolics (Esfanjani and Jafari, 2016).

Nanotherapeutics has enhanced nutrient delivery systems, which has led to significant advancements in food science. These nanomaterials have the ability to prevent food from being digested in the stomach and the mouth. Encapsulation is one method for ensuring effective nutrient delivery, as such preferring nanomaterials as encapsulants to create edible nanoparticles requires careful consideration of each one's unique physicochemical and physical properties along with the molecular interactions with other molecules already present in the nanoparticles (Razavi et al., 2020). Pharmaceutical bioactive molecules such as nucleic acids, peptides, and proteins that are hydrophilic have been defined in certain works as being encapsulated (Smaoui et al., 2021). Regarding their utilization in the food industry, synthetic biopolymers' level of toxicity must also be considered. As a result of this, sophisticated hydrophilic biopolymer molecules have been thoroughly studied. One of the most widely utilized biopolymers for medication delivery and encapsulating bioactive components is polylactic acid (PLA). For instance, chitosan and chitosan-grafted PLA were employed by Di Martino et al. (2015) as a matrix for the entrapment of bovine serum albumin (BSA) in a nanoscale structure that was made using the polyelectrolyte complexation process and dextran sulfate (Valente et al., 2013).

1.3.6 NANOTHERAPEUTICS AS DIAGNOSTIC AGENTS

Recent advances in biological imaging technology have transformed them into a powerful tool for pathological condition progression and diagnosis. It enables us to easily detect and quantify the cells that cause various types of disorders (Han and Zhou, 2016; Lee et al., 2016). The imaging system has undergone significant progress in recent years. When compared to conventional imaging techniques, the NPs coupled with radiolabeling produce effective results. To eliminate nonspecific cell attachment, NPs must have a very precise nature to pinpoint the appropriate region for image-based diagnosis and treatments.

Nanotherapeutics participate in a variety of imaging modalities, such as magnetic resonance imaging and ultrasonography, and are able to provide superior results than conventional imaging systems (Leng et al., 2015). Quantum dots (QDs), which possess the quantum energy to emit light, are one of the significant applications of NPs. They have excellent applicability in the field of more precise techniques to tumor elimination. In magnetic resonance imaging, QD was employed, and it was discovered that they are effective at exhibiting tumor-affected regions (Su et al., 2017). Another study discovered that when exposed to UV light, selenide cadmium enhanced the illumination. These illumination properties facilitate the use of selenide cadmium as imaging agents (Zhu et al., 2017).

Particles such as poly(lactic-*co*-glycolic acid) have been recognized as excellent polymers due to their biocompatibility and biodegradability. According to one study, 5-ethylamino-9-diethylaminobenzo(*a*)henothiazinium (EtNBS) capsuled with PLGA exhibited reducing rates in side effects. Throughout this study, NPs entrapment was used to overcome the toxicity effects and minimal limitations. Surprisingly, they discovered that using EtNBS and poly(lactic-*co*-glycolic acid) as encapsulating materials significantly reduced toxicity. As a result, these methods aid in reducing the toxicity of cancer cell therapy (Hung et al., 2016; Klein et al., 2012).

1.3.7 NANOTHERAPEUTICS AS BIOSENSORS

A biosensor is an electrical device that combines a transducer and a bioconjugation component to evaluate or target various biological desires (Baranwal et al., 2018; Mahato et al., 2018). Organs, antibodies, enzymes, receptors, and nucleic acids are only a few examples of the biological constituents that biosensor devices are responsive to as analytical targets (Holzinger, Goff and Cosnier, 2014). The use of biosensor devices is prevalent in the field of medical diagnostics for rapid analysis of various disorders and microbiological identifications. With the adoption of conducting NPs such as gold nanoparticles (AuNPs), silver nanoparticles (AgNPs), and platinum nanoparticles (PtNPs), which are recognized as appropriate substrates, material technology has developed and strengthened innovative biosensors (Martin et al., 2014). These are useful for biosensor equipment with fast dynamic response (Chen et al., 2011). Figure 1.6 illustrates the various components of a nanobiosensor with their working principle.

Systems for nucleic acid hybridization or biosensors based on gold nanoparticles are demonstrated to have greater sensitivity. Tiny magnetic nanoparticles (<100 nm) have more surface area and silt at slower rates, which enhance tissue diffusion. As a result, they continue to circulate through the capillaries of tissues and organs, preventing vascular embolism following injection. Both magnetic and gold nanoparticles are being used in several immunological chromatographic screenings and lateral circulation assays on the Ebola virus (Illescas et al., 2017). However, due to their highly charged contact area and decreased precipitation rate, NPs with magnetic characteristics and a size of <100 nm are having a significant impact on biosensors (Wang et al., 2010). According to Arruebo et al. (2007), these magnetic NPs-based nanotherapeutics are beneficial for tissue diffusion.

Better biosensors can be designed using the magnetic NPs' circulation phenomenon and capillary system. Researchers have reported on the use of magnetic and AuNPs in combination with immunological chromatography tests to detect the Ebola virus. Due to the use of sensitive colloidal gold strips, they discovered that this combination was far more effective than the standard traditional process (Saha et al., 2016). In parallel, other analytical investigations for the improvement of biosensor technologies have made use of these NPs' enzymatic characteristics to quantify real sample analysis to an exceptional degree and to ascertain their high sensitivity in comparison to conventional processes (Ganguly et al., 2017). Recent studies have shown the value of nanoport technology in the development of analytical detecting devices that convert nucleic acids into electric impulses and subsequently match those signals with traditional databases to enable speedy on-the-spot diagnosis (Zheng et al., 2005). Additionally, leveraging these advancements, a variety of sensor chips have been created to identify biomarkers for diseases like cancer, HIV, Alzheimer's, and Parkinson's (Zhang et al., 2017). A key factor in the development of contemporary diagnostic gadgets is the use of electrochemical processes based on nanobiosensors (Wang et al., 2013).

A very sophisticated biosensor is using the enzymatic function of nanoparticles to achieve a high level of sensitivity. A cutting-edge technique called multicolor optical coding involves designing quantum dots of various sizes on tiny beads that can emit light at various frequencies that can be applied to microarray technology. For the examination of nucleic acids, nanopore technology turns the length of the nucleotides through an electronic signature that can be quickly correlated with the signature already contained in the database. Utilizing only a drop of blood, a sensor chip test can identify disease-related biomarkers in a pathological condition like cancer. The use of nanotechnology and nanotherapeutics in instrumentation is noteworthy. A pencil-sized arthroscope that is utilized in minimally invasive surgical procedures is based on nanotechnology. The general rule in surgery is that the minimum the incision, the speedier and greater the recovery.

A key area of nanodiagnostics that is still under development is nanoelectrochemical based biosensors. Those sensors can be employed to create sophisticated devices and guarantee precise, digital outcomes. The electrochemical-based biosensor is

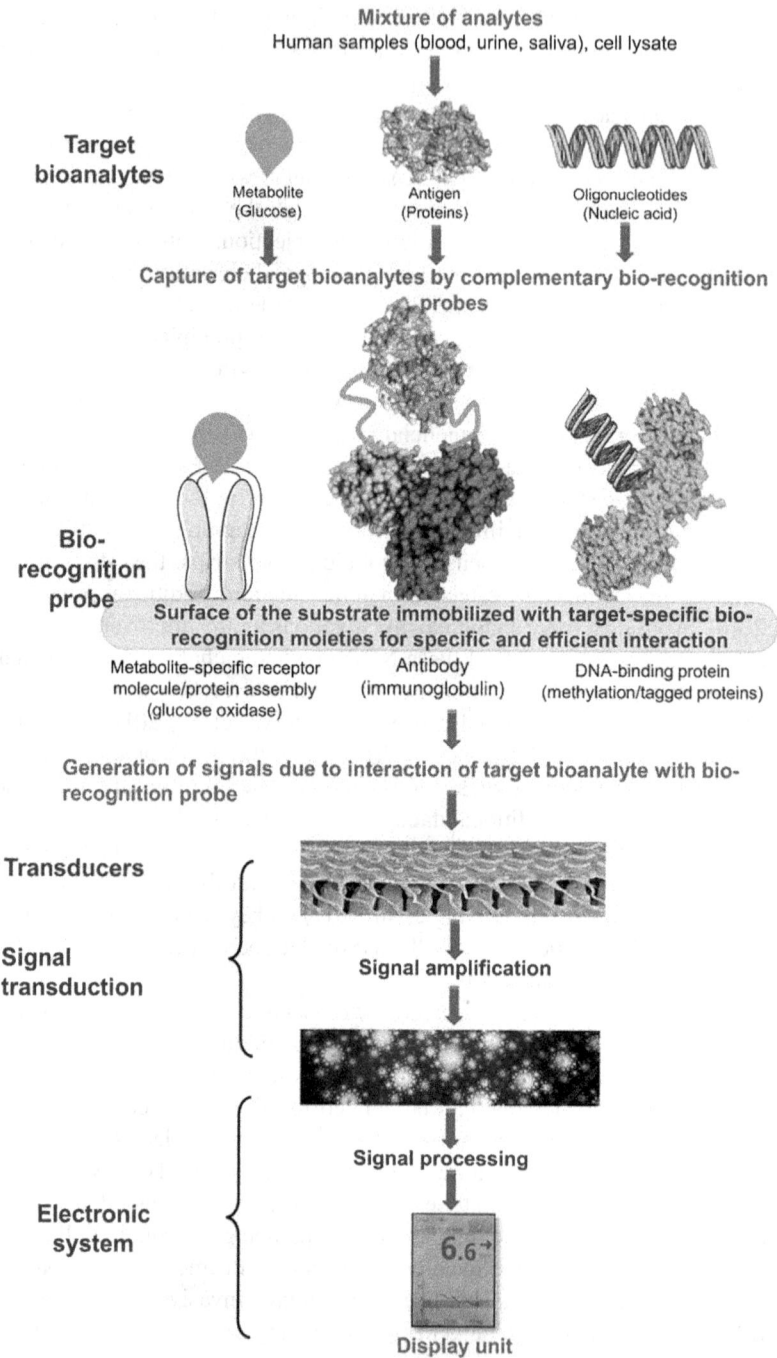

FIGURE 1.6   An illustration of various components of a nanobiosensor with their working principle.

Source: Reproduced with permission from Singhal et al., 2021.

most frequently used for the determination of blood glucose concentration. The best material for such a gadget is a multi-walled carbon nanotube since it uses less blood. Furthermore, using just a drop of peripheral blood over 5 minutes, nanowires can also be utilized to diagnose tumors. One specific sort of targeted marker protein is primed to be detected by each nanowire (Kumar et al., 2019). The expenses for the diagnosis of tumors can be reduced and those remained funds can be allocated for other medical needs by facilitating such simple techniques to detect tumors with aid of the nanotherapeutic approaches. Moreover, the sensitivity is a 1,000-folds of magnitude better in comparison to other diagnostic procedures.

Oncology treatment has become more personalized because of nanotherapeutic-based approaches, enabling each patient to receive a specific diagnosis and treatment plan. Different genetic tests that may be utilized for screening, recognizing, and diagnosing the target body part affected by cancer in an individual have been thoroughly studied (Kumar et al., 2019 Wang et al., 2015).

1.3.8 NANOTHERAPEUTICS AS BLOOD PURIFICATION AGENTS

Blood is composed of a diverse range of cells, proteins, and biological components that can be separated using the traditional magnetic-driven cell separation approach (Kang et al., 2014). Previous studies have demonstrated the removal of several hazardous elements from biological fluid, including microorganisms, toxins, and some pretentious material, with the aid of a circuit architecture resembling the dialysis system (Lunardi et al., 2009). Diffusion and ultrafiltration via a semipermeable membrane are the basis of the dialysis technique (Lunardi et al., 2009). Additionally, covalently attaching various antibodies, protein-specific substances, and synthetic chemicals to these nanoparticles over their exterior surfaces improved blood purification via a microfluidic device (Schumacher et al., 2013). The magnetically reactive NPs attached to distinct functional groups have the ability to bind with a particular item present in body fluids and secretions like the blood circulation. Thereafter, when this fluid was exposed to an external magnetic field, NPs began to accumulate at the magnet's pole, resulting in the way different blood components were separated. In recent research, using magnetic NPs-based purification by focusing on a specific molecule made the purification stage for blood easier (Lee et al., 2013).

Magnetically triggered cell classification or Dynabeads can be used to separate the proteins and cells from a heterogeneous mixture like blood. These materials have been successfully shown to remove a variety of hazardous substances from blood, including toxins, infections, and specific proteins with the aid of a circuit that is similar to the machinery used for the process of dialysis. The fundamental aspect of dialysis is the solute diffusion or ultrafiltration through semipermeable membranes. Nevertheless, the purification method based on nanoparticles targets certain molecules. Iron oxide or carbon-coated metal nanoparticles that are fictitious are employed for this. Iron exhibits both ferromagnetic or supermagnetic properties. On their interfaces, such nanoparticles can be covalently coupled to various proteins, antibodies, antibiotics, or synthetic compounds. In the blood or another intricate body fluid, such functionalized magnetic nanoparticles link with the target substance. The fluid is subsequently exposed to an appropriate external magnetic field, permitting all of the magnetic nanoparticles to accumulate close to the magnetic pole. Particles and impurities from blood or other heterogeneous bodily fluids can be easily isolated in this method. Nanoparticles have a higher loading capacity, are more accessible, have improved selectivity, and diffuse faster than hemoperfusion, a blood purification technology that requires far fewer dosage volumes. This is a unique pharmaceutical effort to treat systemic infections by directly eliminating the bacteria that cause them in conditions like sepsis. It could also drive the elimination of cytokines and endotoxins that promote inflammation and aids in the simplification of laborious conventional procedures like dialysis. This technique is still being developed, despite having many advantages (Kumar et al., 2019).

1.3.9 Nanotherapeutics for Tissue Engineering

Tissue engineering has shown to be a very effective application of nanotherapeutics based on nanotechnology. It has the ability to fully upgrade current treatments, including organ transplants, grafts, and artificial implants, among others. Fabrication of tissue engineering is based on nanoparticles (grapheme, carbon nanotubes, molybdenum disulfide, and tungsten disulfide). Additionally, it effectively enhances the compression and flexion of polymeric nanocomposites, which are essential features of bones. As a result, these kinds of nanocomposites can be employed to create incredibly thin bone implants. The "Flesh welder" method, which is based on nanotechnology, can be used to join the pieces of flesh together. By combining an infrared laser reaction with a suspension of gold-coated nanoshells, it was possible to combine two portions of chicken flesh into one (Gobin et al., 2005). In accident cases, this precise method can be used to cauterize the tissue and rejoin major veins that have been damaged during surgery. Nano-nephrology is a novel concept that has recently been used. This study focuses on the use of nanotechnology in the diagnosis and treatment of kidney disease. The ultimate goal of this branch is to develop a nanoscale artificial kidney to avoid the problems associated with transplant rejection (Sinha et al., 2022).

1.3.10 Nanotherapeutics as Nanorobots

The diseased state can be treated at the submicroscopic level using molecular mechanical assembly based on nanotherapeutics (Prasad et al., 2018). These mechanical systems at the nanoscale are known as nanorobots. They can recognize and fix damage when they are introduced into the body. The field of nanorobotics focuses on creating and building nanorobots made of silicon and carbon nanotubes with a size range of 0.1–10 m. The development of such robots will benefit from future developments in nanomedicine. K. Eric Drexler proposed a cell repair device that would stop cells from aging. However, Freitas conducted the initial scientific and technical research of therapeutic nanorobots (Jones, 2005). The computer systems are able to communicate with the nervous system owing to the neuro-electronic interface clearance, including nanodevices. The computer systems will be able to link to and operate the nervous system using a refutable energy that is supplied by an external sonic, chemical, or magnetic source. Self-sufficient nanodevices have been created that run on biofluid glucose. The drawbacks of this technique include overheating, leakage, or electrostatic discharge from the source of electricity. Because electrical circuits are located in the nervous system, their structure is of vital importance (Kumar et al., 2019).

Nanorobotic technology has effectively exploited the study of microorganisms as a launching pad for the early development of robotic capabilities. Nanorobots can be designed and functionalized for many diseases, however difficulties with delivery and propulsion restrict their usage within the bloodstream. Nanorobots can be propelled effectively when conjugated with magnetotactic bacteria like *Magnetococcus, Magnetospirillum magnetotacticum*, or *Magnetospirillum magneticum*. Furthermore, nanorobots can also be employed in the medicinal field as phagocytic entities. "Nanobivores" is the term coined to these nanorobots. The outer walls of these robots might be assembled with a vast number of programmable receptors for antigens or diseases, ranging from HIV to *Escherichia coli* (Saadeh and Vyas, 2014).

Dentistry is one industry where nanorobots can be used both routinely and specifically. Nanorobots have the potential to improve patient care by being used in almost every aspect of dental hygiene and therapy. Their numerous applications range from basic hygiene to hypersensitivity, cosmetological agents, dental bleaching, and even orthodontics. The preliminary analgesia is one application for nanorobots in dentistry, which a dentist might administer at the beginning of a consultation. Furthermore, the patient is given an oral suspension consisting of millions of nanorobots. These nanorobots are sufficiently tiny to fit within the gingival sulcus and finally pass via tooth tubules that are the dimension of micrometers to get to the pulp. They might be controlled from a central location, enabling the stimulation of bioactivity in targeted locations proximal to the dentist's point of care (Saadeh and Vyas, 2014).

1.3.11 Nanotherapeutics as Nanomotors

Nanolocomotion, which can be described as the mechanism that allows a nanoscale item to move ahead through an anisotropic energy and is typically assisted by an asymmetric architecture, is how nanomotors demonstrate autonomous self-propulsion. Usually, catalysis, biosensing, and site-specific administering medication can be accomplished with nanomotors. The incapability to accomplish motion at a nontoxic and neutral pH as well as the lack of biocompatibility seem to be the main issues with existing micro- and nanomotor platforms, which restrict their potential for use in biological applications (Munaweera et al., 2016).

In this instance, mesoporous silica nanomotors in gold/palladium-coated magnesium nanoparticles have been designed by Munaweera et al. to generate hydrogen gas and carry out nanolocomotion together in neutral pH environment. The outcomes of this research, which used aspirin as a standard medicine, demonstrate that the constructed nanomotor systems offer suitable delivery platforms for the conservation of fuel and payload. High biocompatibility capabilities are present in this concept, and it can store payloads or fuel wherever desired (Munaweera et al., 2016).

REFERENCES

Arruebo, M., Fernandez-Pacheco, R., Ibarra, M. R. and Santamaria, J. (2007) "Magnetic nanoparticles for drug deliver," *Nano Today*, 2, pp. 22–32.

Baranwal, A., Srivastava, A., Kumar, P., Bajpai, V. K., Maurya, P. K. and Chandra, P. (2018) "Prospects of nanostructure materials and their composites as antimicrobial agents," *Frontiers in Microbiology*, 9, p. 422.

Bawa, R. and Bawa, S. R. (2005) "Patents and nanomedicine," in Wagner, C. G. (ed.) *Foresight, innovation, and strategy: Towards a wiser future*. Bethesda, MD: World Future Society, pp. 31–44.

Bharali, D. J. and Mousa, S. A. (2010) "Emerging nanomedicines for early cancer detection and improved treatment: Current perspective and future promise," *Pharmacology & Therapeutics*, 128(2), pp. 324–335.

Bhaskar, S. et al. (2010) "Multifunctional nanocarriers for diagnostics, drug delivery and targeted treatment across blood-brain barrier: Perspectives on tracking and neuroimaging," *Particle and Fibre Toxicology*, 7(1), p. 3.

Birrenbach, G. (1973) *Über Mizellpolymerisate, mögliche Einschlußverbindungen (Nanokapseln) und deren Eignung als Adjuvantien*. PhD thesis ETH: No. 5071, Zurich.

Chen, J.-P., Yang, P.-C., Ma, Y.-H. and Wu, T. (2011) "Characterization of chitosan magnetic nanoparticles for in situ delivery of tissue plasminogen activator," *Carbohydrate Polymers*, 84, pp. 364–372.

Chen, K. and Guan, J. (2011) "A bibliometric investigation of research performance in emerging nanobiopharmaceuticals," *Journal of Informetrics*, 5(2), pp. 233–247.

Cimalla, V. et al. (2007) "Nanoelectromechanical devices for sensing applications," *Sensors and Actuators. B, Chemical*, 126(1), pp. 24–34.

Correia, J. H. et al. (2021) "Photodynamic therapy review: Principles, photosensitizers, applications, and future directions," *Pharmaceutics*, 13(9), p. 1332. doi: 10.3390/pharmaceutics13091332.

Di Martino, A., Kucharczyk, P., Zednik, J. and Sedlarik, V. (2015) "Chitosan grafted low molecular weight polylactic acid for protein encapsulation and burst effect reduction," *International Journal of Pharmaceutics*, 496, pp. 912–921.

Esfanjani, A. F. and Jafari, S. M. (2016) "Biopolymer nano-particles and natural nano-carriers for nano-encapsulation of phenolic compounds," *Colloids Surface B Biointerfaces*, 146, pp. 532–543.

Farokhzad, O. C. and Langer, R. (2006) "Nanomedicine: Developing smarter therapeutic and diagnostic modalities," *Advanced Drug Delivery Reviews*, 58(14), pp. 1456–1459.

Feynman, R. P. (1960) "There's plenty of room at the bottom: An invitation to enter a new field of physics," *Engineering and Science (Caltech)*, 23, pp. 22–36.

Freitas, R. A., Jr. (2005) "What is nanomedicine?," *Nanomedicine: Nanotechnology, Biology, and Medicine*, 1(1), pp. 2–9.

Ganguly, J., Saha, S., Bera, A. and Ghosh, M. (2017) "Exploring electro-optic effect and third-order nonlinear optical susceptibility of impurity doped quantum dots: Interplay between hydrostatic pressure, temperature and noise," *Optics Communications*, 387, pp. 166–173.

Gobin, A. M. et al. (2005) "Near infrared laser-tissue welding using nanoshells as an exogenous absorber," *Lasers in Surgery and Medicine*, 37(2), pp. 123–129. doi: 10.1002/lsm.20206.

Gulati, K. et al. (2023) "Craniofacial therapy: Advanced local therapies from nano-engineered titanium implants to treat craniofacial conditions," *International Journal of Oral Science*, 15(1). doi: 10.1038/s41368-023-00220-9.

Han, L. and Zhou, Z. (2016) "Synthesis and characterization of liposomes nano-composite-particles with hydrophobic magnetite as a MRI probe," *Applied Surface Science*, 376, pp. 252–260.

Herrero, P. E. and Medarde, A. F. (2015) "Advanced targeted therapies in cancer: Drug nano-carriers, the future of chemotherapy," *Eur J. Pharm. Biopharm*, 93, pp. 52–79.

Holzinger, M., Goff, A. L. and Cosnier, S. (2014) "Nanomaterials for biosensing applications: A review," *Frontiers in Chemistry*, 2, p. 63.

Hong, E. J., Choi, D. G. and Shim, M. S. (2016) "Targeted and effective photodynamic therapy for cancer using functionalized nanomaterials," *Acta Pharmaceutica Sinica. B*, 6(4), pp. 297–307. doi: 10.1016/j.apsb.2016.01.007.

Hung, H.-I., Klein, O. J., Peterson, S. W., Rokosh, S. R., Osseiran, S., Nowell, N. H. and Evans, C. L. (2016) "PLGA nanoparticle encapsulation reduces toxicity while retaining the therapeutic efficacy of EtNBS-PDT in vitro," *Scientific Reports*, 6, p. 33234.

Illescas, B. M. et al. (2017) "Multivalent glycosylated nanostructures to inhibit Ebola virus infection," *Journal of the American Chemical Society*, 139(17), pp. 6018–6025. doi: 10.1021/jacs.7b01683.

Jones, R. (2005) "Biology, Drexler, and nanotechnology," *Materials Today (Kidlington, England)*, 8(8), p. 56. doi: 10.1016/s1369–7021(05)71057–9.

Joseph, T. M. et al. (2023) "Nanoparticles: Taking a unique position in medicine," *Nanomaterials (Basel, Switzerland)*, 13(3), p. 574.

Kang, J. H., Super, M., Yung, C. W., Cooper, R. M., Domansky, K., Graveline, A. R., Mammoto, T., Berhet, J. B., Tobin, H., Cartwright, M. J., Watters, A. L., Rottman, M., Waterhouse, A., Mammoto, A., Gamini, N., Roadas, M. J., Kole, A., Jiang, A., Valentin, T. M., Diaz, A., Takahashi, K. and Ingber, D. E. (2014) "An extracorporeal blood-cleansing device for sepsis therapy," *Nature Methodology*, 20, pp. 1211–1216.

Kaspar, A. A. and Reichert, J. M. (2013) "Future directions for peptide therapeutics development," *Drug Discovery Today*, 18, pp. 807–817.

Klein, O. J., Bhayana, B., Park, Y. J. and Evans, C. L. (2012) "In vitro optimization of EtNBS-PDT against hypoxic tumor environments with a tiered, high-content, 3D model optical screening platform," *Molecular Pharmaceutics*, 9, pp. 3171–3182.

Kreuter, J. (2007) "Nanoparticles: A historical perspective," *International Journal of Pharmaceutics*, 331, pp. 1–10.

Krukemeyer, M. G., Krenn, V., Huebner, F., Wagner, W. and Resch, R. (2015) "History and possible uses of nanomedicine based on nanoparticles and nanotechnological progress," *Journal of Nanomedicine & Nanotechnology*, 6, p. 336. doi: 10.4172/2157-7439.1000336.

Kumar, A. et al. (2019) "Nanotherapeutics," In Pawan Kumar Maurya and Sanjay Singh (Eds.), *Nanotechnology in modern animal Biotechnology*. St. Louis, MO: Elsevier, pp. 149–161.

Kumar, P. (2020) "Control of mind using nanotechnology," *Journal of Regenerative Biology and Medicine*, 2(4), pp. 1–14.

Lee, J., Gordon, A. C., Kim, H., Park, W., Cho, S., Lee, B., Larson, A. C., Rozhkova, E. A. and Kim, D.-H. (2016) "Targeted multimodal nano-reporters for pre-procedural MRI and intra-operative image-guidance," *Biomaterials*, 109, pp. 69–77.

Lee, J.-L., Jeong, K. J., Hashimoto, M., Kwon, A. H., Rwei, A., Shankarappa, S. A., Tsui, J. H. and Kohane, D. S. (2013) "Synthetic ligand-coated magnetic nanoparticles for microfluidic bacterial separation from blood," *Nano Letters*, 14, pp. 1–5.

Leng, J., Li, J., Ren, J., Deng, L. and Lin, C. (2015) "Stareblock copolymer micellar nanocomposites with Mn, Zn-doped nanoferrite as superparamagnetic MRI contrast agent for tumor imaging," *Materials Letters*, 152, pp. 185–188.

Lunardi, G., Armirotti, A., Nicodemo, M., Cavallini, L., Demonte, G., Vannozzi, M. O. and Venturini, M. (2009) "Comparison of temsirolimus pharmacokinetics in patients with renal cell carcinoma not receiving dialysis and those receiving hemodialysis: A case series," *Clinical Therapeutics*, 31, pp. 1812–1819.

Mahato, K., Kumar, S., Srivastava, A., Maurya, P. K., Singh, R. and Chandra, P. (2018) "Electrochemical immunosensors: Fundamentals and applications in clinical diagnostics," *Handbook of Immunoassay Technologies*, pp. 359–414.

Market research report, Nanomedicine Market Analysis by Products, (Therapeutics, Regenerative Medicine, Diagnostics), by Application, (Clinical Oncology, Infectious Diseases), by Nanomolecule (Gold, Silver, Iron Oxide, Alumina), & Segment Forecasts, (2017), pp. 2013–2025 Report ID: 978-1-68038-942-5.

Martin, M., Salazar, P., Villalonga, R., Campuzano, S., Pingarron, J. M. and Gonzalez-Mora, J. L. (2014) "Preparation of core-shell Fe_3O_4 @ poly (dopamine) magnetic nanoparticles for biosensor construction," *Journal of Materials Chemistry* B2, pp. 739–746.

Minamihata, K. et al. (2020) "Genetically fused charged peptides induce rapid crystallization of proteins," *Chemical Communications (Cambridge, England)*, 56(27), pp. 3891–3894. doi: 10.1039/c9cc09529b.

Misra, S. K. et al. (2014) "A cationic cholesterol based nanocarrier for the delivery of p53-EGFP-C3 plasmid to cancer cells," *Biomaterials*, 35(4), pp. 1334–1346.

Mitchell, M. J. et al. (2021) "Engineering precision nanoparticles for drug delivery," *Nature Reviews: Drug Discovery*, 20(2), pp. 101–124.

Mujokoro, B. et al. (2016) "Nano-structures mediated co-delivery of therapeutic agents for glioblastoma treatment: A review," *Materials Science & Engineering. C, Materials for Biological Applications*, 69, pp. 1092–1102.

Müller, R. H. and Keck, C. M. (2010) "Pharmaceutical nanoparticles—from their innovative origin to their future," *International Journal of Pharmaceutics*, 390(1), pp. 1–2.

Munaweera, I. et al. (2016) "Chemically powered nanomotor as a delivery vehicle for biologically relevant payloads," *Journal of Nanoscience and Nanotechnology*, 16(9), pp. 9063–9071. doi: 10.1166/jnn.2016.12904.

Nanomedicine Market Analysis By Products, (Therapeutics, Regenerative Medicine, Diagnostics), By Application, (Clinical Oncology, Infectious diseases), By Nanomolecule (Gold, Silver, Iron Oxide, Alumina), & Segment Forecasts, 2013–2025 (2017). Available at: www.reportlinker.com/p04899216/Nanomedicine-Market-Analysis-By-Products-Therapeutics-Regenerative-Medicine-Diagnostics-By-Application-Clinical-Oncology-Infectious-diseases-By-Nanomolecule-Gold-Silver-Iron-Oxide-Alumina-Segment-Forecasts.html.

Ngoc, N. T. et al. (2015) "Application of chitosan-based nanocarriers in tumor-targeted drug delivery," *Reinvention of Chemotherapy: Drug Conjugates and Nanoparticles*, 27, pp. 201–218.

Prasad, M. et al. (2018) "Nanotherapeutics: An insight into healthcare and multi-dimensional applications in medical sector of the modern world," *Biomedecine & pharmacotherapie [Biomedicine & Pharmacotherapy]*, 97, pp. 1521–1537. doi: 10.1016/j.biopha.2017.11.026.

Razavi, R., Kenari, R. E., Farmani, J. and Jahanshahi, M. (2020) "Fabrication of zein/alginate delivery system for nanofood model based on pumpkin," *International Journal of Biological Macromolecules*, 165(Pt B), pp. 3123–3134.

Reibold, M. et al. (2006) "Materials: Carbon nanotubes in an ancient Damascus sabre: Materials," *Nature*, 444(7117), p. 286.

Roorda, W. K. (2001) *Advanced Cardiovascular Systems, Inc. Patent No. US 6283949*.

Saadeh, Y. and Vyas, D. (2014) "Nanorobotic applications in medicine: Current proposals and designs," *American Journal of Robotic Surgery*, 1(1), pp. 4–11. doi: 10.1166/ajrs.2014.1010.

Saha, S., Ganguly, J., Pal, S. and Ghosh, M. (2016) "Influence of anisotropy and position-dependent effective mass on electro-optic effect of impurity doped quantum dots in presence of Gaussian white noise," *Chemical Physics Letters*, 658, pp. 254–258.

Schumacher, C. M., Herrmann, I. K., Bubenhofer, S. B., Gschwind, S., Hirt, A.-M., Beck-Schimmer, B., Gunther, D. and Stark, A. J. (2013) "Quantitative recovery of magnetic nanoparticles from flowing blood: Trace analysis and the role of magnetization," *Advanced Functional Materials*, 23, pp. 4888–4896.

Shah, A. et al. (2021) "Nanocarriers for targeted drug delivery," *Journal of Drug Delivery Science and Technology*, 62(102426), p. 102426.

Singhal, J. et al. (2021) "Recent advances in nano-bio-sensing fabrication technology for the detection of oral cancer," *Molecular Biotechnology*, 63(5), pp. 339–362. doi: 10.1007/s12033-021-00306-x.

Sinha, A. et al. (2022) "The translational paradigm of nanobiomaterials: Biological chemistry to modern applications," *Materials Today: Bio*, 17(100463), p. 100463.

Smaoui, S., Ben Hlima, H., Ben Braïek, O., Ennouri, K., Mellouli, L. and Mousavi Khaneghah, A. (2021) "Recent advancements in encapsulation of bioactive compounds as a promising technique for meat preservation," *Meat Science*, 181, p. 108585.

Su, X., Chan, C., Shi, J., Tsang, M.-K., Pan, Y., Cheng, C., Gerile, O. and Yang, M. (2017) "A graphene quantum dot@ Fe_3O_4@ SiO_2 based nanoprobe for drug delivery sensing and dual-modal fluorescence and MRI imaging in cancer cells," *Biosensors and Bioelectronics*, 92, pp. 489–495.

Tian, J. et al. (2013) "Cell-specific and pH-activatable rubyrin-loaded nanoparticles for highly selective near-infrared photodynamic therapy against cancer," *Journal of the American Chemical Society*, 135(50), pp. 18850–18858. doi: 10.1021/ja408286k.

Valente, J. F. A. et al. (2013) "Microencapsulated chitosan–dextran sulfate nanoparticles for controled delivery of bioactive molecules and cells in bone regeneration," *Polymer*, 54(1), pp. 5–15. doi: 10.1016/j.polymer.2012.10.032.

Ventola, C. L. (2012) "The nanomedicine revolution: Part 1: Emerging concepts," *Pharmacy and Therapeutics*, 1, pp. 512–525.

Wagner, V. et al. (2006) "The emerging nanomedicine landscape," *Nature Biotechnology*, 24(10), pp. 1211–1217.

Wang, A. Z., Langer, R. and Farokhzad, O. C. (2012) "Nanoparticle delivery of cancer drugs," *Annual Review of Medicine*, 63, pp. 185–198.

Wang, F. et al. (2013) "Bioinspired micro/nano fabrication on dental implant—bone interface," *Applied Surface Science*, 265, pp. 480–488. doi: 10.1016/j.apsusc.2012.11.032.

Wang, F., Banerjee, D., Liu, Y., Chen, X. and Liu, X. (2010) "Upconversion nanoparticles in biological labeling, imaging and therapy," *Analyst*, 135, pp. 1839–1854.

Wang, K., Huang, Q., Qiu, F. et al. (2015) "Non-viral delivery systems for the application in p53 cancer gene therapy," *Current Medicinal Chemistry*, 22, pp. 4118–4136.

Wang, Z. et al. (2021) "NanoZnO-modified titanium implants for enhanced anti-bacterial activity, osteogenesis and corrosion resistance," *Journal of Nanobiotechnology*, 19(1), p. 353. doi: 10.1186/s12951-021-01099-6.

Xu, H., Li, S. and Liu, Y.-S. (2022) "Nanoparticles in the diagnosis and treatment of vascular aging and related diseases," *Signal Transduction and Targeted Therapy*, 7(1), p. 231. doi: 10.1038/s41392–022–01082-z.

Xu, Y. et al. (2021) "Photodynamic therapy with tumor cell discrimination through RNA-targeting ability of photosensitizer," *Molecules (Basel, Switzerland)*, 26(19), p. 5990.

Yamamoto, V. et al. (2014) "From nanotechnology to nanoneuroscience/nanoneurosurgery and nanobioelectronics: A historical review of milestones," in Kateb, B. and Heiss, J. D. (eds.) *The textbook of nanoneuroscience and nanoneurosurgery*. Boca Raton, FL: CRC Press.

Yao, N., Epstein, A. and Akey, A. (2006) "Crystal growth via spiral motion in abalone shell nacre," *Journal of Materials Research*, 21(8), pp. 1939–1946.

Zhang, B. et al. (2014) "Charge-reversal polymers for biodelivery," in *Bioinspired and biomimetic polymer systems for drug and gene delivery*. Weinheim, Germany: Wiley-VCH Verlag GmbH & Co. KGaA, pp. 223–242.

Zhang, Y., Wang, L., Yu, J., Yang, H., Pan, G., Miao, L. and Song, Y. (2017) "Three-dimensional macroporous carbon supported hierarchical ZnO-NiO nanosheets for electrochemical glucose sensing," *Journal of Alloys and Compounds*, 698, pp. 800–806.

Zheng, G., Patolsky, F., Cui, Y., Wang, W. U. and Lieber, C. M. (2005) "Multiplexed electrical detection of cancer markers with nanowire sensor arrays," *Nature Biotechnology*, 23, pp. 1294–1301.

Zhu, X., Wu, G., Lu, N., Yuan, X. and Li, B. (2017) "A miniaturized electrochemical toxicity biosensor based on graphene oxide quantum dots/carboxylated carbon nanotubes for assessment of priority pollutants," *Journal of Hazardous Materials*, 324, pp. 272–280.

2 Nanotherapeutics—An Emerging Topic in Health Sciences

2.1 EVOLUTION AND CURRENT STATUS OF NANOTHERAPEUTICS

Nanotherapeutics have become the pillars of numerous successful interventions in the field of health science. They have a few decades of history starting with scanning tunnel microscopes (STM) (Yamamoto et al., 2014). Although nanotherapeutics is a growing field of study, it has already achieved a number of medical milestones. The first nanotechnological approach in the 1950s by Richard P. Feynman, who was a Nobel laureate, is considered as the constitutive force to the establishment of the nanotherapeutics (Feynman, 1960). The book *Unbounding the Future*, by K. Eric Drexler, Chris Peterson, and Gayle Pergamit, discusses the potential applications of "nanobots" or "assemblers" in medicine. It was the first time the interfaces of nano-technology and medicine were combined. The word "nanomedicine" which is also related to nanotherapeutics was allegedly first used in the book *The Nanotechnology Revolution*, which was released in 1991 (Drexler, Peterson and Pergamit, 1991). In addition, the book *Nanomedicine* by Robert A. Freitas, which was released in 1999, has originated the word "Nanomedicine," which has subsequently been used in technical literature. Feynman and Drexler's visions were that nanoscale robots can patrol the body, neutralize disease foci, and detect and repair organs and cells with impaired function. Without this paradigm shift of vision, it is still decades away where nanomedicine is primarily focused on research into the potential for controlling and manipulating cell processes, such as by using genetically modified organisms (Freitas, 1999).

Paul Ehrlich tried to create "magic bullets" at the start of the twentieth century that contained medications that could be used to target diseases and eliminate all pathogenic agents with just one treatment (Kreuter, 2007). He created Salvarsan, which is said to be the first precisely acting treatment of its kind and the birth of che-motherapy. The development of ever-more complex "magic bullets" was made fea-sible by the information obtained over the course of the twentieth century about cells and their components, intra- and intercellular activities, and cell communication, as well as advancements in biochemistry and biotechnology. Peter Paul Speiser created the first nanoparticles that can be used for targeted medicinal therapies at the end of the 1960s. The monoclonal antibodies were successfully produced by Georges Jean Franz Köhler and César Milstein in the 1970s (Köhler and Milstein, 1975). Since then, there had been a lot of investigation into the potential synthesis, applications, and physicochemical functionalization of a variety of nanotechnology-based carrier systems. Nanoparticles were originally modified at the beginning of the 1990s to carry DNA fragments and genes, and they were then sluiced into cells with the help of antibodies (Kateb and Heiss, 2014).

In the late twentieth century, the term "nanotherapeutics" first appeared; nevertheless, the first scientific publications that used this term emerged in 2000, claims the Science Citation Index (Institute for Scientific Information, Thompson, Philadelphia, PA). Since research programs, symposiums, and publications have been concentrating on nanotherapeutics for an array of years, it is apparent that this area of study is more than just a conceptual trend despite the difficulty in defining it precisely given its blurred borders encompassed by biotechnology and microsystems technological advances (Royal Society & Royal Academy of Engineering, 2004).

The rise in "nanotherapeutics" research over the past ten years is being translated into significant commercialization activities on a global scale. Governmental organizations are proposing funding programs to assist this research in response to these changes, and several scientific administrations have commissioned roadmaps and foresight studies to examine the marketable and technological aspects of this expanding industry. Based on a comparison of the amount of journal publications in nanomedicine and nanotechnology (approximately 34,300 papers during 2004), nanotherapeutics currently account for around 4% of all research on nanotechnology carried out globally. According to a study of the geographical distribution of nanotherapeutics research, the largest research communities are in the Boston area, San Francisco, Tokyo, Berlin, and South-east England. Throughout the last ten years, the first nanotherapeutic agents have entered the market. According to the active patenting activity of US scientists and enterprises, the United States has a more advanced commercialization status than other nations (Anselmo and Mitragotri, 2016).

The majority of the time, nanotechnology in medicine serves as an enabler. However, its greatest power comes by its own adaptability. Numerous pharmaceutical products and medical equipment could benefit from the revolutionary features that nanotechnology might experience. Most of the time, it only serves as a useful element of a pharmaceutical agent. Since the beginning of the twentieth century, the interest of pharmaceutical and medical device industries has gradually increased; the last few decades have seen an upsurge in patent activities in particular (Dullaart, Bock and Zweck, 2006).

Anselmo and Mitragotri (2016) described the clinical landscape of nanotherapeutics, which included more than 25 nanotechnological approaches approved by the FDA and 45 nanotherapeutic products that were undergoing clinical studies. Fifty nanotherapeutic formulations were available for patient care in 2019 (Anselmo and Mitragotri, 2019). In addition, 90 clinical trials for nanomedicines used 15 new nanotechnologies (Anselmo and Mitragotri, 2019). In the context of the most recent achievement, the generation of lipid nanoparticles (NPs) for vaccine distribution in the aftermath of COVID-19 (Shin et al., 2020; Khurana et al., 2021) has provided nanotherapeutics the boost they required to demonstrate their higher potential.

The biggest barrier to commercialization of nanotherapeutics is the caution with which firms are still investing in the research of nanotherapeutics. The implementation of unique medical regulations tailored to nanotechnology that can add new requirements to the licensing procedure for nanotherapeutics also hinders the commercialization of these products. For businesses preparing to invest in nanotherapeutics, an early resolution of this matter is crucial. Despite the commercial operations, nanotherapeutics are still a technological field with unmet scientific needs. Since the chemistry of nanosized molecules is still poorly understood, it is expensive to produce nanomaterials like dendrimers or pharmaceutical-grade liposomes.

Hence there is an ongoing debate among regulators, industry, and scientists about whether or not new laws are required to take into consideration the unique pharmacokinetic characteristics of nanotherapeutics. These qualitative discussions will enable the entry of nanotherapeutics from the benchtop of the laboratory to the real world (Dullaart, Bock and Zweck, 2006).

2.2 FORMULATION OF NANOTHERAPEUTICS

Nanotechnology and nanotherapeutics have undergone an entire revolution recently. From 1980, there has occurred a significant growth in the number of authorized nano-based therapeutic formulations. These innovative nano-based platforms may function as therapeutic substances in their own proper capacity or serve as vehicles for delivering various active pharmacological drugs to specific regions of the body. Nanocrystals, micelles, liposomes and lipid nanoparticles, nanoemulsions, PEGylated polymeric nanodrugs, bioconjugates, other polymers, dendrimers, protein-based nanoparticles, organic nanoparticles, and metal-based nanoparticles are currently commercialized nanoformulations. In order to develop these nanostructures, a number of obstacles must be dealt with. Some critical problems in developing of nanotherapeutics include ethical issues, market share, the likelihood of market abandonment, price, and commercialization. Only a few of the aforementioned nanoformulations received marketing approval following all ethical and biological tests and fulfilling investors about future profitability (Ahmed et al., 2022).

Despite the fact that different nanocarriers are utilized in the fabrication of antitumor nano-therapeutics, the majority of these compounds depend on two basic fundamental principles. They include increasing tumor tissue concentration by exploiting the high penetrating ability of the tumor and retention impact (EPR) for enhanced efficacy; minimizing the clearance of nanotherapeutic agent by the reticuloendothelial system in the human body; and improving the amount present in plasma, thus decreasing the intake of nanotherapeutic agent by regular tissues and decreasing adverse reactions, while strengthening nanotherapeutic agent has efficacy in tumor EPR to increase therapeutic effect. Despite the fact that these two concepts have been consistently validated in animal tumor models, the majority of antitumor nanotherapeutic drugs did not increase effectiveness in clinical trials, leading to failure (Colombo et al., 2018).

Furthermore, nanotherapeutic formulations ought to be drug- and nanocarrier-specific in the design of formulation. To fully comprehend the unique effectiveness and security of nanotherapeutic agents, it is vital to thoroughly examine their pharmacokinetic profiles, which may boost the success percentage of clinical modification in preclinical laboratory animal models. Figure 2.1 shows generalization of a

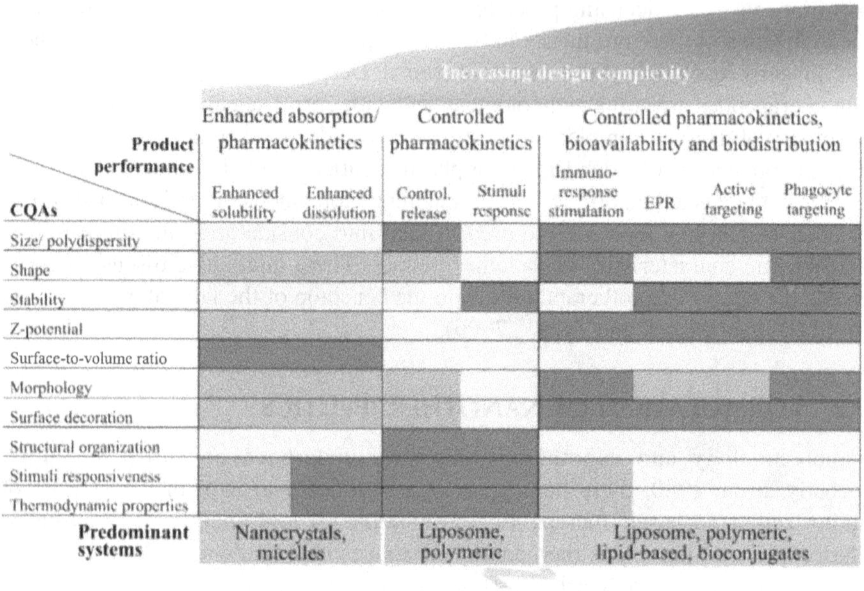

Increasing design complexity

Product performance / CQAs	Enhanced absorption/ pharmacokinetics		Controlled pharmacokinetics		Controlled pharmacokinetics, bioavailability and biodistribution			
	Enhanced solubility	Enhanced dissolution	Control. release	Stimuli response	Immuno-response stimulation	EPR	Active targeting	Phagocyte targeting
Size/ polydispersity								
Shape								
Stability								
Z-potential								
Surface-to-volume ratio								
Morphology								
Surface decoration								
Structural organization								
Stimuli responsiveness								
Thermodynamic properties								
Predominant systems	Nanocrystals, micelles		Liposome, polymeric		Liposome, polymeric, lipid-based, bioconjugates			

FIGURE 2.1 Generalization of a formulation model allows clustering of existing nanomedicine products by principle of action, where each group identified by a limited number of critical quality attributes (CQA) is related to the primary seminal invention principles.

Source: Reproduced with permission from Colombo et al., 2018.

formulation model allows clustering of existing nanomedicine products by principle of action, where each group identified by a limited number of critical quality attributes (CQA) is related to the primary seminal invention principles (Colombo et al., 2018).

A number of researchers have offered novel suggestions or recommendations for the current research interests in nanotherapeutics formulation and design. Those suggestions and recommendations can be summarized as follows: assess the special chemical and physical characteristics, pharmacokinetic profiles, and possible drawbacks of each medication, and their associated efficacy and toxic characteristics, aim designing of nanoformulations, investigate the properties of nanocarrier circulation in the human body along with how to adjust medications to target various tissues to establish safety and effectiveness. They have highlighted that the transport of nanotherapeutic drugs to infected target tissues is however not a sufficient prerequisite, and finally to increase their curative impact. Moreover, nanotherapeutic agents must distribute medications to multiple targeted tissues in the pathological tissue microenvironment.

2.3 PHARMACOKINETICS OF NANOTHERAPEUTICS

The main aim of nanotherapeutics is the development of next-generation medicines with improved safety, bioavailability, pharmacological activity, biocompatibility, and biological adherence while reducing the dosage, clearance, and metabolism

(Sahoo, Parveen and Panda, 2007). Advanced drug pharmacology engineering has been made possible by nanoscale formulations, which have improved release of therapeutics, absorption, distribution, metabolism and excretion, and duration of drug residence (Suk et al., 2016). PEGylation of nanotherapeutics to extend their duration of circulation and to postpone immune identification and metabolism has strongly mediated these advancements (Suk et al., 2016).

Improved modeling and screening of nanotechnology platforms, targeting to intracellular compartments, sensor-based drug release, as well as the utilization of nanotechnology toward a wider range of therapeutic categories, along with drug release that are based on sensors and focusing to intracellular compartments are some of the nanotherapeutic advancements (Sindhwani and Chan, 2021). Current developments demonstrated the wide-ranging effects of nanomaterials on medication absorption, distribution, metabolism, and excretion as well as the significance of regulatory frameworks (Zolnik and Sadrieh, 2009).

In order to change the pharmacology of the nanotherapeutics being transported, nanotherapeutics use the properties of various nanomaterials. This results in alterations in the biological accumulation of nanotherapeutics (absorption, distribution, cellular uptake, metabolism, and elimination), and finally, their pharmacological effect. It offers a chance to improve the pharmacological actions of nanotherapeutics, especially which rely on hepatic activity. Future use of nanotherapeutics in humans will depend on the gathering of evidences regarding the clearance and safety of nanotherapeutics, which must be weighed against the toxicity of nanoparticles.

2.3.1 Pharmacokinetic Mechanisms of Nanotherapeutics

There are major mechanisms of pharmacokinetics which are responsible for the pharmacological action of the nanotherapeutics. They can be categorized as absorption, distribution, cellular uptake, clearance, and elimination (Figure 2.2).

Absorption of Nanotherapeutics

When taken orally, absorption takes place through the gastrointestinal tract and stomach. Therapeutics administered subcutaneously or intraperitoneally are absorbed through the circulation, whereas those administered intravenously are injected directly into the systemic circulation. The percentage of a nanotherapeutic that reaches the systemic circulation is known as bioavailability; therefore, pharmaceuticals administered intravenously will have a 100% bioavailability. When administered using various injection methods (subcutaneous, intramuscular, intraperitoneal, intravenous, or intradermal), the kinetics of lipid NPs carrying mRNA (Pardi et al., 2015) resulted in quick systemic absorption and diffusion. One significant distinction was that intravenous injections had a C_{max} (peak concentration) that was ten times higher than that of all other injection techniques, although T_{max} (time to reach the peak concentration) occurred simultaneously for all delivery techniques. The shortest half-life was seen with intravenous injections, which were twofold shorter than subcutaneous, intraperitoneal, and intramuscular injections and threefold shorter than intradermal and intramuscular injections (Pardi et al., 2015).

A. Zhang et al. / Advances in Colloid and Interface Science 284 (2020) 102261

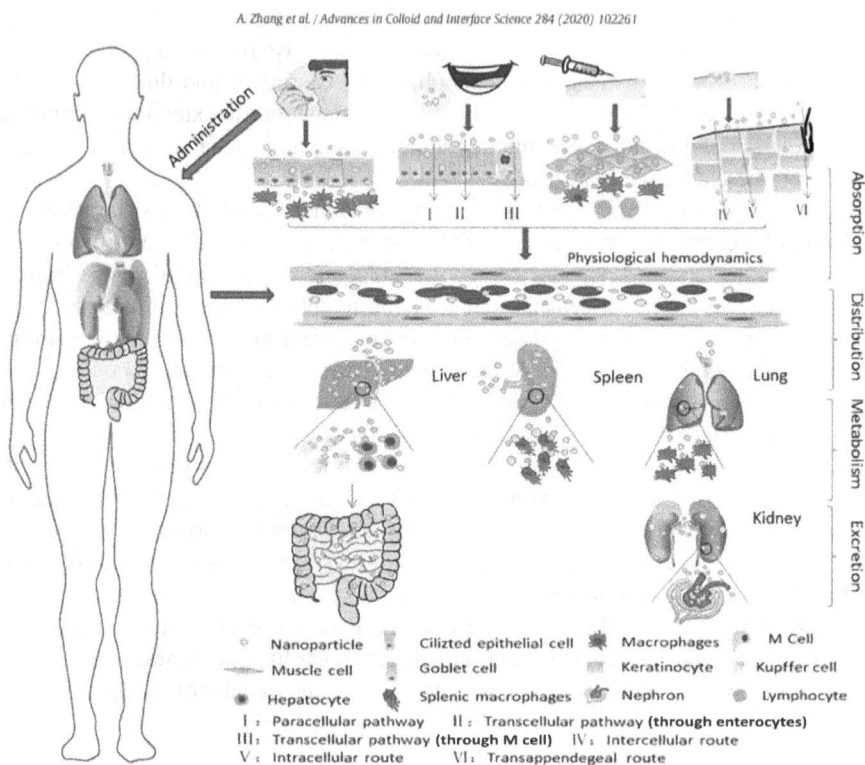

FIGURE 2.2 Absorption, distribution, metabolism, elimination (ADME) of nanotherapeutics *in vivo*.

Source: Reproduced with permission from A. Zhang et al., 2020.

Utilizing both *in vitro* and *in vivo* techniques, the assessing of the absorption by the oral route of nanotherapeutics demonstrate the significance of using different techniques to estimate the bioavailability percentage throughout the early stages of nanotherapeutics research (Faria et al., 2018). Peyer's patches or accumulated lymphoid nodules, M cells, and enterocytes all aid in the absorption of nanotherapeutics that are administered via the oral route into the gastrointestinal tract (Schimpel et al., 2014). Although lymphatic drainage patches have been investigated for immune modulation strategies and have been demonstrated to enhance the uptake of a variety of nanomaterials that are in different dimensions from 50 nm to 200 m, the absorption via lymphatics does not necessarily translate to enhanced bioavailability (Borges et al., 2006). Intestinal enterocytes may uptake an additional restricted range of nanostructures (50–500 nm), along with uptake rising with decreases in NP dimensions (Yao, McClements and Xiao, 2015).

In-depth analyses of enterocyte uptake for dendrimers (Kitchens et al., 2007), solid lipid nanoparticles (SLN), organics nanoparticles (Behrens et al., 2002; Coyuco et al., 2011), metal nanoparticles all have been conducted using Caco-2 cells (Chai et al.,

2016). To observe and analyze the dynamics of NP transfer, Caco-2 cells and co-cultures of Caco-2/HT29-MTX (enterocyte, mucus-secreting goblet, and M cells) are used (Schimpel et al., 2014). The utilization of inhibitors of endocytosis have shown that the uptake of metal nanoparticles, dendrimers, and organics NPs can be occurred through various particular and nonspecific methods, such as micropinocytosis and clathrin- and caveolin-mediated endocytosis (Kitchens et al., 2007; Chai et al., 2016).

These transcytosis and endocytosis routes are transport mechanisms that occur actively in the liver as well as in the GI tract, where they are used to remove systemically circulating nanomaterials directly. Several researches have used explants in the small intestine to examine the taking up of NPs. Those explants are more analogous toward the *in vivo* environment than *in vitro* cell cultures, allowing for easier and more flexible uptake studies (Kothari and Rajagopalan, 2019). By employing explants, it revealed that inhibitors of macropinocytosis, clathrin- and caveolin-mediated endocytosis, and macropinocytosis inhibited the nonspecific uptake of metal quantum dots (QDs) into small intestine explants (Hunt et al., 2020). By covering the surfaces of QDs with different polymers, receptor-specific endocytosis routes were made easier. The results of determination of the *in vivo* bioavailability of typical and polymer-coated QDs were consistent with those of the explant investigations (Hunt et al., 2020).

These investigations demonstrate that a variety of transporters actively take up nanoparticles rather than absorbing them passively. Usually, nanotherapeutics that are xenobiotic in their nature largely rely on active transport channels, especially the superfamilies of membrane transporters known as solute carriers (SLC) and solute carrier organic anions (SLCO). This pathway is not specific to nanomaterials with medicines (Döring and Petzinger, 2014).

It has been widely researched how to target certain nutrient-transporting vehicles (SLC5A6, SCL10A2, and SLC22A5) using surface coatings, selective dendrimers, and nanotherapeutic formulations to increase the oral bioavailability of distribution nanotherapeutic medication systems (Kou et al., 2018). The bioavailability of insulins and heparin that are administered orally has been enhanced by using biotin, tetra DOCA, deoxycholic acid, taurocholic acid, and L-carnitine (Lee et al., 2001; Lee et al., 2005; Lee et al., 2006). Several studies have revealed that the medication and the nanomaterials both are quickly transported to the liver and processed after ingestion. This clearly illustrates how these nanotherapeutic drug delivery systems may be used to specifically target hepatic drug receptors.

Interest in the way that gut microbial flora effects on the metabolism of xenobiotic agents (including NPs) has recently grown. Through azo reduction, amide generation, hydrolysis, nitro reduction, acetylation, deamination, sulfoxide/oxide reduction, and thiazide ring formation, microbiota aid in metabolism of nanotherapeutics (Jourova, Anzenbacher and Anzenbacherova, 2016). AgNP degradation has been extensively studied and is influenced by the microbiome and gastric pH (Bi et al., 2020). Nanotherapeutics, the intestinal microbiota, and the mucus secreted by epithelia all have intricated and multidirectional connections. NPs cause a rise in mucosal secretions, which restricts their ability to interact with cell membranes and prevents uptake. It has been reported that AgNPs may also have an immediate effect on the microbiome's composition, reducing populations of the microorganisms: Firmicutes and Lactobacillus (Bi et al., 2020). Figure 2.3 exhibits the cellular mechanisms of the absorption of nanotherapeutics which is administered via parenteral route.

Distribution of Nanotherapeutics

Distribution is the ratio of the steady-state concentration of a nanotherapeutic agent in the region where the drug is activated to the concentration of the circulation or the accumulation inside peripheral compartments. After the impacts of absorption, bioavailability, and first pass metabolism, the influence of drug transportation via the circulatory system is typically observed (Doogue and Polasek, 2013).

Nanotherapeutics usually face some issues with the distribution. Regardless of their composition, typical metal-based or uncoated nanoparticles exhibit extremely poor distribution and bioavailability since they are typically eliminated from the bloodstream after 10 minutes of systemic injection (Yoo, Chambers and Mitragotri, 2010; Suk et al., 2016). The liver is the site of most of this rapid accumulation and uptake takes place which is caused by the liver's extraordinary capacity for the first pass metabolism of xenobiotics, such as nanotherapeutics, and by the mononuclear phagocytic system (MPS). This absorption into the liver has been limited, and also MPS and first pass metabolism have been bypassed. Although NP hepatic absorption

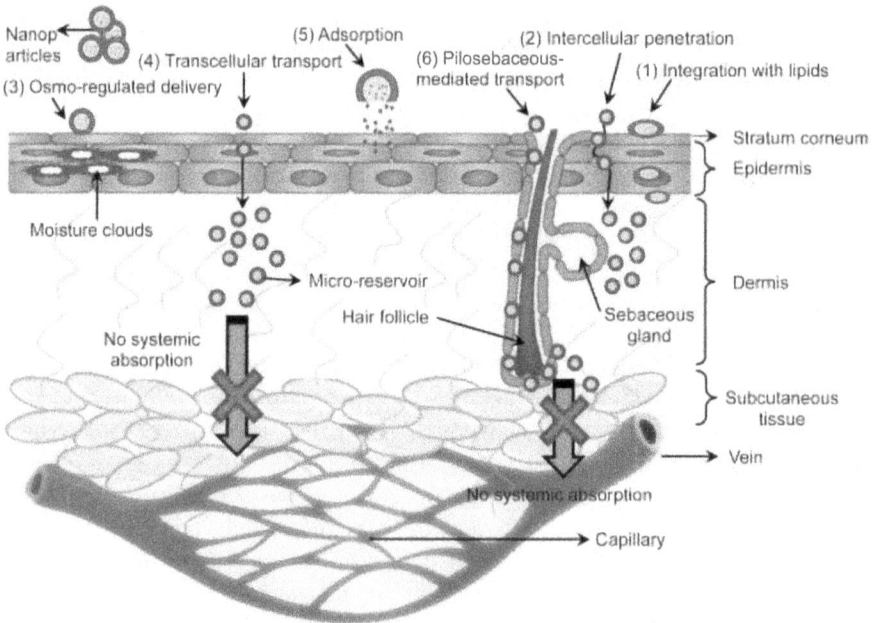

FIGURE 2.3 Pictorial representation of nanoparticles-based nanotherapeutics absorption from the skin to the circulatory system.

Source: Reproduced with permission from Raza et al., 2017.

and MPS are covered within the section on cellular uptake of nanotherapeutics, it is crucial to consider about the function of the cardiovascular system in supporting these clearance routes.

The circulating proteins include serum albumin, glycoproteins, complement, lipoproteins, coagulants, and immunoglobulins which can be rapidly bound to NPs Madathiparambil Visalakshan et al. (2020). As soon as entering those nanotherapeutics into body which are administered to the circulatory system, proteins bound to NPs and then soft and hard protein coronas made up of 10–1,000 proteins begin to form as a result of this phenomenon (Ke et al., 2017). Considering their constitutes, morphologies, and surface chemistry, those proteins can bind to NPs in a wide variety of ways, with alterations in hard and soft protein coronas controlling the duration taken for the circulation along with a differential cellular uptake (García-Álvarez et al., 2018; Richtering, Alberg and Zentel, 2020). A crucial tactic for targeted drug administration is to conceal NPs from protein corona formation (Oh et al., 2018; Alberg et al., 2020). One technique used to prevent MPS uptake is the prefabricated serum albumin attachment to NPs (Pitek et al., 2016). Several researches have focused their attention on reduction of MPS uptake in order to enhance the uptake of nanotherapeutics in order to obtain an effective distribution of nanotherapeutics.

Cellular Uptake of Nanotherapeutics

Mononuclear phagocyte system (MPS) plays a crucial role in cellular uptake of nanotherapeutics. Monocytes and macrophages from the spleen and lymph, as well as Kupffer cells (KCs) in the liver, make up the MPS. The scavenger endothelial cells located in the liver, or scavenger endothelial cells in the liver (LSECs), represent the second hurdle that NPs should get past to enter the circulatory system after encompassing the KCs (Poon et al., 2019). After optimization or attachment by the complement system, MPS cell types and LSECs are predominantly responsible for NP absorption; nevertheless, other passive and active transporting vehicles also contribute to NP clearance. Through nanopores in the LSECs known as fenestrations (below 120 nm), NPs are passively cleared from the circulation. Once in the space of Disse, they can be picked up by hepatocytes and guided toward the bile (Cogger, Hunt and Le Couteur, 2020).

Although KCs play a significant role in NP phagocytosis (Tsoi et al., 2016), those KCs also carry out a variety of other tasks, some of which may have an impact on nanotherapeutics. Through the inhibition of T regulatory cells and activation of IL-10 production, they contribute to the regulation of tolerogenic processes (Breous et al., 2009). Dendritic cells (DCs), natural killer cells, and natural killer T cells can all communicate with one another more easily, thanks to KCs (Nguyen-Lefebvre and Horuzsko, 2015). As a result of the C3 complement products' high activation of KCs, phagocytosis is triggered and NP absorption is increased (Nguyen-Lefebvre and Horuzsko, 2015). On the other hand, NP absorption by macrophages, especially KCs, is decreased by CD47-mediated immune suppression (Yong et al., 2017).

Protein coronas that encase NPs frequently contain the portions of C3a and C3b. The initial binding of immunoglobulin attaching to nanomaterials, especially IgG, is necessary for the binding of C3a and C3b to NPs. The epitope for NP attachment has not yet been found, however IgG served as a scaffold for C3b binding (Vu et al., 2019). Not surprisingly, IgG is utilized as a control in flow cytometry for its inherent ability to nonspecifically bind to a variety of diseases, surfaces, antigens, and proteins (Vu et al., 2019) IgG can bind to liposomes, superparamagnetic iron oxide NPs (SPIONs), FeNPs, and AuNPs. The presence of fibronectin or Fc on NPs helps macrophages to identify them as well (Neuberger et al., 2005). Additionally, NP clearance is aided by the opsonin-independent scavenger receptors on macrophages (Walkey et al., 2012). LSECs also carry out this task. The LSEC receptors implicated in NP consumption are still investigated, despite the fact that numerous receptors are likely to contribute to intake with varying degrees of efficiency. Stabilin-2 is of particular relevance because it is known to endocytose liposome-based NPs in alternative animal model for laboratory animals—zebra fish (Campbell et al., 2018).

In order to properly understand scavenging and phagocytosis in the context of nanotherapeutics clearance, it is necessary to describe the function of the scavenger endothelium. Phagocytosis is a process carried out by KCs, dendritic cells (DCs), and mononuclear cells, whereas clathrin-mediated scavenging represents a combination of transcytosis/endocytosis and pinocytosis (cellular drinking) that promotes the intake of sub-200 nm materials that are soluble (Sørensen et al., 2012). This distinction plays a significant role because nanotherapeutics scavenged by clathrin-mediated endocytosis are subjected to degrade, undergo exocytosis, and are cleared from this urine or bile within few days to a few weeks, whereas nanotherapeutics that remained within phagocytic cells have extended retention time duration (months to years) (Zhang et al., 2016; Hunt et al., 2020). This gives designers of nanotherapeutics a justification for choosing scavenging over phagocytosis as their preferred mode of targeting.

Pits that have been coated with clathrin mediate the endothelial transcytosis and endocytosis. This complex had been internalized, moved through tubules and vesicles, and then exocytosed toward the Disse space, which is the region located between LSECs and hepatocytes. Either receptors are involved in transcytosis and endocytosis, or they are not. Independent transcytosis performs for solutes in the plasma and macromolecules (restricted to 70 nm by the dimensions of clathrin-coated pits) like glycogen, dextran, and ferritin (Simionescu, Popov and Sima, 2009). The transportation of LDL, ceraloplasmin, transferrin, ceraloplasmin, insulin, and albumin (alb) is facilitated by clathrin-mediated transcytosis (Simionescu, Popov and Sima, 2009). Glycated proteins, as well as the chemokines CXCL10 and MCP-1, have recently been added to this list (Li et al., 2013; Shetty, Lalor and Adams, 2018). IL-1, p75 (death receptors), insulin, AGE, CP, Tf, Alb, EGF, HDL, and LDL receptors, as well as other receptors for receptor-mediated transcytosis, are present in the clathrin-coated pits (Simionescu, Popov and Sima, 2009).

Metabolism of Nanotherapeutics

An active drug is typically rendered inactive and water soluble through drug metabolism, enabling excretion of the drug via urine or bile. Phase I mechanisms and routes (e.g., oxidation and reduction, hydrolysis) and phase II mechanisms and routes (conjugation with water-soluble constituents such as glutathione, acetate, sulfate, and glucuronide) are the two processes by which nanotherapeutics are metabolized (Klotz, 2009). Despite the fact that the liver is where the most metabolism takes place, CYP3A4 can also be found in the colon, kidneys, brain, lung, placenta, and lymphocytes. P450 enzymes CYP3A4 (52%), CYP2D6 (30%), and CYP2C9/10/19 (11%) account for the majority of hepatic metabolism (Anzenbacher and Anzenbacherová, 2001). When it comes to metabolism, nanotherapeutics and NPs present a unique difficulty because of their quick cellular absorption by MPS (phagocytic cells) and LSECs, right after phagolysosome/lysosome-driven destruction. In this phase, enzyme metabolism also takes place, and nanotherapeutics are reduced and oxidized to increase their solubility for renal and biliary clearance.

The opsonization aided by C3b or/and IgG, phagocytic cells (MPS) are encouraged to degrade nanotherapeutics. These opsonin proteins encourage phagocytosis in KCs, neutrophils, and macrophages via either complement receptor or Fc receptor (FcR) signaling. The two signaling cascades produce phagosomes in distinctly different ways. In contrast to FcR signaling, which stimulates the Src family of kinases—SFKs (non-receptor tyrosine kinases) cause the activation of PI3K, PKC, Rac, and ERK and complement receptor signaling that facilitates activation of Rho GTPase and Arp 2/3 complexes (Uribe-Querol and Rosales, 2020). The actin cytoskeleton is altered by the phagosome to aid internalization. Once absorbed, the phagosome changes into a phagolysosome as lysozymes, myeloperoxidase, lipases, oxidase complexes of NADPH, and V-ATPase accumulate (Uribe-Querol and Rosales, 2020). V-ATPase supports an acidic surrounding (pH 4.5), and oxidase complexes generate reactive oxygen species (ROS) and superoxide (O^{2-}). Hydrogen peroxide is produced when oxygen dismutates, and it is based on coenzymes. O^{2-} dismutates to hydrogen peroxide, which in turn can form additional radical ions (Cl^-) based on coenzymes (myeloperoxidase) (Nauseef, 2014). In contrast to the phagolysosome, phagocytic cells also produce cytokines, ROS, secrete inflammatory mediators, degranulate antimicrobial compounds, and generate inflammatory mediators (Uribe-Querol and Rosales, 2020).

There have been reports of many nanotherapeutics degrading via phagolysosomes. Myeloperoxidase-induced hypochlorite and peroxynitrite pathways mediate the degradation of carbon nanotubes (Ding et al., 2017). Complete decomposition of MnO_2 NPs results in the formation of free Mn^{2+} ions, which are easily eliminated by the kidneys (Liu et al., 2017). Calcium-based nanotherapeutics breakdown at pH 5, but remain stable under neutral pH. Myeloperoxidases are produced when polystyrene- and TiO_2-based nanotherapeutics are added to the blend (Sanfins et al., 2018).

Compared to other nanotherapeutics, AuNPs incorporated nanotherapeutics pose a difficulty for degradation because, while being chemically inert, Au was demonstrated to stimulate a localized inflammatory response (Oh and Park, 2014). By trying to break down AuNPs, the phagocytic cell triggers this inflammatory reaction. The presence of coatings over the surface (such as PEGylation) or, with standard AuNPs, their prolonged retention within the phagocytic cell mediates the exocytosis of non-degraded AuNPs from macrophages (Oh and Park, 2014). Clinically, ferric carboxymaltose, ferric dextran, and ferric sucrose are forms of FeNPs that are utilized as treatments for iron shortage and are destroyed by phagocytic cells (Lyseng-Williamson and Keating, 2009). Fe sucrose exhibits complement-mediated absorption; however, other compounds differ in how their cellular take-up into phagocytic cells is carried out (Faria et al., 2019). The aforementioned findings emphasize the significance of the metal propensity of NPs-based nanotherapeutics to degrade.

Due to their enormous endocytic capability, LSECs play a crucial part in the degradation of nanotherapeutic agents (Poon et al., 2019). LSECs recognize and internalize immune complexes, such as small circulating IgG complexes, pathogen-associated molecular patterns, and cellular debris employing a number of receptors, including the mannose receptor, stabilins 1/2 (SRH1/2), and the endocytic Fc2B receptor. For instance, LSEC remove gram quantities of denatured collagen and procollagen I N-terminal peptides resulting from bone turnover via the mannose receptor and stabilin-2/SRH-2, respectively (Mousavi et al., 2007). BK polyoma virus, bacteriophages, and adenoviruses are also eliminated by LSECs (Øie et al., 2020). The ability of LSECs to degrade endocytosed proteins, lipids, and nucleic acids depends on the availability of circulating lysosomal enzymes that are taken up by LSECs by mannose receptor-mediated endocytosis (Elvevold et al., 2008). It has demonstrated that Ag_2S QDs coupled to a scavenger receptor binding ligand can be selectively degraded by LSECs *in vivo* (Hunt et al., 2020). In comparison to unconjugated Ag_2S QDs, the endocytic absorption rate increased by five times when this ligand was attached, but there were no variations in the volume or rate of excretion from the entire animal. Figure 2.4 illustrates the pathways of hepatic clearance of nanotherapeutics.

It is crucial to note that phagocytic cells and NPs-based nanotherapeutics that are broken down or saturated by LSECs result in soluble and excretable agent that can either be eliminated via the kidneys or carried to the bile by soluble carriers (SLCs and SLCOs). Problematically, the base of the nanotherapeutic can continue to be reactive and capable of causing cellular stress and harm even after it has been destroyed. The categorical sequence of metals that cause toxic effects highlights this effect, which is most obviously associated with metal nanoparticles-based nanotherapeutics. For instance, compared to Ag- and carbon-based nanotherapeutics, CeSe/ZnS induce high amounts of oxidative stress, cellular damage, and DNA damage (Malaviya, Shukal and Vasavada, 2019).

Elimination of Nanotherapeutics

Activated or passive mechanisms can cleanse the urine in order to eliminate the metabolized nanotherapeutics from the body. The solubility of the medicine or nanotherapeutic size (hydrodynamic diameter which is lesser than 6 nm), and protein binding status (albumin or corona-coated materials are difficult to eject) all affect passive clearance, which takes place via glomerular filtration. Glomerular filtration rate (GFR) which can be referred to as the plasma flow from the glomerulus toward the Bowman's space determines passive clearance.

Nanotherapeutics might even cross the renal proximal tubule cells and reach the renal tubules via active secretion, which is made possible by solute carriers (SLC) and ATP-binding cassette (ABC) transporters (Yin and Wang, 2016). Active urine secretion transporters and biliary excretion transporters have a lot in common. Waste is transported into the bile cannula through hepatic biliary transport, which is handled by several mediators (Jetter and Kullak-Ublick, 2020). Hepatic bile, which

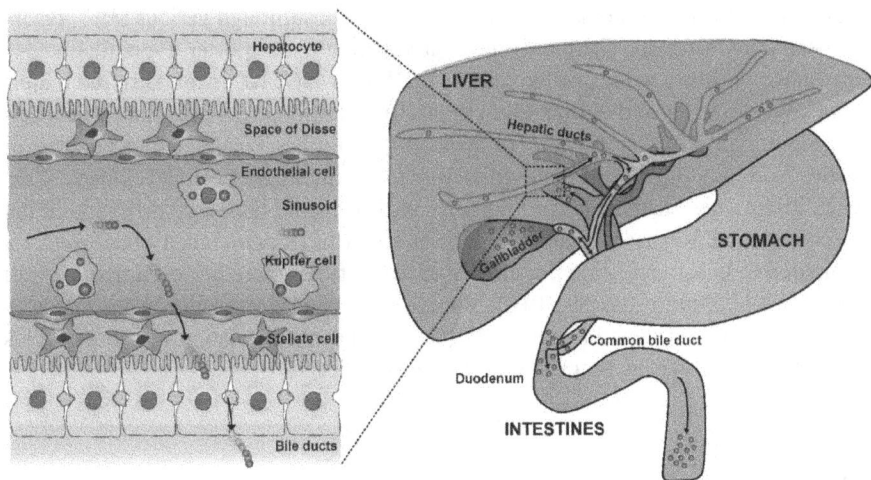

FIGURE 2.4 Schematic of the hepatobiliary processing and clearance of nanoparticles. (1) Nanoparticles enter the liver via the portal vein. (2) Nanoparticles traverse the hepatic sinusoid and (3) may be taken up and sequestered in liver resident Kupffer cells. (4) Depending on their physicochemical properties, nanoparticles may filter out into the space of Disse and be endocytosed by hepatocytes. (5) Nanoparticles transcytose through the hepatocytes and enter the bile duct via bile canaliculi. (6) Nanoparticles travel through the hepatic ducts. (7) Depending on digestive state and bile production, nanoparticles may first collect inside the gallbladder or (8) nanoparticles may enter into the common bile duct. (9) Nanoparticles are excreted into the duodenum of the small intestines via the sphincter of Oddi. (10) Nanoparticles eventually traverse the entire gastrointestinal tract and are eliminated in feces.

Source: Reproduced with permission from Zhang et al., 2016.

is produced by the CYP450-mediated metabolism of cholesterol, bilirubin, and lipids, is made up of water, bile cholic acid, salts, and chenodexycholic acid.

The enzymatic decomposition that happens in an extensive spectrum of tissues causes an intersection across the two locations, with soluble blood-born solid wastes being eliminated from the body frequently. Collectively, these channels play a part toward the active excretion of drugs, xenobiotics, as well as nanotherapeutics. It has been demonstrated that AuNP-based nanotherapeutics cause size-dependent NP excretion via the urinary and biliary systems. AuNPs less than 6 nm are more easily excreted through the urine (Poon et al., 2019). The NPs with dimensions in the range of 7–8 nm have greater biliary clearance due to the fact that they contain reduced KC uptake and also perform passive filtration via the projected surface of the liver endothelium. This is truly the case for NPs which have larger dimensions than this, which shows a size-dependent correlation with active excretion through biliary clearance (Tsoi et al., 2016; Poon et al., 2019).

Many different NP subtypes have incredibly high biliary clearance. Mesoporous silica NPs coupled with indocyanine were used by Souris et al. (2010) to show excellent biliary clearance. Last but not least, it has been shown that 7-nm Ag_2S QDs administered orally have a high biliary clearance (Hunt et al., 2020).

Active removal of xenobiotics and nanotherapeutics through various transporters has been demonstrated. The most prevalent xenobiotic transporter, P-gp, that is also known as multidrug resistance protein 1 (MDR1) or ABCB1, is found in the majority of organs (Jetter and Kullak-Ublick, 2020). Additionally, some cancerous cells have significant P-gp expression. To avoid P-gp-facilitated clearance of nanotherapeutics from specific malignancies, different techniques have been developed (Niazi et al., 2016). These tactics' lower long-term clearance and increased diffusion of the aforementioned NP-based nanotherapeutics could have unintended consequences. Compared to hepatocytes, P-gp is expressed seven times more in the GI tract as well as in the blood–brain barrier (BBB). Impaired P-gp clearance may be a factor in NP toxicity and protracted retention. Figure 2.5 shows elimination of nanoparticles through different organs according to their properties.

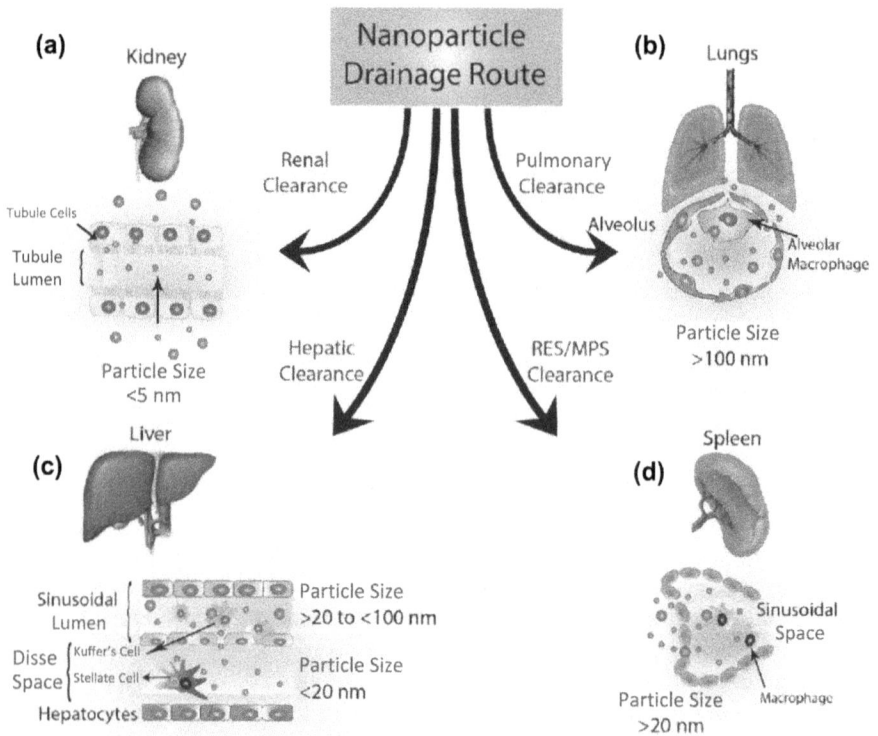

FIGURE 2.5 Elimination of nanoparticles through different organs according to their properties. The kidney is the most traditional drainage system eliminating the particles <5 nm (a) and the particles <5 nm are easily eliminated from the blood. Although the lungs (b) are not a conventional eliminatory system, they can help in filtering aerosolic nanoparticle elimination with sizes >100 nm. A second level of elimination is done through the liver (c) where particles of size 20–100 nm can pass through. The larger particles (<200 nm) which are not eliminated through the kidney or liver are eventually eliminated by the RES, e.g., lymph node and spleen (d).

Source: Reproduced with permission from Bose et al., 2014.

The GI tract and liver have the highest concentrations of these active absorption routes, particularly the SLC channels. This widely accepted presence draws attention to a crucial problem with identifying and using these channels to promote bioavailability because it shows a probably higher clearance with more exact targeting of those transporters. Nevertheless, if the nanotherapeutic agent can be discharged within a short period of time, drug administration may be facilitated during this quick clearance.

REFERENCES

Ahmed, T. et al. (2022) "Advances in nanomedicine design: Multidisciplinary strategies for unmet medical needs," *Molecular Pharmaceutics*, 19(6), pp. 1722–1765. doi: 10.1021/acs.molpharmaceut.2c00038.

Alberg, I., Kramer, S., Schinnerer, M., Hu, Q., Seidl, C., Leps, C. et al. (2020) "Polymeric nanoparticles with neglectable protein corona," *Small*, 16, p. 1907574. doi: 10.1002/smll.201907574.

Anselmo, A. C. and Mitragotri, S. (2016) "Nanoparticles in the clinic," *Bioengineering & Translational Medicine*, 1, pp. 10–29. doi: 10.1002/btm2.10003.

Anselmo, A. C. and Mitragotri, S. (2019) "Nanoparticles in the clinic: An update," *Bioengineering & Translational Medicine*, 4(3). doi: 10.1002/btm2.10143.

Anzenbacher, P. and Anzenbacherová, E. (2001) "Cytochromes P450 and metabolism of xenobiotics," *Cellular and Molecular Life Sciences*, 58, pp. 737–747. doi: 10.1007/pl00000897.

Behrens, I., Pena, A. I. V., Alonso, M. J. and Kissel, T. (2002) "Comparative uptake studies of bioadhesive and non-bioadhesive nanoparticles in human intestinal cell lines and rats: The effect of mucus on particle adsorption and transport," *Pharm. Res.*, 19, pp. 1185–1193. doi: 10.1023/a:1019854327540.

Bi, Y., Marcus, A. K., Robert, H., Krajmalnik-Brown, R., Rittmann, B. E., Westerhoff, P. et al. (2020) "The complex puzzle of dietary silver nanoparticles, mucus and microbiota in the gut," *J. Toxicol. Environ. Health B*, 23, pp. 69–89. doi: 10.1080/10937404.2019.1710914.

Borges, O., Cordeiro-Da-Silva, A., Romeijn, S. G., Amidi, M., De Sousa, A., Borchard, G. et al. (2006) "Uptake studies in rat peyer's patches, cytotoxicity and release studies of alginate coated chitosan nanoparticles for mucosal vaccination," *J. Controlled Release*, 114, pp. 348–358. doi: 10.1016/j.jconrel.2006.06.011.

Bose, T. et al. (2014) "Overview of nano-drugs characteristics for clinical application: The journey from the entry to the exit point," *Journal of Nanoparticle Research: An Interdisciplinary Forum for Nanoscale Science and Technology*, 16(8). doi: 10.1007/s11051-014-2527-7.

Breous, E., Somanathan, S., Vandenberghe, L. H. and Wilson, J. M. (2009) "Hepatic regulatory T cells and Kupffer cells are crucial mediators of systemic T cell tolerance to antigens targeting murine liver," *Hepatology*, 50, pp. 612–621. doi: 10.1002/hep.23043.

Campbell, F., Bos, F. L., Sieber, S., Arias-Alpizar, G., Koch, B. E., Huwyler, J. et al. (2018) "Directing nanoparticle biodistribution through evasion and exploitation of Stab2-dependent nanoparticle uptake," *ACS Nano*, 12, pp. 2138–2150. doi: 10.1021/acsnano.7b06995.

Chai, G.-H., Xu, Y., Chen, S.-Q., Cheng, B., Hu, F.-Q., You, J. et al. (2016) "Transport mechanisms of solid lipid nanoparticles across Caco-2 cell monolayers and their related cytotoxicology," *ACS Appl. Mater. Inter.*, 8, pp. 5929–5940. doi: 10.1021/acsami.6b00821.

Cogger, V. C., Hunt, N. J. and Le Couteur, D. G. (2020) "Fenestrations in the liver sinusoidalendothelial cell," *The Liver*, pp. 435–443. doi: 10.1002/9781119436812.ch35.

Colombo, S. et al. (2018) "Transforming nanomedicine manufacturing toward quality by design and microfluidics," *Advanced Drug Delivery Reviews*, 128, pp. 115–131. doi: 10.1016/j.addr.2018.04.004.

Coyuco, J. C., Liu, Y., Tan, B. J. and Chiu, G. N. (2011) "Functionalized carbon nanomaterials: Exploring the interactions with Caco-2 cells for potential oral drug delivery," *Int. J. Nanomedicine*, 6, pp. 2253–2263. doi: 10.2147/IJN.S23962.

Ding, Y., Tian, R., Yang, Z., Chen, J. and Lu, N. (2017) "NADPH oxidasedependent degradation of single-walled carbon nanotubes in macrophages," *J. Mater. Sci. Mater. Med.*, 28, p. 7. doi: 10.1007/s10856-016-5817-z.

Doogue, M. P. and Polasek, T. M. (2013) "The ABCD of clinical pharmacokinetics," *Ther. Adv. Drug Saf.*, 4, pp. 5–7. doi: 10.1177/2042098612469335.

Döring, B. and Petzinger, E. (2014) "Phase 0 and Phase III transport in various organs: Combined concept of phases in xenobiotic transport and metabolism," *Drug Metab. Rev.*, 46, pp. 261–282. doi: 10.3109/03602532.2014.882353.

Drexler, K. E., Peterson, C. and Pergamit, G. (1991) *Unbounding the future: The nanotechnology revolution*. New York: Morrow.

Dullaart, A., Bock, A.-K. and Zweck, A. (eds.) (2006) "The emerging nanomedicine landscape Volker Wagner, Anwyn Dullaart," *Nature Biotechnology*, 24(10).

Elvevold, K., Simon-Santamaria, J., Hasvold, H., Mccourt, P., Smedsrød, B. and Sørensen, K. K. (2008) "Liver sinusoidal endothelial cells depend on mannose receptor-mediated recruitment of lysosomal enzymes for normal degradation capacity," *Hepatology*, 48, pp. 2007–2015. doi: 10.1002/hep.22527.

Faria, B., Gaya Da Costa, M., Poppelaars, F., Franssen, C. F. M., Pestana, M., Berger, S. P. et al. (2019) "Administration of intravenous iron formulations induces complement activation in-vivo," *Front. Immunol.*, 10, p. 1885. doi: 10.3389/fimmu.2019.01885.

Faria, M., Björnmalm, M., Thurecht, K. J., Kent, S. J., Parton, R. G., Kavallaris, M. et al. (2018) "Minimum information reporting in bio-nano experimental literature," *Nat. Nanotech*, 13, pp. 777–785. doi: 10.1038/s41565-018-0246-4.

Feynman, R. P. (1960) "There's plenty of room at the bottom: An invitation to enter a new field of physics," *Engineering and Science (Caltech)*, 23, pp. 22–36.

Freitas, Jr., R. A. (1999) *Nanomedicine, vol. I: Basic capabilities*. Georgetown, TX, USA: Landes Bioscience.

García-Álvarez, R., Hadjidemetriou, M., Sánchez-Iglesias, A., Liz-Marzán, L. M. and Kostarelos, K. (2018) "In vivo formation of protein corona on gold nanoparticles: The effect of their size and shape," *Nanoscale*, 10, pp. 1256–1264. doi: 10.1039/c7nr08322j.

Hunt, N. J., Lockwood, G. P., Le Couteur, F. H., Mccourt, P. A. G., Singla, N., Kang, S. W. S. et al. (2020) "Rapid intestinal uptake and targeted delivery to the liver endothelium using orally administered silver sulfide quantum dots," *ACS Nano*, 14, pp. 1492–1507. doi: 10.1021/acsnano.9b06071.

Jetter, A. and Kullak-Ublick, G. A. (2020) "Drugs and hepatic transporters: A review," *Pharmacol. Res.*, 154, p. 104234. doi: 10.1016/j.phrs.2019.04.018.

Jourova, L., Anzenbacher, P. and Anzenbacherova, E. (2016) "Human gut microbiota plays a role in the metabolism of drugs," *Biomed. Pap.*, 160, pp. 317–326. doi: 10.5507/bp.2016.039.

Kateb, B. and Heiss, J. D. (2014) *The textbook of nanoneuroscience and nanoneurosurgery*. Boca Raton, FL: CRC Press.

Ke, P. C., Lin, S., Parak, W. J., Davis, T. P. and Caruso, F. (2017) "A decade of the protein corona," *ACS Nano*, 11, pp. 11773–11776. doi: 10.1021/acsnano.7b08008.

Khurana, A., Allawadhi, P., Khurana, I., Allwadhi, S., Weiskirchen, R., Banothu, A. K. et al. (2021) "Role of nanotechnology behind the success of mRNA vaccines for COVID-19," *Nano Today*, 38, p. 101142. doi: 10.1016/j.nantod.2021.101142.

Kitchens, K. M., Foraker, A. B., Kolhatkar, R. B., Swaan, P. W. and Ghandehari, H. (2007) "Endocytosis and interaction of poly (amidoamine) dendrimers with Caco-2 cells," *Pharm. Res.*, 24, pp. 2138–2145. doi: 10.1007/s11095-007-9415-0.

Klotz, U. (2009) "Pharmacokinetics and drug metabolism in the elderly," *Drug Metab. Rev.*, 41, pp. 67–76. doi: 10.1080/03602530902722679.

Köhler, G. and Milstein, C. (1975) "Continuous cultures of fused cells secreting antibody of predefined specificity," *Nature*, 256(5517), pp. 495–497. doi: 10.1038/256495a0.

Kothari, A. and Rajagopalan, P. (2019) "Isolating rat intestinal explants for in vitro cultures," *Curr. Protoc. Toxicol.*, 80, p. e79. doi: 10.1002/cptx.79.

Kou, L., Bhutia, Y. D., Yao, Q., He, Z., Sun, J. and Ganapathy, V. (2018) "Transporter-guided delivery of nanoparticles to improve drug permeation across cellular barriers and drug exposure to selective cell types," *Front. Pharmacol.*, 9, p. 27. doi: 10.3389/fphar.2018.00027.

Kreuter, J. (2007) "Nanoparticles—a historical perspective," *International Journal of Pharmaceutics*, 331(1), pp. 1–10. doi: 10.1016/j.ijpharm.2006.10.021.

Lee, S., Lee, J., Lee, D. Y., Kim, S. K., Lee, Y. and Byun, Y. (2005) "A new drug carrier, N?-deoxycholyl-l-lysyl-methylester, for enhancing insulin absorption in the intestine," *Diabetologia*, 48, pp. 405–411. doi: 10.1007/s00125-004-1658-2.

Lee, Y.-K., Kim, S. K., Lee, D. Y., Lee, S., Kim, C.-Y., Shin, H.-C. et al. (2006) "Efficacy of orally active chemical conjugate of low molecular weight heparin and deoxycholic acid in rats, mice and monkeys," *J. Controlled Release*, 111, pp. 290–298. doi: 10.1016/j.jconrel.2005.12.011.

Lee, Y.-K., Nam, J. H., Shin, H.-C. and Byun, Y. (2001) "Conjugation of low molecular-weight heparin and deoxycholic acid for the development of new oral anticoagulant agent," *Circulation*, 104, pp. 3116–3120. doi: 10.1161/hc5001.100627.

Li, H.-H., Li, J., Wasserloos, K. J., Wallace, C., Sullivan, M. G., Bauer, P. M. et al. (2013) "Caveolae-dependent and -independent uptake of albumin in cultured rodent pulmonary endothelial cells," *PLoS One*, 8, e81903. doi: 10.1371/journal.pone.0081903.

Liu, J., Chen, Q., Zhu, W., Yi, X., Yang, Y., Dong, Z. et al. (2017) "Nanoscale coordination-polymer-shelled manganese dioxide composite nanoparticles: A multistage redox/pH/H_2O_2-responsive cancer theranostic nanoplatform," *Adv. Funct. Mater.*, 27, p. 1605926. doi: 10.1002/adfm.201605926.

Lyseng-Williamson, K. A. and Keating, G. M. (2009) "Ferric carboxymaltose," *Drugs*, 69, pp. 739–756. doi: 10.2165/00003495-200969060-00007.

Madathiparambil Visalakshan, R., González García, L. E., Benzigar, M. R., Ghazaryan, A., Simon, J., Mierczynska-Vasilev, A. et al. (2020) "The influence of nanoparticle shape on protein corona formation," *Small*, 16, 2000285. doi: 10.1002/smll.202000285.

Malaviya, P., Shukal, D. and Vasavada, A. R. (2019) "Nanotechnology-based drug delivery, metabolism and toxicity," *Curr. Drug Metab.*, 20, pp. 1167–1190. doi: 10.2174/1389200221666200103091753.

Mousavi, S. A., Sporstøl, M., Fladeby, C., Kjeken, R., Barois, N. and Berg, T. (2007) "Receptor-mediated endocytosis of immune complexes in rat liver sinusoidal endothelial cells is mediated by FcγRIIb2," *Hepatology*, 46, pp. 871–884. doi: 10.1002/hep.21748.

Nauseef, W. M. (2014) "Myeloperoxidase in human neutrophil host defence," *Cell Microbiol.*, 16, pp. 1146–1155. doi: 10.1111/cmi.12312.

Neuberger, T., Schöpf, B., Hofmann, H., Hofmann, M. and Von Rechenberg, B. (2005) "Superparamagnetic nanoparticles for biomedical applications: Possibilities and limitations of a new drug delivery system," *J. Magnetism Magn. Mater.* 293, pp. 483–496. doi: 10.1016/j.jmmm.2005.01.064.

Nguyen-Lefebvre, A. T. and Horuzsko, A. (2015) "Kupffer cell metabolism and function," *Journal of Enzymology and Metabolism*, 1, p. 101.

Niazi, M., Zakeri-Milani, P., Najafi Hajivar, S., Soleymani Goloujeh, M., Ghobakhlou, N., Shahbazi Mojarrad, J. et al. (2016) "Nano-based strategies to overcome P-glycoprotein-mediated drug resistance," *Expert Opin. Drug Metab. Toxicol.*, 12, pp. 1021–1033. doi: 10.1080/17425255.2016.1196186.

Oh, J. Y., Kim, H. S., Palanikumar, L., Go, E. M., Jana, B., Park, S. A. et al. (2018) "Cloaking nanoparticles with protein corona shield for targeted drug delivery," *Nat. Commun.*, 9, p. 4548. doi: 10.1038/s41467-018-06979-4.

Oh, N. and Park, J.-H. (2014) "Surface chemistry of gold nanoparticles mediates their exocytosis in macrophages," *ACS Nano*, 8, pp. 6232–6241. doi: 10.1021/nn501668a.

Øie, C. I. et al. (2020) "Liver sinusoidal endothelial cells contribute to the uptake and degradation of entero bacterial viruses," *Scientific Reports*, 10(1). doi: 10.1038/s41598-020-57652-0.

Pardi, N., Tuyishime, S., Muramatsu, H., Kariko, K., Mui, B. L., Tam, Y. K. et al. (2015) "Expression kinetics of nucleoside-modified mRNA delivered in lipid nanoparticles to mice by various routes," *J. Controlled Release*, 217, pp. 345–351. doi: 10.1016/j.jconrel.2015.08.007.

Pitek, A. S., Jameson, S. A., Veliz, F. A., Shukla, S. and Steinmetz, N. F. (2016) "Serum albumin 'camouflage' of plant virus based nanoparticles prevents their antibody recognition and enhances pharmacokinetics," *Biomaterials*, 89, pp. 89–97. doi: 10.1016/j.biomaterials.2016.02.032.

Poon, W., Zhang, Y.-N., Ouyang, B., Kingston, B. R., Wu, J. L. Y., Wilhelm, S. et al. (2019) "Elimination pathways of nanoparticles," *ACS Nano*, 13, pp. 5785–5798. doi: 10.1021/acsnano.9b01383.

Raza, K. et al. (2017) "Pharmacokinetics and biodistribution of the nanoparticles," In Surendra Nimesh, Ramesh Chandra and Nidhi Gupta (Eds.), *Advances in nanomedicine for the delivery of therapeutic nucleic acids*. Duxford: Elsevier, pp. 165–186.

Richtering, W., Alberg, I. and Zentel, R. (2020) "Nanoparticles in the biological context: Surface morphology and protein corona formation," *Small*, 16, p. 2002162. doi: 10.1002/smll.202002162.

Royal Society & Royal Academy of Engineering (2004) *Nanoscience and nanotechnologies: Opportunities and uncertainties*. Royal Society of Chemistry City: London, UK, pp. 485–488.

Sahoo, S. K., Parveen, S. and Panda, J. J. (2007) "The present and future of nanotechnology in human health care," *Nanomedicine: Nanotechnology, Biol. Med.*, 3, pp. 20–31. doi: 10.1016/j.nano.2006.11.008.

Sanfins, E., Correia, A., Gunnarsson, S. B., Cedervall, T. and Cedervall, T. (2018) "Nanoparticle effect on neutrophil produced myeloperoxidase," *PLoS One*, 13, p. e0191445. doi: 10.1371/journal.pone.0191445.

Schimpel, C., Teubl, B., Absenger, M., Meindl, C., Fröhlich, E., Leitinger, G. et al. (2014) "Development of an advanced intestinal in vitro triple culture permeability model to study transport of nanoparticles," *Mol. Pharmaceutics*, 11, pp. 808–818. doi: 10.1021/mp400507g.

Shetty, S., Lalor, P. F. and Adams, D. H. (2018) "Liver sinusoidal endothelial cells—gatekeepers of hepatic immunity," *Nat. Rev. Gastroenterol. Hepatol.*, 15, pp. 555–567. doi: 10.1038/s41575-018-0020-y.

Shin, M. D., Shukla, S., Chung, Y. H., Beiss, V., Chan, S. K., Ortega-Rivera, O. A. et al. (2020) "COVID-19 vaccine development and a potential nanomaterial path forward," *Nat. Nanotechnol.* 15, pp. 646–655. doi: 10.1038/s41565-020-0737-y.

Simionescu, M., Popov, D. and Sima, A. (2009) "Endothelial transcytosis in health and disease," *Cell Tissue Res.*, 335, pp. 27–40. doi: 10.1007/s00441-008-0688-3.

Sindhwani, S. and Chan, W. C. W. (2021) "Nanotechnology for modern medicine: Next step towards clinical translation," *J. Intern. Med.*, 290, pp. 486–498. doi: 10.1111/joim.13254.

Sørensen, K. K., Mccourt, P., Berg, T., Crossley, C., Le Couteur, D., Wake, K. et al. (2012) "The scavenger endothelial cell: A new player in homeostasis and immunity," *Am. J. Physiol. Regul. Integr. Comp. Physiol.*, 303, R1217–R1230. doi: 10.1152/ajpregu.00686.2011.

Souris, J. S., Lee, C.-H., Cheng, S.-H., Chen, C.-T., Yang, C.-S., Ho, J.-a. A. et al. (2010) "Surface charge-mediated rapid hepatobiliary excretion of mesoporous silica nanoparticles," *Biomaterials*, 31, pp. 5564–5574. doi: 10.1016/j.biomaterials.2010.03.048.

Suk, J. S., Xu, Q., Kim, N., Hanes, J. and Ensign, L. M. (2016) "PEGylation as a strategy for improving nanoparticle-based drug and gene delivery," *Adv. Drug Deliv. Rev.*, 99, pp. 28–51. doi: 10.1016/j.addr.2015.09.012.

Tsoi, K. M., Macparland, S. A., Ma, X.-Z., Spetzler, V. N., Echeverri, J., Ouyang, B. et al. (2016) "Mechanism of hard-nanomaterial clearance by the liver," *Nat. Mater*, 15, pp. 1212–1221. doi: 10.1038/nmat4718.

Uribe-Querol, E. and Rosales, C. (2020) "Phagocytosis: Our current understanding of a universal biological process," *Front. Immunol.*, 11, p. 1066. doi: 10.3389/fimmu.2020.01066.

Vu, V. P., Gifford, G. B., Chen, F., Benasutti, H., Wang, G., Groman, E. V. et al. (2019) "Immunoglobulin deposition on biomolecule corona determines frontiers in nanotechnology," *Nat. Nanotechnol.*, 14, pp. 260–268. doi: 10.1038/s41565-018-0344-3.

Walkey, C. D., Olsen, J. B., Guo, H., Emili, A. and Chan, W. C. W. (2012) "Nanoparticle size and surface chemistry determine serum protein adsorption and macrophage uptake," *J. Am. Chem. Soc.*, 134, pp. 2139–2147. doi: 10.1021/ja2084338.

Yamamoto, V., Suffredini, G., Nikzad, S., Hoenk, M. E., Boer, M. S. et al. (2014) "From nanotechnology to nanoneuroscience/nanoneurosurgery and nanobioelectronics: A historical review of milestones," in Kateb, B. and Heiss, J. D. (eds.) *The textbook of nanoneuroscience and nanoneurosurgery*. Boca Raton, FL: CRC Press.

Yao, M., McClements, D. J. and Xiao, H. (2015) "Improving oral bioavailability of nutraceuticals by engineered nanoparticle-based delivery systems," *Current Opinion in Food Science*, 2, pp. 14–19. doi: 10.1016/j.cofs.2014.12.005.

Yin, J. and Wang, J. (2016) "Renal drug transporters and their significance in drug-drug interactions," *Acta Pharmaceutica Sinica B*, 6, pp. 363–373. doi: 10.1016/j.apsb.2016.07.013.

Yong, S.-B., Song, Y., Kim, H. J., Ain, Q. U. and Kim, Y.-H. (2017) "Mononuclear phagocytes as a target, not a barrier, for drug delivery," *J. Controlled Release*, 259, pp. 53–61. doi: 10.1016/j.jconrel.2017.01.024.

Yoo, J.-W., Chambers, E. and Mitragotri, S. (2010) "Factors that control the circulation time of nanoparticles in blood: Challenges, solutions and future prospects," *Cpd*, 16, pp. 2298–2307. doi: 10.2174/138161210791920496.

Zhang, A. et al. (2020) "Absorption, distribution, metabolism, and excretion of nanocarriers in vivo and their influences," *Advances in Colloid and Interface Science*, 284(102261), p. 102261. doi: 10.1016/j.cis.2020.102261.

Zhang, Y.-N. et al. (2016) "Nanoparticle—liver interactions: Cellular uptake and hepatobiliary elimination," *Journal of Controlled Release: Official Journal of the Controlled Release Society*, 240, pp. 332–348. doi: 10.1016/j.jconrel.2016.01.020.

Zolnik, B. S. and Sadrieh, N. (2009) "Regulatory perspective on the importance of ADME assessment of nanoscale material containing drugs," *Adv. Drug Deliv. Rev.* 61, pp. 422–427. doi: 10.1016/j.addr.2009.03.006.

3 Nanotheranostics

3.1 WHAT ARE NANOTHERANOSTICS?

Nanotheranostics integrates diagnostic and therapeutic performance in a single system with the recent advances of nanotechnology in nanotherapeutics. It has become the most exciting technological horizons in the treatment of various medical disorders with the advancements of nanotheranostics. Current research aims at applying these technologies with many purposes, including multimodal imaging, targeting, and synergistic treatments, with the goal of developing nanocarriers with both diagnostic and therapeutic characteristics. Advanced nanotheranostics perform by activating their therapeutic and diagnostic capabilities only at the affected pathological site through the utilization of physical, chemical, and/or biological stimuli (Kim, Lee and Chen, 2013).

The discipline of nanotheranostic advancement, which aims to combine therapeutic and diagnostic capabilities in a single delivery platform, may represent the nanotherapeutic industry's utmost stage of technological progress (Wong et al., 2020). Nanotheranostics as one of the ultimate frontiers in personalized medicine, can be referred to as nanoparticles developed to offer factual information regarding drug distribution, release of various agents in the body, and focused treatment *in vivo* (Jo et al., 2016). Complicated synthetic methods are typically used to synthesize nanotheranostics in order to assign numerous functions to the same distribution platform. As a result, in some instances, the targeting of nanotheranostics relies solely on the passive accumulation of particle in the infected tissue via increased permeability and retention effect (EPR), which is typically accomplished with biological coating (such as albumin and peptides), or polyethylene glycol (PEG) interfacial modification (Silva et al., 2019).

Nanodimensions, therapeutic impact, and diagnostic component are the three main characteristics of nanotheranostics. Additionally, due to their capacity to sense a variety of ailment markers and secrete a variety of therapeutic substances, additional biological systems, such as microorganisms and mammalian cells, can be engineered using nanotechnologies and have a significant potential to be utilized in the invention of novel nanotheranostic systems. Nano theranostics boost the solubilization and discharge of cargoes to favor several functions into one particle and enhance the deposition of both contrast and therapeutic substances at the ailment site (Catalano, 2018).

Nanotheranostics are also able to be utilized as a contrast media for photoacoustic tomography, fluorescence imaging, and positron emission tomography (PET) to provide prolonged, regulated, and targeted administration of therapeutic and diagnostic substances for greater theranostic benefits with minimal detrimental reactions. Additionally, nanotheranostics can facilitate transport across the blood–brain

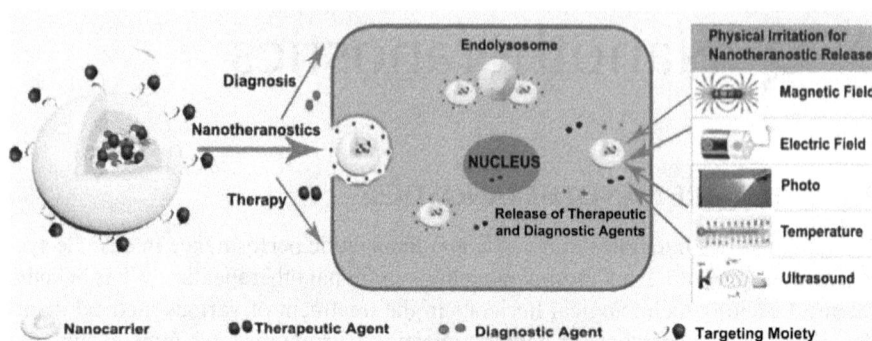

FIGURE 3.1 A pictorial description of a nanocarrier which includes both diagnostic and therapeutic agents and how it acts at the cellular and molecular levels.

Source: Reproduced with permission from Opoku-Damoah et al., 2016.

barrier, siRNA co-delivery, stimuli-responsive release, oral delivery, multimodality therapies, and synergetic and combinatory therapy. Diseases associated with aging may also be treated using nanotheranostics. In order to diagnose and treat the ailment at the molecular and cell level, they can attain systemic circulation, elude host defenses, and distribute the therapeutic and diagnostic components at the targeted place. According to unique disease state of each patient, nanotheranostics allows accurate spatiotemporal regulation of the production and release of bioactive molecules, optimizing the therapeutic benefit while reducing negative impacts (Funkhouser, 2002). Figure 3.1 shows a general representation of a nanocarrier which includes both diagnostic and therapeutic agents and how it acts at the cellular and molecular levels.

3.2 IMPORTANCE OF SUCCESSFUL DIAGNOSIS OF DISEASES

Nanotheranostics will be expanded in a larger perspective to enable therapy and diagnostics to coexist. *In vitro* diagnostics could be combined with particular medications to more precisely guide clinical decision. In this case, biomarkers play a crucial role as diagnostic agents of numerous pathological conditions, especially in detection of various cancers. A particular biomarker cannot serve as the only predictor addressing the cancer category, despite the fact that biomarkers are currently being associated with stages of the disease. The interaction of particular biomarkers can provide more insights about the disease status and, additionally, the responses to treatments. The growth of state-of-the-art molecular profiling approaches will be necessary to better understand the relationship between various biomarkers and the ailment category. These biomarker discoveries will encourage multiplexing in diagnostic system design as well as effective therapy monitoring. It will be much easier to find, plan, and monitor therapies if several biomarkers are analyzed and their relationships to one another are determined. Substantial changes in policy may be necessary for such biomarker discovery and correlation advancements. To avoid a backlog of information, it would be necessary to correctly assemble and evaluate any genetic or such types of biomarker evidence gleaned from a patient (Liotta and Petricoin, 2000).

Based on the above facts, it is essential to research different nanotheranostics strategies. Targeted imaging and therapy, activable therapy, activable probes, and molecular and biomarker analysis are the drive shafts of this phenomenon. Any form of biomolecule, including proteins, carbohydrates, lipids, amino acids, enzymes, genes, and metabolites, can serve as a biomarker by indicating the presence or alteration of significant physiological states in the body. The most popular method of identifying gene biomarkers by DNA arrays and correlating them with various cancer types employing clustering algorithms is known as molecular profiling. It really has allowed for the identification of distinct cancer signatures and the identification of classes of cancers to specific patients. With the present understanding of the human genome, specific details about a genotype of a patient and clinical information can be utilized to choose medicines, therapies, or preventative measures that are specifically tailored to that patient during the time of therapy (Sadée and Dai, 2005).

Antibodies, peptides, amino acids, and aptamers can target certain protein biomarkers that have been discovered and verified at the ailment region in addition to recognizing genes in a disease state. These biomarkers are primarily ligands that are typically expressed in numerous cells; however, they are overexpressed in pathological conditions. For the purpose of choosing a biomarker, flow cytometry, immunohistochemistry, and mRNA expression profiles of tumor proteins are necessary. Once a biomarker is revealed, it could be tailored to distribute conjugated medicinal agents or imaging probes to treat and monitor the specific site of the ailment or targeted to be obstructed for inhibition (Sievers and Senter, 2013).

Tackling more complicated targets of pathological conditions could pursue many mechanisms, including apoptosis, proliferation, hypoxia, angiogenesis, inflammatory reactions, and metastasis. In this case nanotherapeutics-based activatable probes achieve more *in vitro* diagnostics and identify major pathological conditions *in vivo*, whereas molecular beacons primarily identify oligonucleotides solely for *in vitro* applications (Tyagi and Kramer, 1996). Utilizing inorganic nanoparticles as fluorescence-activatable probes is another tactic. These particles, including gold, iron oxide, silica, QDs, and silica nanoparticles, have been widely used in the development of multimodal molecular imaging probes, such as the iron oxide NPs used as magnetic resonance imaging (MRI) contrast agents (Swierczewska, Lee and Chen, 2011). The *in vivo* capability of these metal nanoparticles-based activatable probes can be developed for activatable imaging and therapy when integrated with suitable biomolecules.

Current therapeutical approaches for treatments consist of "activated" therapy, such as enzyme-cleavable prodrug, which is comparable to activatable probes that may diagnose and identify pathological conditions. Only when these medications gain a certain biomarker in the cellular level, they become therapeutically effective. The original form of drug is released at the site of the stimulus following conversion from an enzyme, a chemical, or an environmental stimulus. As a result, there are less hazardous side effects in the body's healthy regions and the treatment can only function at the spot in which the altered biomarker is present (Huang et al., 2012).

Targeted molecular imaging, which is a crucial component of a nanotheranostic framework, can target, noninvasively image, and trace biomarkers responsible for disease pathogenesis. Because it offers a complete physical examination of molecular activities in real time, this kind of information can be used for purposes other than only diagnosing a rare mutation. Clinical professionals can use targeted molecular imaging to assess the extent to which specific biomarkers are present in the body. This information is crucial for disease staging and treatment planning, including drug dose and timing. In order to specifically design imaging probes that target genes, nucleic acids, including mRNA, DNA, metabolites, proteins, amino acids, and protein–protein interactions, biomarkers in the initial stages of disease pathological conditions must be identified (Eckelman, Reba and Kelloff, 2008).

Additionally, *in vivo* molecular imaging can be incorporated into diagnostic systems to upgrade them. Instead of selecting a small portion of a wide variety of tissues, targeted molecular imaging might provide additional information on the heterogeneity of the disorder. Activatable probes might improve the dispersion of tailored medication delivery as well as the spatial interpretation of biomarkers. The particular capabilities of nanotechnology will be crucial to the ability of diagnostic systems to increase sensitivity and multiplexity.

There is great potential for nanotheranostics in medicine, despite the fact that these approaches remain far from being used in clinical settings and need more in-depth analysis among biomarkers and the heterogeneity of malignancies in addition to various biomarkers. When designing nanotheranostic systems for the detection of diseases, it is important to understand and manage the type of targeted moiety, imaging modalities, therapy, and stimulation. Research is also required for advanced systems that incorporate nanohybrids for multiplexing and multifunctionality. The most crucial preclinical considerations for any prospects of nanotheranostics include pharmacokinetic tests, acute and long-term toxicity investigations, and quality control during production (Rai and Jamil, 2019).

Besides the biomarkers, the "responsiveness" of the transporters to a particular external stimulus can contribute to the selection of nanotheranostic for the affected site (Sneider et al., 2017). This "activation trigger" is typically administered remotely and rapidly in the area of interest, which has the advantage of being noninvasive. According to Zhao et al. (2017), standard diagnostic or therapeutic vehicles are typically in the "on" state, and both detection and cargo release start as soon as they are administered. However, the formulation of vehicles with "off–on" theranostic capabilities (Yu et al., 2018) can support a tailored evaluation of the quantity of medication that really reaches the diseased site. Due to this, sensitive nanotheranostics may provide new opportunities for adjusting and regulating the frequency and dose of treatment (Fan et al., 2016) in several therapies. Nanotheranostics, often known as "smart" nanotheranostics, that respond to stimuli typically rely on chemical linkers or functional molecules to arrange the nanoparticle systems.

Various chemical synchronization primitives and pH-sensitive materials can be used to impart pH responsiveness, which will activate the therapeutic and/or imaging features. The sensitivity of their structure and composition to pH determines how responsive the majority of these technologies are. Furthermore, the pH-responsiveness has the potential to improve radiation effectiveness or chemodynamic therapy (CDT) in hypoxic tumor circumstances by raising tumor oxygen supply. Last but not least, pH-sensitivity can be integrated with other responsiveness mechanisms that depend on external stimuli to enhance the carrier's therapeutic and diagnostic characteristics.

In preclinical drug screening, the generation of reactive oxygen species (ROS) compounds yield satisfactory results in the field of theranostics. They can be utilized as *in vivo* nanotheranostics to quantify ROS formation despite having theranostic features. Current ultrasound diagnostic techniques can be improved by making use of the ability of particular material to respond to ROS by producing CO_2. Additionally, these approaches can be used to treat a variety of diseases because the formation of ROS is a trait of many pathological conditions.

Theranostic enzyme responsiveness often relies on hydrolytic enzymes that promote the degradation of carrier or peptide synchronization primitives. The medicinal or diagnostic chemicals contained in the coatings of various particles, which stabilize them, can also be employed to take advantage of this phenomenon. The overexpression of a few enzymes that can identify various clinical states is strictly necessary for the effective use of enzyme-responsive nanotheranostics. They are produced by designing biological substrates, which are typically functionalized with other molecules (including targeting modifications) (Karimi et al., 2016).

Besides enzymes and ROS as diagnostic triggers, a reactive substance called glutathione (GSH) regulates the redox equilibrium within cells. This molecule is markedly expressed exclusively in cancer cells, suggesting that it could serve as a targetable trigger for the creation of sophisticated nanotheranostics (Liu et al., 2017). The goal of many of these alterations of biomarkers and other parameters is to increase biocompatibility and biological interaction, which will open up new research avenues in the study of biologically inspired nanotherapeutics.

3.3   EMERGING NANOTHERANOSTICS AS DIAGNOSTIC TOOLS

To get around the constraints of routine therapy and diagnosis for much more proper governance of diverse pathological illnesses, the nanotheranostic framework is a promising strategy that is desperately required. Through the utilization of biologically compatible nanoparticles that concurrently carry out both diagnostic and therapeutic tasks, nanotheranostic modalities offer a viable answer to the diagnostic and therapeutic issues encountered in a number of disorders. Through the use of nanoparticles that can be made to recognize particular biomarkers of the target diseased region, enable real-time scanning or visual analytics of the target, and then distribute therapeutic methods of treatment with greater accuracy, this strategy may offer a more individualized and targeted strategy to many treatment options. Nanosensors and nanomedicine technologies have made significant strides in recent years, paving the way for prospective ways to integrate nanotheranostics in the management of numerous pathological conditions.

Therefore, the objectives of nanotheranostics include not only improving detection of pathological conditions and treatment effectiveness but also limiting the cytotoxic effects related to this therapy (Muthu et al., 2014). In order to anticipate the next treatment or determine whether to continue the same therapeutic treatment, it may be possible to rapidly examine the results of a treatment in specific patients owing to nanotheranostics (personalized medicine).

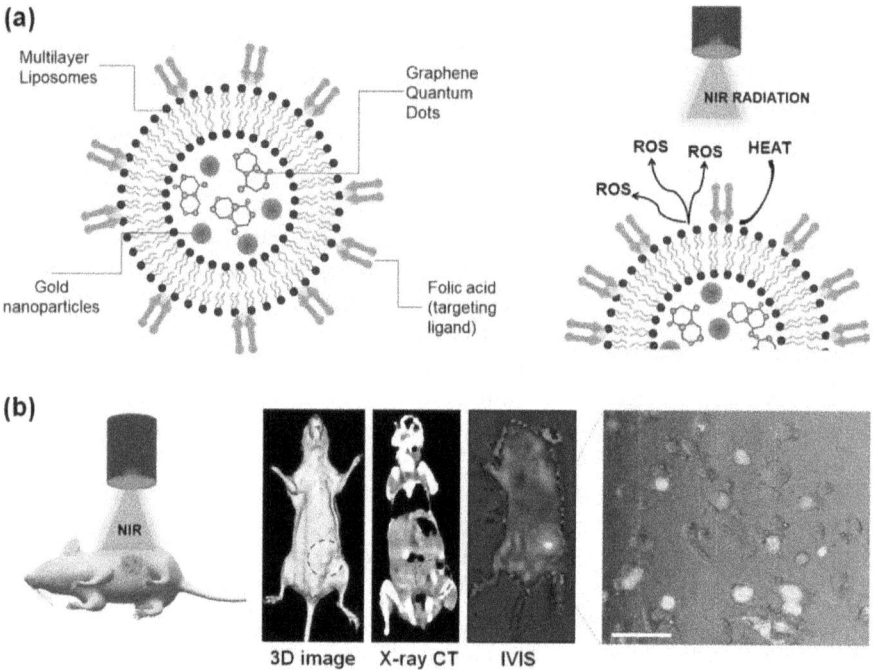

FIGURE 3.2 Schematic representation of liposomal nanotheranostics for multimode-targeted bioimaging and photo-triggered cancer therapy. (a) Folic acid targeting ligand-decorated self-assembled liposomal nanohybrid-loaded multimode imaging probes, viz., gold nanoparticles (AuNPs as radiocontrast for X-ray computed tomography and reactive oxygen species scavenger) and graphene quantum dots (GQDs as fluorescent contrast for near-infrared fluorescence imaging and photothermal agent). Designed functional liposomal nanohybrids demonstrating photothermal response/heat and the generation of reactive oxygen species (ROS, considered as the side product of photothermal therapy) under near-infrared (NIR) light exposure. (b) NIR light-mediated cancer therapeutic representation with tumor-bearing mice model using engineered liposomal nanotheranostic agents and targeted imaging bimodality of breast cancer through X-ray computed tomography (X-ray CT) and *in vivo* imaging system (IVIS). Liposomal nanotheranostics-treated cancer cells displaying the production of ROS (green emission represents the presence of ROS captured by DCFDA (2′,7′-dichlorofluorescin diacetate) dye staining) during NIR light exposure, scale bar = 20 μm.

Source: Reproduced with permission from Prasad et al., 2020.

Figure 3.2 depicted a schematic representation of liposomal nanotheranostics for multimode-targeted bioimaging and photo-triggered cancer therapy. Considering the major threats to health worldwide, cancers are the leading threat that surge day by day. Regarding the photothermal cancer therapy, the quantity of photoenergy that is delivered directly to the tumor location can be controlled to maximize the therapeutic effectiveness while minimizing harm to the neighboring normal tissues in a healthy state. Precious metal-based nanostructures have been well-synthesized and have shown strong near-infrared (NIR) laser-induced photothermal therapy (PTT) efficacy. Furthermore, because of the inherent toxicity and uncertain long-term toxicity of the aforementioned PTT drugs, their potential therapeutic applications were mainly constrained. In addition to using magnetic nanotherapeutics, modified mammalian cell-based nanotherapeutics and magnetic hyperthermal therapies based on nanotherapeutics all play a significant part in cancer therapies that are strengthened with nanotherapeutics (Prasad et al., 2020).

One of the other major sources of the most important public health problem across the world is cardiovascular diseases (CVD). Different preclinical results with nanotheranostic applications for CVD have been achieved, and they could be applied to prospective noninvasive real-time cardiovascular investigation and clinical translation strategies. At this time, there are no standardized test methods available to assess the efficacy of NP therapies in general or their use for CVD especially (Fitzgerald et al., 2011). Ultrasmall iron oxide particles (IOPs), one of the pioneering nanotheranostics for atherosclerosis, were employed as a noninvasive imaging method based on NPs to assess the medication therapy in atherosclerosis patients (Tang et al., 2009).

Targeted theranostic nano- and microbubbles are also a type of theranostics which can be employed for CVDs. They can be used to pinpoint the location of clot which is concentrated with fibrinolytic activity associated with the avoidance of thrombus and clogs in the bloodstreams because they attach to platelets and enable ultrasound molecular scanning of thrombi *in vivo* (Wang et al., 2016). The discovery of novel therapeutic approaches and the evaluation of the efficacy and safety of fibrinolytic and thrombolytic therapy for CVDs can be both accelerated and improved by nanotheranostics.

Diseases inherited to the central and peripheral nerve systems caused by injury, infection, or neurodegenerative conditions pose a serious problem in contemporary cultures having numerous, concurrent needs and expectations. The disease's progression cannot be even slowed down by current treatments, which cannot even address or lessen the symptoms of brain damage or neurodegeneration. Important advancements were made in the introduction of therapeutic or diagnostic contrast probes into the nervous system, such as in the case of glioblastoma, while preserving the capability to realize tailored delivery to particular brain or spinal cord subregions (Alam et al., 2010). The use of nanotechnology-based methodologies and nanotheranostics as a resource to enhance the practical efficacy of the scanning of central nervous system processes, explore severe pathological states, and promote neurosurgical practice has great development potential. The application that is most useful is bioimaging. MRI is the most crucial tool for diagnosing brain diseases. By employing positron emission tomography (PET) imaging, it will not be long to track the progression of various nervous system problems and to better understand the biology of Alzheimer's disease. For this purpose, the use of radiolabeled amyloid ligands has been suggested (Jack et al., 2013). For scientists and medical professionals in the field, it is still difficult to fully comprehend the processes and pathophysiology of neurodegenerative illnesses and to build synergy to identify neurological diseases at their earliest stages and before overt symptoms appear. Such clinical issues can be resolved more easily with the help of nanotherapeutics and nanotheranostics.

REFERENCES

Alam, M. I., Beg, S., Samad, A., Baboota, S., Kohli, K., Ali, J. et al. (2010) "Strategy for effective brain drug delivery," *European Journal of Pharmaceutical Sciences*, 40, p. 385403.

Catalano, E. (2018) "Nanotheranostics and theranostic nanomedicine for diseases and cancer treatment," Alexandru Mihai Grumezescu (Ed.), *Design of nanostructures for theranostics applications.* Oxford: Elsevier, pp. 41–68.

Eckelman, W. C., Reba, R. C. and Kelloff, G. J. (2008) "Targeted imaging: An important biomarker for understanding disease progression in the era of personalized medicine," *Drug Discovery Today*, 13(17–18), pp. 748–759.

Fan, Z., Sun, L., Huang, Y., Wang, Y. and Zhang, M. (2016) "Bioinspired fluorescent dipeptide nanoparticles for targeted cancer cell imaging and real-time monitoring of drug release," *Nature Nanotechnology*, 11, pp. 388–394.

Fitzgerald, K. T., Holladay, C. A., McCarthy, C., Power, K. A., Pandit, A. and Gallagher, W. M. (2011) "Standardization of models and methods used to assess nanoparticles in cardiovascular applications," *Small*, 7(6), p. 705717.

Funkhouser, J. (2002) "Reinventing pharma: The theranostic revolution," *Current Drug Discovery Technologies,* 2, p. 1719.

Huang, X. et al. (2012) "Multiplex imaging of an intracellular proteolytic cascade by using a broad-spectrum nanoquencher," *Angewandte Chemie (Weinheim an der Bergstrasse, Germany)*, 124(7), pp. 1657–1662. doi: 10.1002/ange.201107795.

Jack, Jr., C. R., Knopman, D. S., Jagust, W. J., Petersen, R. C., Weiner, M. W., Aisen, P. S. et al. (2013) "Tracking pathophysiological processes in Alzheimer's disease: An updated hypothetical model of dynamic biomarkers," *Lancet Neurology*, 12, p. 207216.

Jo, S. D., Ku, S. H., Won, Y.-Y., Kim, S. H. and Kwon, I. C. (2016) "Targeted nanotheranostics for future personalized medicine: Recent progress in cancer therapy," *Theranostics*, 6, pp. 1362–1377.

Karimi, M., Ghasemi, A., Zangabad, P. S., Rahighi, R., Basri, S. M. M., Mirshekari, H. et al. (2016) "Smart micro/nanoparticles in stimulus-responsive drug/gene delivery systems," *Chemical Society Reviews*, 45, pp. 1457–1501.

Kim, T. H., Lee, S. and Chen, X. (2013) "Nanotheranostics for personalized medicine," *Expert Review of Molecular Diagnostics*, 13(3), pp. 257–269.

Liotta, L. and Petricoin, E. (2000) "Molecular profiling of human cancer," *Nature Reviews, Genetics*, 1(1), pp. 48–56.

Liu, Z., Chen, X., Zhang, X., Gooding, J. J. and Zhou, Y. (2017) "Carbon-quantum-dots-loaded mesoporous silica nanocarriers with pH-switchable zwitterionic surface and enzyme-responsive pore-cap for targeted imaging and drug delivery to tumor," *Advanced Healthcare Materials*, 5, pp. 1401–1407.

Muthu, M. S., Leong, D. T., Mei, L. and Feng, S. S. (2014) "Nanotheranostics—application and further development of nanomedicine strategies for advanced theranostics," *Theranostics*, 4(6), p. 660677.

Opoku-Damoah, Y. et al. (2016) "Versatile nanosystem-based cancer theranostics: Design inspiration and predetermined routing," *Theranostics*, 6(7), pp. 986–1003.

Prasad, R. et al. (2020) "Liposomal nanotheranostics for multimode targeted in vivo bioimaging and near-infrared light mediated cancer therapy," *Communications Biology*, 3(1), p. 284. doi: 10.1038/s42003-020-1016-z.

Rai, M. and Jamil, B. (eds.) (2019) *Nanotheranostics: Applications and limitations*. 1st ed. Cham, Switzerland: Springer Nature.

Sadée, W. and Dai, Z. (2005) "Pharmacogenetics/genomics and personalized medicine," *Human Molecular Genetics*, 14(Spec No. 2) (suppl_2), pp. R207–R214.

Sievers, E. L. and Senter, P. D. (2013) "Antibody-drug conjugates in cancer therapy," *Annual Review of Medicine*, 64(1), pp. 15–29.

Silva, C. O., Pinho, J. O., Lopes, J. M., Almeida, A. J., Gaspar, M. M. and Reis, C. (2019) "Current trends in cancer nanotheranostics: Metallic, polymeric, and lipid-based systems," *Pharmaceutics*, 11, p. 22.

Sneider, A., Vandyke, D., Paliwal, S. and Rai, P. (2017) "Remotely triggered nano-theranostics for cancer applications," *Nanotheranostics*, 1, pp. 1–22.

Swierczewska, M., Lee, S. and Chen, X. (2011) "Inorganic nanoparticles for multimodal molecular imaging," *Molecular Imaging*, 10(1), p. 7290.2011.00001.

Tang, T. Y., Howarth, S. P., Miller, S. R., Graves, M. J., Patterson, A. J., U-King-Im, J. M. et al. (2009) "The ATHEROMA (atorvastatin therapy: Effects on reduction of macrophage activity) study: Evaluation using ultrasmall superparamagnetic iron oxide-enhanced magnetic resonance imaging in carotid disease. *Journal of American College of Cardiology*, 53(22), p. 20392050.

Tyagi, S. and Kramer, F. R. (1996) "Molecular beacons: Probes that fluoresce upon hybridization," *Nature Biotechnology*, 14(3), pp. 303–308.

Wang, X., Gkanatsas, Y., Palasubramaniam, J., Hohmann, J. D., Chen, Y. C., Lim, B. et al. (2016) "Thrombus-targeted theranostic microbubbles: A new technology towards concurrent rapid ultrasound diagnosis and bleeding-free fibrinolytic treatment of thrombosis," *Theranostics*, 6(5), p. 72673.

Wong, X. Y., Sena-Torralba, A., Alvarez-Diduk, R., Muthoosamy, K. and Merkoçi, A. (2020) "Nanomaterials for nanotheranostics: Tuning their properties according to disease needs," *ACS Nano*, 14, pp. 2585–2627.

Yu, G., Yung, B. C., Zhou, Z., Mao, Z. and Chen, X. (2018) "Artificial molecular machines in nanotheranostics," *ACS Nano*, 12, pp. 7–12.

Zhao, X., Yang, C.-X., Chen, L.-G. and Yan, X.-P. (2017) "Dual-stimuli responsive and reversibly activatable theranostic nanoprobe for precision tumor-targeting and fluorescence-guided photothermal therapy," *Nature Communications*, 8, p. 14998.

4 Nanotherapeutics in Monitoring Therapies

4.1 INTRODUCTION TO NANOTHERAPEUTICS IN MONITORING THERAPIES

Nanotherapeutics are being used more frequently for imaging applications to monitor drug delivery, release, and efficacy in addition to therapeutic applications of nanotherapeutic agents. The use of nanotherapeutics for evaluating and enhancing the characteristics of medication delivery platforms, as well as their capacity to be utilized for the purpose of patient pre-screening and facilitating personalized treatment, is the (pre)clinically foremost significant implementation of nanotherapeutics for monitoring purposes (Lammers et al., 2011).

The determination of concentration levels of drugs in biomaterials as a basis for drug therapy monitoring is definitely a crucial tool for tailored dosing to each individual patient as well as adjustment of doses within a wide range of therapeutics. Its function is constrained since it does not take into account pharmacodynamic and toxicodynamic interactions like those brought on by individualized and environmental factors. Nonetheless, those reactions continue to be crucial in the effectiveness and safety measurements of the medication treatments. As a result, there has been a rise in the favor of personalized medication treatment strategy recently, as evidenced by the advancement and utilization of molecular "biomarkers" which serve as either direct or proximate indicators of therapeutic properties in clinical settings (pharmacodynamic therapeutic drug monitoring, PD TDM). Additionally, the aforementioned approach is fueled through recent advancements in computational biology/pharmacology, data bases, and bioinformatics as well as apparatus with nanotechnology, including mass spectrometry, MRI, and array techniques (Shipkova and Christians, 2019).

Real-time commentary on the pharmacokinetic profiles, target site placement, as well as deposition of nanomedicines in healthy tissues (off-target) is offered by nanotherapeutics used in monitoring purposes. There are numerous examples for this, including the fact that via noninvasively observing the degree of which the delivery substances are capable of delivering therapeutically active entities to the diseased location and the degree of those entities are capable of preventing those substances from depositing in typical tissues that are healthy. It facilitates obtaining crucial information for improving the fundamental characteristics of drug delivery platforms and for striking a better balance between the effectiveness and the toxic effects of the drug (Davis, Chen and Shin, 2008).

Considering personalized medicine, it stands to reason that targeted therapy should be proceeded only in individuals who exhibit greater amounts of target location segregation and who respond favorably to the initial few therapy sessions. Thus, alternative therapeutic strategies should be taken into account regarding this. Nanotherapeutics make it easier to monitor cell therapies in addition to the active moiety release from the

DOI: 10.1201/9781003442202-5

principal drug, drug delivery to the targeted site, and the effectiveness of the treatment. Organ and cell line transplants are a part of these cell therapies. By exposing promising strategies to overcome the problems in cell therapies, monitoring cell therapies improves the quality of life for patients who have received cell therapies and ensures the benefits of nanotherapeutics as monitoring agents (Davis, Chen and Shin, 2008).

4.2 TYPES OF MONITORING THERAPIES

The pharmacokinetics monitoring is undoubtedly a crucial step in adjusting doses to account for inter- and intra-patient pharmacokinetics variations, as well as monitoring the adherence of the patient to treatment and especially avoiding side effects associated with accidental overdose as well as drug–drug interactions. Thus, this is constrained by the point that it cannot represent pharmacodynamics and toxic and dynamic interplay including those due to individual and exterior surrounding-related influences, which are crucial in therapeutic success. These factors may include, but are not constrained to a sensitivity of a person to a specific therapeutic agent and/or its undesired harmful reactions, the progression of tolerance, the possible impact of coexisting morbidity, the degree of immunological responsiveness, age, patient stature, nutritional and dietary habits, as well as general lifestyle habits (Dreesen and Gils, 2019). On a cellular scale, *in vivo* influences like the number of cell surface receptors, the efficiency of second messengers in signaling, stability, the regulatory aspects that regulate the translation of genetic materials and protein expression, and translational alterations affect drug reaction and have an influence on the interaction among drug kinetics and the respective pharmacodynamics or toxic and dynamic impacts. Considering the above-mentioned factors, it is crucial to monitor those facts to gain the maximum benefit from nanotherapeutics through effective monitoring aspects (Dreesen and Gils, 2019).

4.2.1 MONITORING THE RELEASE OF DRUGS

In addition to building up at the diseased site, the medicine must also be released effectively for therapy to be effective. It is crucial to observe and evaluate drug release not only under semi-artificial *in vitro* systems but also under physiologically suitable *in vivo* systems because drug release patterns differ significantly between formulations. Also, significant differences in the liberation models of drugs are available. As examples liposomes, polymers, and micelles can be mentioned (Lammers et al., 2005). *In vivo* drug liberation analysis is far more restricted than it is *in vitro*. As fact, after extracting the target tissue, the substance usually requires to be homogenized and the cellular material require being degraded in order to liberate the substances from particular intracellular compartments. Numerous types of carrier agents are disrupted during these procedures, particularly during cell lysis (using detergents). For instance, mostly in case of liposomes, they become harder to distinguish among the quantity of medication that was continued to be contained in the liposomes at the time of extraction and the quantity that had been discharged into the extracellular and intracellular surroundings (Lammers et al., 2010).

Nanotherapeutic preparations, in which medications and imaging compounds are incorporated inside them as a single delivery platform, have been created to address this limitation as well as to facilitate noninvasive *in vivo* investigations on (the pharmacokinetics of) drug release. These imaging modalities are not appropriate for monitoring medication release since radionuclides provide comparable signals when bound or entrapped and when unbound or free. On the other hand, MR compounds like gadolinium and manganese also rely on their interaction with molecules of water around them to produce a signal, and this interaction differs significantly depending on whether the materials are inside or outside of vesicles that are water-impermeable like liposomes. For monitoring the release of medications, MR probes are a very valuable material (Terreno, Uggeri and Aime, 2012).

The therapeutic dosage being released from nanotherapeutic systems at the target location is equally important to attaining optimal biodistribution and accumulation in the target site. Cancer nanotherapeutics, in which imaging compounds and chemotherapeutic medications are incorporated within a single distribution system, have been created to allow noninvasive imaging and quantification of drug release. When an imaging compound is attached or trapped in a nanomaterial, it represents in unbound or liberated phase after discharge. Thus, it must produce a distinct signal. Because of this, probes relying on positron emission tomography (PET) and single photon emission computed tomography (SPECT) have become less appropriate for drug release monitoring. Figure 4.1 shows the monitoring of drug release by QDs. Nevertheless, MRI-based contrast agents and optical mediators have properties that are appropriate for this application (Lv et al., 2023).

4.2.2   MONITORING DRUG RELEASE BY MAGNETIC RESONANCE IMAGING

Drug release monitoring techniques based on MRI are routinely used. Entrapped paramagnetic MR compound that is within a water-impermeable nanovehicle which carries drugs only provokes a minor T_1 reduction, which is discharged into an aqueous media outcome in hyperintense impulses in T_1-weighted MRI, representing as a marker for assessing drug discharge. This is because the image processing signal by MR contrast agent tends to depend on the contact with bulk water (Onuki et al., 2010).

High spatial resolution provided by MRI enables the analysis of drug distribution within tumors following nanocarrier-triggered drug release. Using imaging to control locally initiated drug release also has the benefit of allowing the stimulus (such as heat) to be applied at the precise moments when nanocarrier aggregation at the target region is greatest. This may be accomplished, for instance, by combining two distinct MRI contrast compounds into a single nanovehicle. For instance, Onuki et al. used multiplexed MRI to monitor cancer and malignancies formation and drug liberation while co-entrapping iron oxide (IO) nanoparticles, Gd-DTPA (diethylene-triamine penta-acetic acid), and 5-fluorouracil (5-FU) inside polylactic-*co*-glycolic acid (PLGA) nanoparticles. The discharge of Gd-DTPA, which was utilized as a stand-in marker to see the liberation of 5-FU from the nanoparticles, was tracked through T_1-weighted imaging after the intravenous administration of the encapsulated IO nanoparticles to measure cancer cell accumulation (de Smet et al., 2011).

4.2.3   MONITORING DRUG RELEASE BY OPTICAL IMAGING

For monitoring drug release in addition to MRI, optical imaging techniques which is relied on quenching/de-quenching and FRET (fluorescence resonance energy

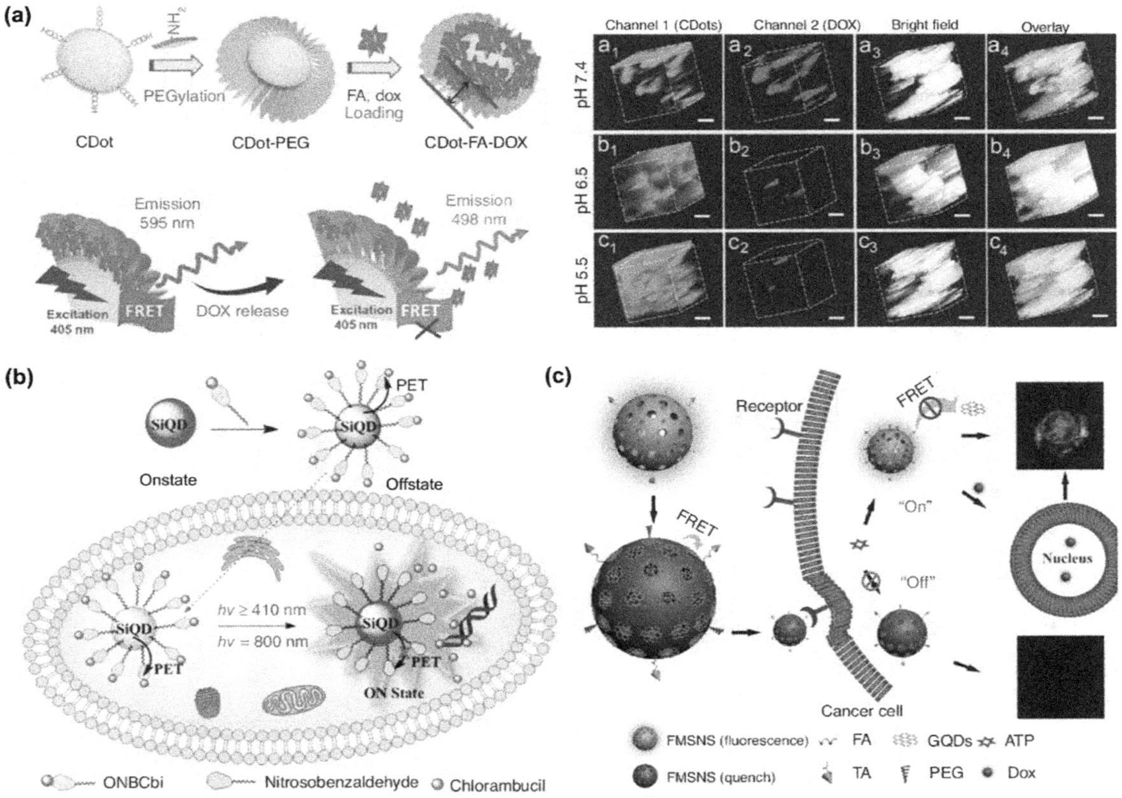

FIGURE 4.1 Monitoring drug release by QDs. (a) Schematic representation of the FRET-CDot-DDS for drug delivery. Also, 3D two-photon confocal fluorescence images (under 810 nm excitation) of CDot-FA-Dox conjugate-incubated glomerular tissues, accumulated along the z-direction at a depth of 65–300 µm, incubated under pH of (i) 7.4, (ii) 6.5, and (iii) 5.5. (b) Schematic representation of controlled release and real-time monitoring of the anticancer drug chlorambucil from ONBCbl-SiQDs. (c) Preparation and application of ATP-responsive GQDs-based nanocarriers.

Source: Reproduced with permission from Zheng et al., 2019.

transfer) have also been employed. These findings demonstrate how MR and OI agents can be used for *in vivo* nanocarrier-drug attachment and dissociation, as well as for real-time monitoring and direction of stimulated drug liberation. These instruments are useful for streamlining treatment regimens and thoroughly researching the stability, drug release, and therapeutic efficacy of nanotherapeutics (Mitra et al., 2012; Zou et al., 2013).

4.3 MONITORING OF BIODISTRIBUTION OF THE DRUGS

Imaging compounds have been encapsulated into or coupled to nanoparticle systems to enable noninvasive imaging approaches to study the circulatory behavior, distribution within the biological systems, and target location deposition of medicines. In this regard, the biodistribution of medications and tumor growth have been monitored using imaging techniques, including optical imaging (OI) and radionuclide imaging, along with more recently adopted noninvasive imaging technologies (Lammers et al., 2010).

Radionuclides have typically been employed for these objectives. Over the years, a significant number of radionuclide-labeled nanomaterials have been the focus of biodistribution assessments in both animal models and human patients. It is now evident that these experiments have a significant impact on the processes of delivery systems and the ability to predict the therapeutic aspects of targeted nanotherapeutics (Kunjachan et al., 2013).

Anshuman and the research team have developed hybrid CT-FMT (computed tomography–fluorescence molecular tomography) for optical imaging in monitoring delivery of drugs into the targeted site. This technology enables CT-based evaluation of laboratory mouse and anatomy of organs along with FMT-based measurement of near-infrared fluorophore (NIRF) tagged polymeric nanovehicles relied on poly(*N*-(2 hydroxypropyl)methacrylamide (pHPMA). Also, they attempted scattering and absorption remodeling to take into account the various optical features of anatomical structures, which noted the significant light absorption in the heart, liver, kidney, and other organs with high blood flow being the main *in vivo* absorber of near-infrared radiation (Rawashdeh et al., 2017). This method has shown to be highly helpful in evaluating the biodistribution of medications in preclinical studies (Xie, Lee and Chen, 2010). Such insights highlight the significance of combining medications and imaging entities in a same formulation when aiming to achieve actually relevant outcomes when it comes to the noninvasive evaluation of the distribution and the aimed location deposition of medicines. They are crucial for enhancing comprehension and prioritizing the efficacy of cutting-edge focused therapeutic techniques. Figure 4.2 depicts noninvasive monitoring therapy for evaluating the drug delivery in a patient with a breast cancer (Harrington et al., 2001).

In addition to the aforementioned recognized imaging modalities, novel noninvasive imaging techniques utilizing magnetic particle imaging (MPI), photoacoustic imaging (PAI), and multispectral optoacoustic tomography (MSOT) are innovative as monitoring techniques in regard to nanotherapeutics. The contrast agents in several of these novel modalities is nanoparticles. Even just a small number of research have conducted up-to-date systematically examined nanoparticle delivery and target

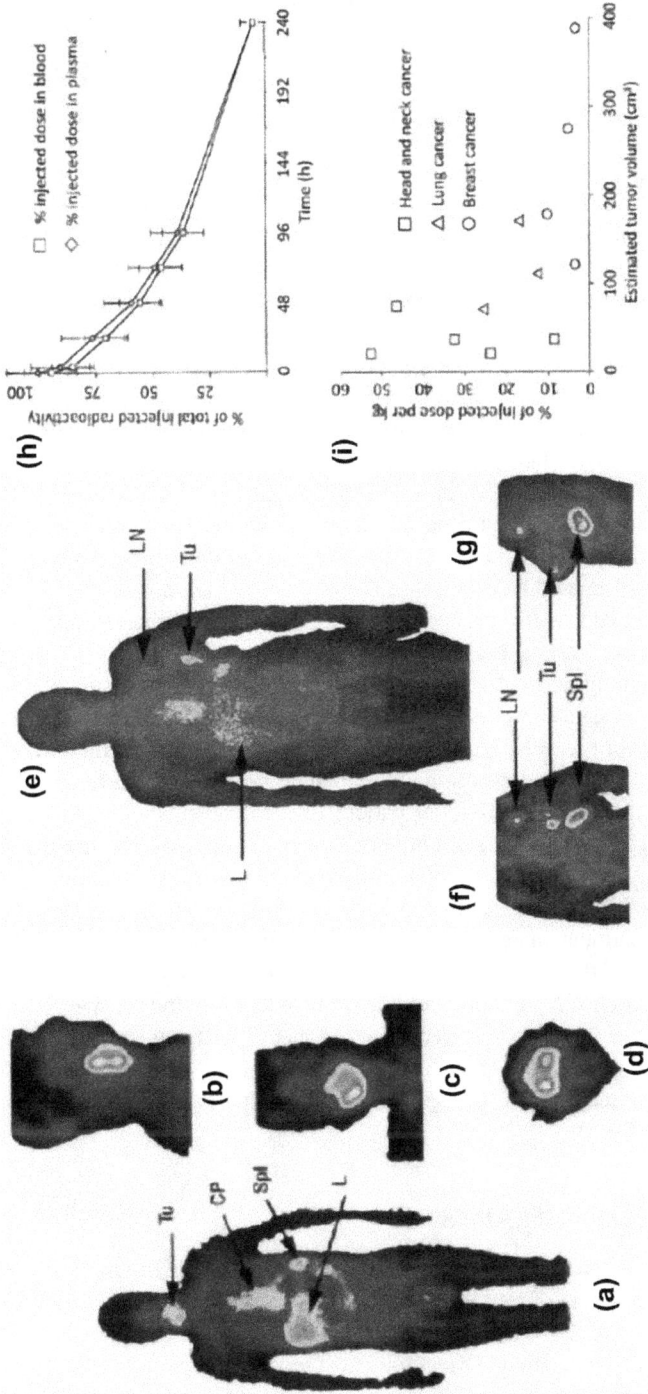

FIGURE 4.2 Noninvasive imaging of drug delivery. (a–g) Gamma camera images showing the biodistribution of indium-111-labeled PEGylated liposomes at 72 hours after i.v. injection into a grade 3 squamous cell carcinoma (a–d) and a grade 4 ductal breast carcinoma (e–g) patient. (a–d) In the SCC patient, it can be seen that, even after three days, a substantial amount of liposomes is still present in the systemic circulation (i.e., in the cardiac blood pool; CP), while a significant amount has also accumulated at the target site (i.e., in a tumor localized at the tongue base; Tu). Significant accumulation was also observed in organs of the reticulo-endothelial system, like liver (L) and spleen (Spl), which are known to be involved in the clearance of long-circulating nanomedicines. (e–g) In the DBC patient, besides localization to blood, tumor (Tu), liver (L), and spleen (Spl), accumulation in left axillary lymph node (LN) could also be clearly observed, indicative of metastasis and of effective drug targeting to this pathological site. (h and i) Besides, for assessing target site accumulation, theranostic nanomedicines are also highly useful for analyzing pharmacokinetics (h), as well as for prescreening patients and identifying tumor types (and sizes) amenable to EPR-mediated drug targeting (i).

Source: Reproduced with permission from Lammers et al., 2011.

site deposition. The use of MPI to investigate the distribution of superparamagnetic iron oxide nanoparticles (SPION) and PAI and MSOT to assess the *in vivo* outcome of gold- and carbon-based nanomaterials and also nanomaterials containing hemoglobin, melanin, and porphyrin is expected to increase in the future (Arami et al., 2015; Poon et al., 2015; Wang et al., 2015).

4.4 DRUG EFFICACY MONITORING

Nanotherapeutic preparations are excellent for predicting and observing treatment responses in addition to noninvasively measuring drug distribution and drug release. These nanotherapeutic preparations may be capable, for example, of being tagged with radionuclides in order to gain several preliminary noninvasive data regarding target site deposition for the predicting of therapeutic reactions, as previously mentioned, throughout phase I and phase II clinical trials. The prospective efficacy of novel therapeutic approaches based on nanotherapeutics might then be predicted logically on the basis of this. A radiolabeled form of the aforementioned inactively tumor-aimed prodrug which is polymeric in its nature might have been utilized for monitoring patients referred to PK1 in the initiation clinical trial—phase I for HPMA-copolymer-based doxorubicin (i.e., PK1). For example, to determine which tumors are susceptible to EPR-mediated targeted therapy and which are not, and thereby to anticipate which patients are susceptible to responding to PK1 therapy and which people with the disease are not (Lammers et al., 2011).

Comparable to this, the integration of functional SPECT imaging and anatomical CT imaging may be employed in the clinical trials—phase I or phase II trying to focus on hepatic-targeted PK1 (i.e., PK2) to identify which hepatocellular carcinoma (HCC) patients exhibit better tumor deposition and which do not, and to determine on the basic principle of this which individual patient PK2 therapies should proceed in. Additionally, by repetitively exposing individuals to anatomical CT imaging along with 2D scintigraphy or 3D PET and blending in smaller levels of nanomaterials that are radiolabeled with medical therapy, it could be feasible to evaluate the effectiveness of the treatment in real time and give crucial data for aiding in taking decisions regardless of the choice to continue treatments and whether or not to modify dosage of medications. Nanotherapeutics may help to attain the prospects of "personalized medicine," or customized treatment for specific patients, which is dependent on research into genetic polymorphisms and biomarkers, as well as the advancement of monitoring techniques for assessing and anticipating responses to treatment (Lammers et al., 2011).

4.5 MONITORING CELL THERAPIES

Exogenous transplant is a potential to transform medications by reviving function of anatomical structures by replacing or repairing damaged or defective cells. The site, distribution, and extended stability of transplanted cells should be assessed in order to create an efficient cell treatment. Imaging techniques based on nanoparticles (NP) have the potential to provide noninvasive cell tracking. The physicochemical characteristics of the NPs-based nanotherapeutics must be accurately regulated throughout production to facilitate sensitive and specific recognition with great spatial resolution *in vivo*. The biological processes of the transplanted cells should remain unaffected by the NPs and cell tagging process in order to clearly understand the complicated spatial-temporal dynamics of the cells.

Fluorescence monitoring with QDs, MRI monitoring with magnetic NPs, and PET imaging with radioisotope-comprised NPs are all current methods for cell monitoring. The following generation of intelligent imaging agents should support a variety of imaging techniques and allow reporting on both location of the cellular materials and activity. It can be concluded that additional characterization is necessary to understand and counteract compounds transfer, signal dilution, and a number of negative effects labeling chemicals may have on cells. The advancement of novel compounds and a deeper comprehension of the reactions between cells and labels would considerably increase the utility of NP-based tracking of cells and avoid over-interpreting imaging (Xu et al., 2011).

4.6 EMERGING NANOTHERAPEUTICS FOR MONITORING THERAPIES

Nanotherapeutics can be applied in a variety of ways in monitoring therapies. They enable the refinement of drug delivery platforms by permitting a noninvasive evaluation of the pharmacokinetic profiles, the distribution within the biological tissues, and the localization of target of coupled or enclosed pharmacologically active compounds. Nanotherapeutics may also be utilized to anticipate treatment outcomes by fusing data on entire target site localization with imaging techniques insights on the local delivery of the drug and/or the vehicle which delivered material at the target location.

Additionally, several fundamental characteristics of drug delivery platforms could be seen and examined by noninvasively monitoring drug liberation *in vivo*, and efforts could be taken to reconcile the *in vitro* qualities of transporting agents with their *in vivo* abilities. The effectiveness of triggerable drug delivery platforms can also be improved by employing contrast materials to track the liberation of drugs which are pharmacologically active from stimuli-sensitive nanomaterials, as demonstrated by numerous research on thermosensitive liposomes. Moreover, nanotherapeutics may be utilized to accelerate (pre-) clinical effectiveness analyses, to monitor individuals, as well as to harness the benefits of customized medications by offering real-time assessment on the effectiveness of focused therapeutic interventions (Dasgupta et al., 2020).

REFERENCES

Arami, H. et al. (2015) "Invivo multimodal magnetic particle imaging (MPI) with tailored magneto/optical contrast agents," *Biomaterials*, 52(1), pp. 251–261.

Dasgupta, A. et al. (2020) "Imaging-assisted anticancer nanotherapy," *Theranostics*, 10(3), pp. 956–967.

Davis, M. E., Chen, Z. G. and Shin, D. M. (2008) "Nanoparticle therapeutics: An emerging treatment modality for cancer," *Nature Reviews: Drug Discovery*, 7(9), pp. 771–782. doi: 10.1038/nrd2614.

de Smet, M. et al. (2011) "Magnetic resonance imaging of high intensity focused ultrasound mediated drug delivery from temperature-sensitive liposomes: An *in vivo* proof-of-concept study," *Journal of Controlled Release: Official Journal of the Controlled Release Society*, 150(1), pp. 102–110.

Dreesen, E. and Gils, A. (2019) "Pharmacodynamic monitoring of biological therapies in chronic inflammatory diseases," *Therapeutic Drug Monitoring*, 41(2), pp. 131–141.

Harrington, K. J. et al. (2001) "Effective targeting of solid tumors in patients with locally advanced cancers by radiolabeled pegylated liposomes," *Clinical Cancer Research: An Official Journal of the American Association for Cancer Research*, 7(2), pp. 243–254.

Kunjachan, S. et al. (2013) "Noninvasive optical imaging of nanomedicine biodistribution," *ACS Nano*, 7(1), pp. 252–262.

Lammers, T. et al. (2005) "Effect of physicochemical modification on the biodistribution and tumor accumulation of HPMA copolymers," *Journal of Controlled Release: Official Journal of the Controlled Release Society*, 110(1), pp. 103–118.

Lammers, T. et al. (2010) "Nanotheranostics and image-guided drug delivery: Current concepts and future directions," *Molecular Pharmaceutics*, 7(6), pp. 1899–1912.

Lammers, T. et al. (2011) "Theranostic nanomedicine," *Accounts of Chemical Research*, 44(10), pp. 1029–1038.

Lv, J. et al. (2023) "Contrast agents of magnetic resonance imaging and future perspective," *Nanomaterials (Basel, Switzerland)*, 13(13), p. 2003. doi: 10.3390/nano13132003.

Mitra, R. N. et al. (2012) "An activatable multimodal/multifunctional nanoprobe for direct imaging of intracellular drug delivery," *Biomaterials*, 33(5), pp. 1500–1508.

Onuki, Y. et al. (2010) "Noninvasive visualization of *in vivo* release and intratumoral distribution of surrogate MR contrast agent using the dual MR contrast technique," *Biomaterials*, 31(27), pp. 7132–7138.

Poon, W. et al. (2015) "Determination of biodistribution of ultrasmall, near-infrared emitting gold nanoparticles by photoacoustic and fluorescence imaging," *Journal of Biomedical Optics*, 20(6), p. 066007.

Rawashdeh, W. A. et al. (2017) "Noninvasive assessment of elimination and retention using CT-FMT and kinetic whole-body modeling," *Theranostics*, 7(6), pp. 1499–1510.

Shipkova, M. and Christians, U. (2019) "Improving therapeutic decisions: Pharmacodynamic monitoring as an integral part of therapeutic drug monitoring," *Therapeutic Drug Monitoring*, 41(2), pp. 111–114.

Terreno, E., Uggeri, F. and Aime, S. (2012) "Image guided therapy: The advent of theranostic agents," *Journal of Controlled Release: Official Journal of the Controlled Release Society*, 161(2), pp. 328–337. doi: 10.1016/j.jconrel.2012.05.028.

Wang, J. et al. (2015) "*In vivo* pharmacokinetic features and biodistribution of star and rod shaped gold nanoparticles by multispectral optoacoustic tomography," *RSC Advances*, 5(10), pp. 7529–7538.

Xie, J., Lee, S. and Chen, X. (2010) "Nanoparticle-based theranostic agents," *Advanced Drug Delivery Reviews*, 62(11), pp. 1064–1079.

Xu, C. et al. (2011) "Nanoparticle-based monitoring of cell therapy," *Nanotechnology*, 22(49), p. 494001.

Zheng, F. et al. (2019) "Recent advances in drug release monitoring," *Nanophotonics*, 8(3), pp. 391–413.

Zou, P. et al. (2013) "Noninvasive fluorescence resonance energy transfer imaging of *in vivo* premature drug release from polymeric nanoparticles," *Molecular Pharmaceutics*, 10(11), pp. 4185–4194.

5 Nanotherapeutics in Drug Discovery and Development

5.1 PROCESS OF DRUG DISCOVERY AND DEVELOPMENT

Drug discovery is an expensive process that typically takes ten years from discovery to commercialization. Importantly, the expense and approval time vary based on the ailment being treated and the medicine being developed. In contrast to a treatment that is urgently required and would typically go through a prioritized review procedure, a drug that offers only modest enhancements over currently marketed treatments will have a significantly longer review process. Research across all therapeutic domains shows that it typically takes substantially longer than 12 years to produce a new drug, from target identification through clinical trials to marketing approval (DiMasi et al., 2010). The expense of developing an entirely novel molecular entity (NME), which can be described as a tiny molecule compound, or a new biological entity (NBE), which can be exemplified as an antibody, gene, protein, drug molecule, etc., is unquestionably greater than $1 billion. On average, it has been approximated to be around $2.6 billion (DiMasi, Grabowski and Hansen, 2016). However, generating an orphan drug (a medication used to treat uncommon and undertreated medical illnesses) is substantially less expensive altogether than developing a nonorphan medication. The drug development procedure is intended to "fail fast, fail early," especially during the clinical development phase, in order to eliminate significant threats before making a costly late-stage expenditure (Cook et al., 2014; Owens et al., 2015).

The key pin of a preclinical drug discovery project is to formulate one or many clinical drug candidate molecules where every single one of which demonstrates enough biological activity at an ailment-relevant target with sufficient safety and drug-like qualities that are intended to test in humans. Although numerous molecules do not proceed through the overall procedure due to issues with safety measurements, toxicity, pharmacokinetic profiles, potency, intellectual property considerations, or other facts. Moreover, the majority of discovery programs aim to develop more than one candidate compound. The wide-ranging chemistry, biology, molecular sciences, toxicology, and collaborative effort of pharmacokinetic aspects are almost always the standard in advanced drug development initiatives. Thus, there is no easy solution for developing an effective clinical candidate chemical compound. New molecular drug discovery projects typically produce enormous quantities of information by utilizing high-throughput screening strategies that assess many molecules at many dose levels against several assay methods (Sams-Dodd, 2005).

The advanced process of drug discovery generally entails the following steps: detecting the disorder to be treated as well as its unsolved medical requirement,

DOI: 10.1201/9781003442202-6

choosing a druggable molecular aim and validating it, developing *in vitro* assays, accompanied by high-throughput screening of molecules against the aim to recognize hits, and hit optimization to produce lead compounds which possess satisfactory potency and selectivity against the targeted biomolecule *in vitro* and that exemplify effectiveness in an experimental animals. Before moving on with drug development, the lead compounds are then further refined to increase their effectiveness and pharmacokinetics (Figure 5.1) (Sinha and Vohora, 2018).

Preclinical and clinical stages of development could be distinguished in the procedure for drug development (Figure 5.2). Pharmacological safety and toxicological investigations of the candidate are carried out during preclinical development in the future desires of determining the optimized and secured dosages in laboratory animals and evaluate the potential for undesired harmful effects of the drug-in-development. Moreover, research is done to determine the most cost-effective manufacturing procedures needed for the particular medication as well as the ideal formulation. If the candidate demonstrates enough safety and effectiveness in preclinical testing, clearance from drug regulatory bodies is requested to begin the clinical development of those drugs, during which their safety and effectiveness are evaluated in pilot and pivotal trials. The number of cutting-edge medications getting marketing approval has been declining over time. This is a result of critical examination by regulatory bodies about the efficiency and safety of new pharmaceuticals, which raises costs and extends development time frames (Sinha and Vohora, 2018).

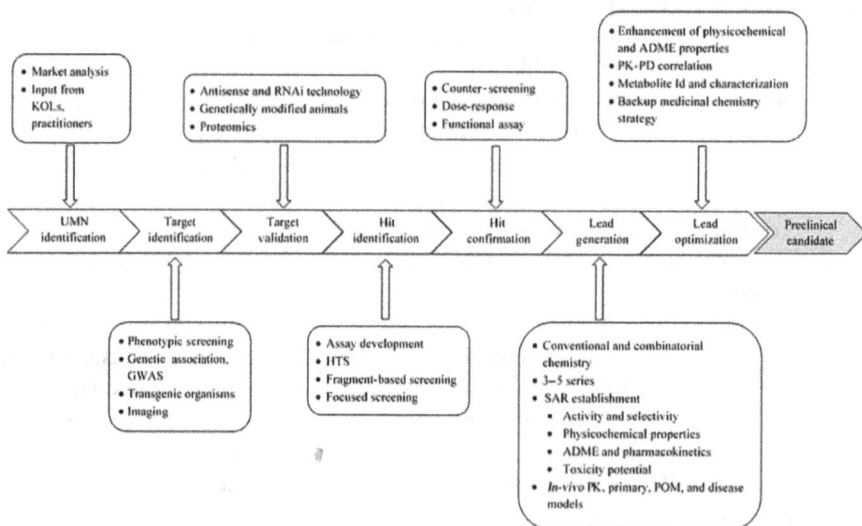

FIGURE 5.1 Overview of drug-discovery process. UMN, unmet medical needs; KOL, key opinion leader; SAR, structure–activity relationship; GWAS, genome-wide association studies; HTS, high-throughput screening; POM, proof of mechanism; PK, pharmacokinetics; PD, pharmacodynamics.

Source: Reproduced with permission from Sinha and Vohora, 2018.

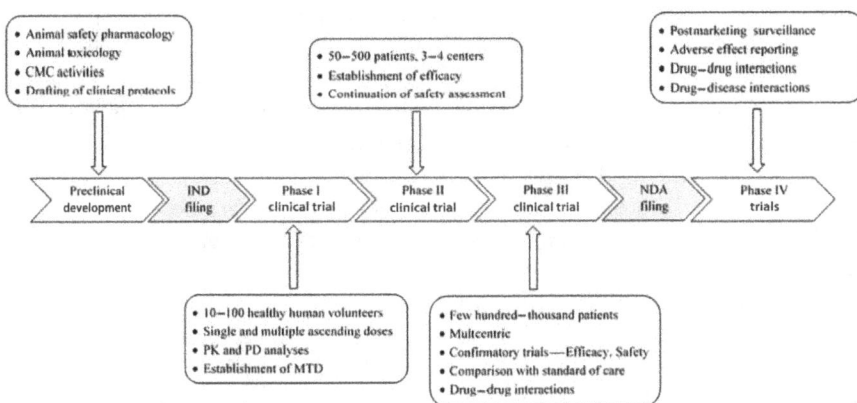

FIGURE 5.2 Overview of drug development process. CMC, chemistry, manufacturing, and controls; MTD, maximum tolerated dose; IND, investigated new drug application; NDA, new drug application.

Source: Reproduced with permission from Sinha and Vohora, 2018.

Furthermore, the senior management of pharmaceutical firms strives to reduce the risks connected to medication development and discovery. Also, the burden on national health systems brought on by the price of medications has a negative effect on their pricing. However, the profitability of pharmaceutical industry and their subsequent growth have decreased due to patent expirations and generic substitutes, which has led to less amounts of capital being invested in cutting-edge research. More mergers and acquisitions in the field of medicines, with the initial goal of lowering R&D expenses and developing synergies, are a direct result of the depressing decline in productivity. It is doubtful that industry consolidation will enhance productivity because post-mergers and acquisitions and pipeline developments spending in creative research have actually declined. Despite the decline in R&D productivity brought on by the aforementioned issues, there continues to be a significant unmet need in the treatment of cancer, infectious diseases, Alzheimer's disease, Parkinson, diabetes, etc. (Mohs and Greig, 2017).

Additionally, there is an immediate necessity of novel medications due to the global upsurge of multidrug-resistant infectious diseases. Today, almost all pharmaceutical companies use the same technical procedures to find new medications. They include the use of combinatorial chemistries, automated screening, nanotechnology-based techniques, and the cloning and expression of receptors and enzymes in arrangements that enable high-throughput. To overcome the above-mentioned bottlenecks, nanotechnology and nanotherapeutics can be implemented as successful efforts in drug discovery and development (Matthews et al., 2012).

5.2 ROLE OF NANOTHERAPEUTICS IN DRUG DISCOVERY

The recent use of nanotechnology and nanotherapeutics in the process of drug discovery and development involves producing superior diagnostic procedures, improved medication formulations, and improved systems for delivering drugs for treating diseases. Innovating solutions are provided by the groundbreaking design of nanotechnology-based nanotherapeutics, which increases analytical capabilities of research scientists, improves the quality of their data, and requires relatively small sample volume for the preservation and screening of molecular, cellular, and tissue banks. The original difficulties of inadequate throughput, inaccurate data, and several other problems are now starting to be overcome through nanotechnological advancements (Berdigaliyev and Aljofan, 2020).

Technology advancements over the past ten years have allowed the drug discovery process to advance into a platform where innovative lead compounds could be discovered quickly toward novel and occasionally challenging aims. Despite the fact that techniques based on nanorobotics and automation advances toward miniaturization have considerably enhanced throughputs in drug formulation and screening, they have only just begun to scratch the surface. The method of discovering new drugs has already undergone a revolution with the development of microarray analysis and lab-on-a-chip (LOC) technology (Pradeep, Raveendran and Babu, 2022).

These cutting-edge techniques reduce the amount of uncertainty required in choosing targets, leads, and therapeutic candidates by producing high-value information quickly. However, nowadays, even more cutting-edge technologies, including nanotechnology, are poised to further automate, speed up, and improve the reliability of tests by functioning at scales which are far smaller than traditional microarrays (Govindarajan et al., 2012).

Cross-disciplinary scientists have the chance to design and create multifunctional nanoparticles which can target, detect, and treat disorders in this quickly expanding field of nanotherapeutics. The primary goals of nanotechnology in the field of drug discovery and development are to strengthen disease therapy through the development of improved diagnostic procedures, therapeutic preparations, and delivery systems for drugs. For the purpose of creating novel utilizations to enhance human healthcare, the research arena is focusing drastically on the novel chemical and physical features of materials in nanodimensions.

The atomic force microscope (AFM) was the first commercial nanotechnology utilized for therapeutic purposes (Butt, Cappella and Kappl, 2005). This method was first utilized to map the topographical features of surfaces in atoms or molecules accuracy using a silicon-based needle with a sharpness at atomic scale. The sample is scanned by the incredibly thin tip, which produces a three-dimensional surface representation. With its ability to directly examine individual atoms or molecules and handle a numerous sample at the nanoscale scale, the AFM is quickly replacing other technologies as the main tool used by scientists and researchers. Although AFM is immensely valuable for visualizing particles that possess nanodimensions in fields like life science, materials science, electrochemistry, polymer science, and biophysics, they have been used only very recently in methods to obtain better chemical complexities of the methods that cells response to stimuli, which might also confirm specifically important for drug discovery (Butt, Cappella and Kappl, 2005).

Identification of various protein content in typical healthy and pathological tissues, characterization of these proteins, and identification of the protein's function in biochemical processes have been the main goals of proteomics investigations. Then, these proteins can be used as prospective therapeutic targets and diagnostic indicators. Protein and DNA microarrays, which enable the greater selective capture and evaluation of numerous proteins expressed in distinct cell types subjected to specific perturbations in a high-throughput manner, remain at the forefront of these developing and emerging advances. The complete suite of drug discovery applications cannot be utilized due to various restrictions in the currently available microarray techniques. Nanoarrays, an ultra-miniaturized variation that belongs to the conventional microarray which enable monitor interactions among atoms and molecules below to nanometer resolutions, are the product of the next stage of evolution. Very small amounts of protein molecules can be successfully tested against a wide range of pharmacological targets using nanoarray technology. Moreover, nanoarrays may be used as sensors in dimensions that large microarrays cannot. Figure 5.3 shows 2D protein nanoarray as a carrier of sensing elements for gold-based immunosensing systems (Tang et al., 2022).

To fulfill the demand for improved specificity in high-throughput screening, nanotherapeutics are being developed. Quantum dots, nanobars, nanodendrimers, or colloids that are nanoscale in size offer extremely stable, easily multiplexable molecular labels that are approximately comparable to the biomolecules of interest. Nanomaterials are useful for bio tagging or labeling since nanoparticles can be found in the same size range as proteins. Nevertheless, a biological or molecular encapsulating or membrane acting as a bioinorganic interface should be linked to the nanoparticle in order to incorporate with a suitable target (Yamankurt et al., 2019).

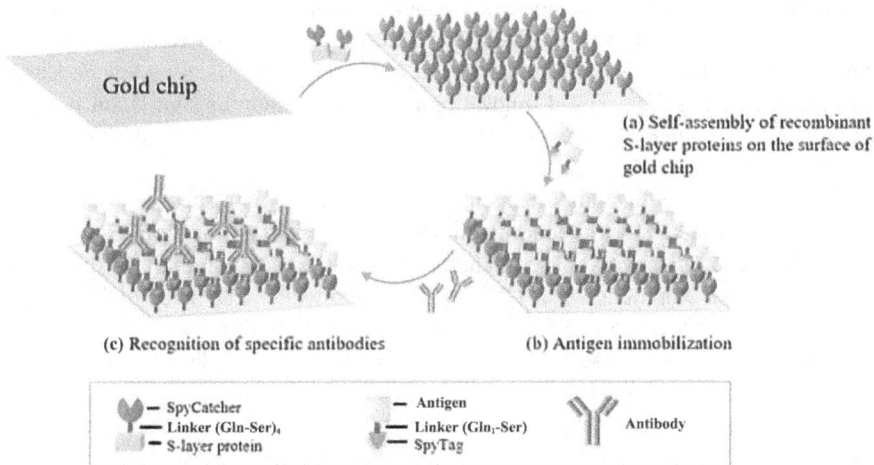

FIGURE 5.3 Two-dimensional protein nanoarray as a carrier of sensing elements for gold-based immunosensing systems.

Source: Reproduced with permission from Tang et al., 2022.

The vast majority of the industrial nanoparticle implementations in medicinal field focus on the development and delivery of new drugs. In applications requiring great photo-stability and multiplexing properties, nanoparticles are gradually replacing organic dyes. Nanobars, a different type of molecular tagging, are made of alternating slabs of reflective metals and may be optically scanned like real bar codes to distinguish various molecular species. These frameworks have several merits upon traditional labeling, including the ability to construct a wide variety of labels, the ability to multiplex, and the persistence of the signal (Bhirde et al., 2011).

The emergence of new chemical compositions, the ability to regulate and track molecules on the nanoscale as a result of advancements in microscopy, upsurged government funding designated for nanotechnology, notable as well as future perspectives provided by the private investment community, and the explosive growth of nanotechnology start-up businesses are primary factors influencing the expansion of nanotherapeutic advancements in drug discovery. The whole marketplace for nanotechnology-related approaches in drug discovery was predicted to have earned lower than $700 million in revenues in 2005, despite a global expenditure of slightly over $8.5 billion. By 2012, the market was projected to increase by double digits and reach a startling $2.5 billion (*The role of nanotechnology in drug discovery*, 2006).

Most of the prospects will be presented by nanoparticle solutions, nano-enabled pharmaceuticals, and many other nano-enabled devices like nanoarrays as well as nano-mass spectrometry. Financing for new technology has historically been a challenge to the industrial firm. Many industries that specialize in the area of nanotherapeutic solutions have been established in response to the desire for fast drug development and enhanced drug treatments. Major microfluidics and LOC firms are in the greatest position to profit from the shift toward nanotechnology-based approaches in drug development, despite the fact that the market now includes a large number of start-ups as a result of the emergence of nanotherapeutics. Aclara Biosciences, Agilent Technologies, Cepheid, Caliper Life Sciences, Eksigent Technologies, CombiMatrix Corporation, Nanogen, Gyros, and Nanostream are a few examples of such firms (Samuel Reich, 2011). The latter is a worldwide leader in semiconducting nanocrystal innovation and holds numerous significant international patents. Its main technology, Qdots®, is utilized for high-throughput screening (Samuel Reich, 2011).

It is worth noting that nanotherapeutic solutions are by no respects a "sure thing" since it remains a very high ladder to climb in order to obtain the Holy Grail. Thus, the bulk of drug discovery–based nanotherapeutic treatments remain in the initial research and development stages (R&D). Nanotherapeutics may need to function at greater precision levels and achieve higher levels of throughput when compared to conventional micro- or macroscale, automatic equipment in order to be considered for commercial implementation.

It is undeniable that any brand-new, cutting-edge technology raises aspirations and expectations. While this may allow the company spend more money and resources, a lack of visible progress, commercial delays, or additional regulatory hurdles may crush the expectations and credibility. Similar to how high-throughput screening (HTS) was heralded as the solution for increasing drug discovery efficiency decades ago, causing a surge in ultra-HTS (UHTS) and high-speed automation, which has since begun to fall after failing to live up to its own expectations. The health science industrial field is just recently starting to embrace micro-fabrication as a means of miniaturizing interdisciplinary (Fox, Filichkin and Mockler, 2009).

In particular, nanoparticle-based nanotherapeutics utilized for drug discovery tasks can raise issues if they break down too rapidly or stay in the body compartments for prolonged periods; as a result, they need to maintain the highest levels of stability. Although nanomaterials can interact with living organisms, there is risk that they will be harmful to both human and the environment. Despite the enormous advantages of nanotechnology, there are undoubtedly numerous obstacles to overcome. Drug discovery strategies based on nanotechnology are starting to reveal substantial fresh insights toward how biological systems work, and they will also enable the development of totally new categories of micro- and nano-fabricated equipment and systems.

REFERENCES

Berdigaliyev, N. and Aljofan, M. (2020) "An overview of drug discovery and development," *Future Medicinal Chemistry*, 12(10), pp. 939–947.

Bhirde, A. et al. (2011) "Nanoparticles for cell labeling," *Nanoscale*, 3(1), pp. 142–153.

Butt, H.-J., Cappella, B. and Kappl, M. (2005) "Force measurements with the atomic force microscope: Technique, interpretation and applications," *Surface Science Reports*, 59(1–6), pp. 1–152.

Cook, D. et al. (2014) "Lessons learned from the fate of Astra Zeneca's drug pipeline: A five-dimensional framework," *Nature Reviews: Drug Discovery*, 13(6), pp. 419–431.

DiMasi, J. A. et al. (2010) "Trends in risks associated with new drug development: Success rates for investigational drugs," *Clinical Pharmacology and Therapeutics*, 87(3), pp. 272–277.

DiMasi, J. A., Grabowski, H. G. and Hansen, R. W. (2016) "Innovation in the pharmaceutical industry: New estimates of R&D costs," *Journal of Health Economics*, 47, pp. 20–33.

Drug Discovery World (DDW). (2006) *The role of nanotechnology in drug discovery*. Available at: https://www.ddw-online.com/the-role-of-nanotechnology-in-drug-discovery-948-200604/ (Accessed: October 24, 2023).

Fox, S., Filichkin, S. and Mockler, T. C. (2009) "Applications of ultra-high-throughput sequencing," *Methods in Molecular Biology (Clifton, N.J.)*, 553, pp. 79–108.

Govindarajan, R. et al. (2012) "Microarray and its applications," *Journal of Pharmacy & Bioallied Sciences*, 4(Suppl 2), pp. S310–S312.

Matthews, P. M. et al. (2012) "Positron emission tomography molecular imaging for drug development: PET for drug development," *British Journal of Clinical Pharmacology*, 73(2), pp. 175–186.

Mohs, R. C. and Greig, N. H. (2017) "Drug discovery and development: Role of basic biological research," *Alzheimer's & Dementia (New York, N. Y.)*, 3(4), pp. 651–657.

Owens, P. K. et al. (2015) "A decade of innovation in pharmaceutical R&D: The Chorus model," *Nature Reviews: Drug Discovery*, 14(1), pp. 17–28.

Pradeep, A., Raveendran, J. and Babu, T. G. S. (2022) "Design, fabrication and assembly of lab-on-a-chip and its uses," *Progress in Molecular Biology and Translational Science*, 187(1), pp. 121–162. doi: 10.1016/bs.pmbts.2021.07.021.

Sams-Dodd, F. (2005) "Target-based drug discovery: Is something wrong?," *Drug Discovery Today*, 10(2), pp. 139–147.

Samuel Reich, E. (2011) "Nano rules fall foul of data gap," *Nature*, 480(7376), pp. 160–161. doi: 10.1038/480160a.

Sinha, S. and Vohora, D. (2018) "Drug discovery and development," Divya Vohora and Gursharan Singh (Eds.), *Pharmaceutical medicine and translational clinical research.* London: Elsevier, pp. 19–32.

Tang, J. et al. (2022) "Two-dimensional protein nanoarray as a carrier of sensing elements for gold-based immunosensing systems," *Analytical Chemistry*, 94(26), pp. 9355–9362.

Yamankurt, G. et al. (2019) "Exploration of the nanomedicine-design space with high-throughput screening and machine learning," *Nature Biomedical Engineering*, 3(4), pp. 318–327.

6 Nanotherapeutics in Drug Delivery

INTRODUCTION

Nanotechnology claims to be the preferred drug delivery method, particularly for the more problematic traditional medications that are utilized in the care of many diseases. Drug aiming and sustained release are the key primary elements required for tailoring an effective and optimized drug delivery system (DDS). The carrier element should arrive the region where the anticipated medicine would reach, and the other elements within the carrier pertain to do with the rate and duration of the drug release.

Moreover, there are several kingpins in employing the targeting of distribution of shabbily water-soluble medicines to a specific site to decrease the deposition of drug within normal tissues. They include assisting in maintaining half-life of the drug and optimized duration of activated drug which gives an effective treatment, extending the therapeutic action of the drug by acting as a shield to protect the drug from biological barriers, and enabling drug delivery throughout epithelial and anatomical barriers. These are considered as advantages of using nanotechnology-based nanotherapeutics in DDS (Patra et al., 2018). Figure 6.1 shows a comprehensive description of different nanoformulations in DDS and their merit points (Rana and Sharma, 2019).

6.1 LIPID-BASED NANOCARRIERS

Lipid-based nanocarriers can be further divided to nanoemulsions, solid lipid nanoparticles, and nanostructured lipid carriers. Nanoemulsions are an intriguing approach of delivering various drugs as a colloidal solution that may be sterilized through filtering. These nanoemulsions which are formulated as nanoscale oil droplets within an aqueous base are heterogeneous in their nature, culminating in a combination of nanodroplets with a narrow particle distribution. The resulting nanoemulsions are homogeneous, opaque or transparent, and well-supported by surfactant. According to their formulation methods, three types of nanoemulsions exist: a nanoemulsion in which water is dispersed in oil, a nanoemulsion in which oil is dispersed in water, and a bicontinuous nanoemulsion (D'Souza et al., 2002; Gao et al., 2011).

The ability of nanoemulsions to mask the unpleasant flavor of greasy drug formulations is their most important feature. Moreover, they extend the activity of medications and shield them from chemical reactions such as oxidation and hydrolysis. Thus, certain nanoformulations of nanoemulsions may be proven to be a highly bioavailable and effective delivery method. To lessen inflammatory responses in vascular environment, Simion et al. developed P-selectin targeted dexamethasone-reinforced lipid nanoemulsions in 2016. Physicochemical evaluations on the produced formulations were performed and the research revealed that the nano-formulation worked both *in vitro* as well as *in vivo*. It preferentially reduces endothelial activation and,

DOI: 10.1201/9781003442202-7

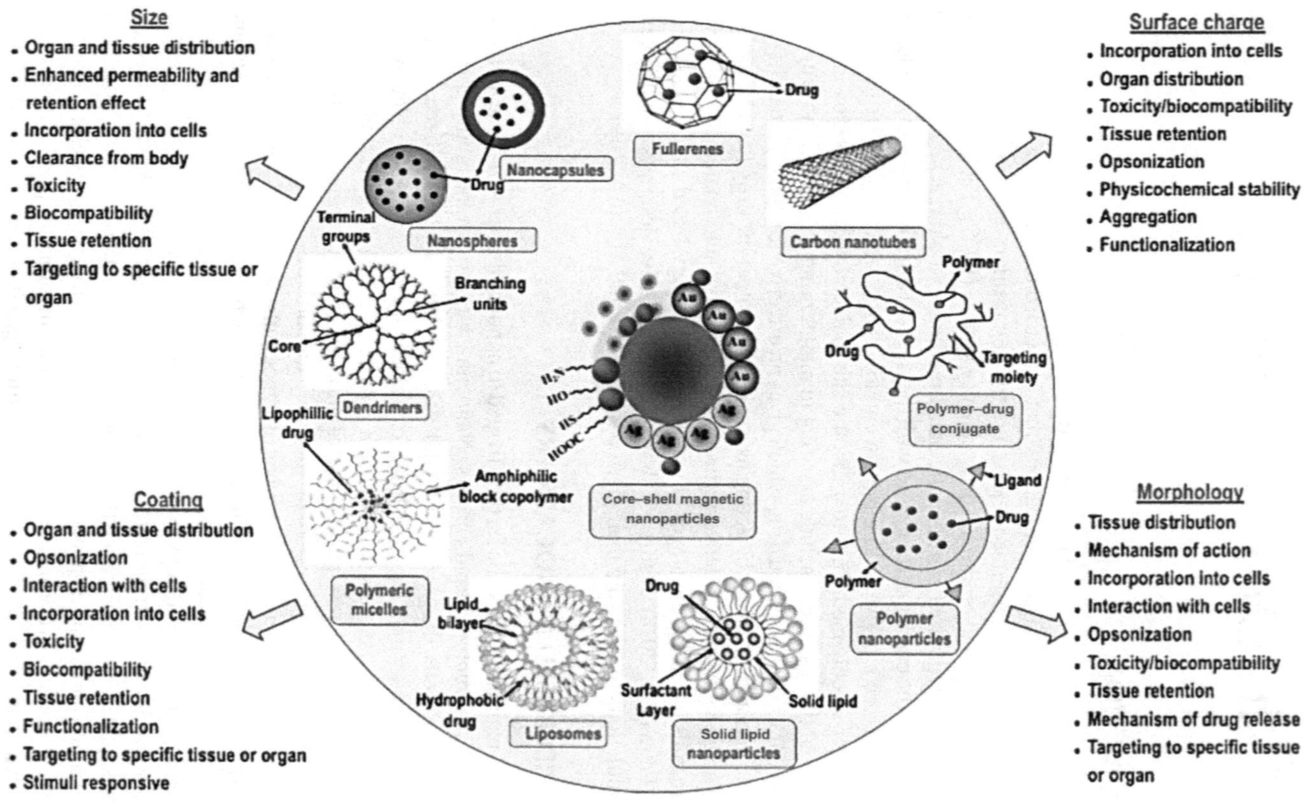

FIGURE 6.1 Different nanoformulations in drug delivery system.

Source: Reproduced with permission from Rana and Sharma, 2019.

as a corollary, monocyte infiltration, which significantly reduces lung inflammation in mice as the utilized laboratory animal model in the study (Simion et al., 2016).

Solid lipid nanoparticles (SLNs) are lipid nanoparticles that have been formulated in a solid material. They are developed by employing a lipid in the solid state to create oil-in-water nanoemulsions. The initial prototypes of SLNs were developed around 1990. Inexpensive raw materials, formulating methods that are carried in the absence of organic solvents, the utilization of biological lipids, simplicity of scaling up, compatible with biological materials, enhancement in bioavailability, shielding delicate moieties from environmental risks, and sustained drug-release are some benefits attributed with SLNs. Solid lipids are less suited for drug delivery systems due to their polymorphic transition, drug ejection problems, inconsistent gelation propensity, and limited drug integration (Fang, Al-Suwayeh and Fang, 2013). Ciprofloxacin-loaded SLNs were recently developed with enhanced antimicrobial properties by employing melt-emulsification approach assisted with ultrasonic technique. With various lipids, release of ciprofloxacin displayed a sustained-release nature. Stearic acid-prepared ciprofloxacin SLNs (CIPSTE) demonstrated the highest burst effect, leading to quick drug release (Shazly, 2017).

The second generation of drug delivery platforms of lipid nanosystems after the initial prototypes, known as nonstructured lipid carriers, is composed of lipids in the liquid state blended with solid lipids (Souto and Muller, 2007). In contrast to emulsions, these drug carriers in nanoscale strongly immobilize therapeutic medicines and inhibit particle agglomeration (Zauner, Farrow and Haines, 2001). Moreover, compared to SLNs, their cargo capacity for drug molecules is higher owing to the oil droplets in the liquid phase incorporated in a solid matrix. Biodegradability, comparably negligible toxicological effects, sustained release, drug stability, and organic solvents-free synthesis are benefits of NLCs against other nanomaterials. NLCs have been thoroughly studied over the past few decades for the delivery of both hydrophobic and hydrophilic medicines. The NLCs were designed with the goal of satisfying industry demands for certification and validation, uncomplicated technology, scalability, and affordability (Shidhaye, Vaidya and Sutar, 2008).

6.2 POLYMER-BASED NANOCARRIERS

Polymer-based nanocarriers are further categorized into four subcategories: self-assemble nanocarriers that include dendrimers and micelles, particulate nanocarriers that include polymeric nanoparticles, capsular and vesicular nanocarriers that include nanocapsules and nanobubbles, and finally cyclodextrin-based nanocarriers that include nanosponges.

Exceptional three-dimensional, spherical, densely branched nanopolymeric frameworks are called dendrimers. They stand out from other nanosystems of drug delivery owing to interesting properties: aqueous solubility, nanoscale size, narrow polydispersity index, customizable structural properties in molecules, presence of niches in the interior, and numerous functional moieties at the exterior. The framework for conjugation and targeting of drugs is provided by terminal characteristics. These auxiliary functional moieties also provide them bespoke features, increasing their adaptability (Patri, Majoros and Baker, 2002). The most extensively researched dendrimer for medication delivery is polyamidoamine. According to a study conducted recently, sonophoresis and terminated by arginine peptide dendrimers may be able to increase the transdermal permeability of ketoprofen (Manikkath et al., 2017).

Multicompartment micelles (MCMs) and associated block copolymer architectures with superior structural features have become a fascinating category of sophisticated self-assemblies belonging to soft-matter nanotechnology that enable a basic understanding of the bottom-up construction of solution-based hierarchies. They are an attractive type of responsive nanotherapeutics because they permit the concomitant delivery of multiple medications and combine much like proteins in various physical nanoenvironments in well-separated compartments (Gröschel et al., 2012).

Polymers that are synthesized are utilized to create the most prominent polymeric nanoparticles. Polymers that have a natural inheritance have inconsistent purity and batch-to-batch uniformity, which cause poor reproducible and controlled release nature for the medicine that is being entrapped in them. The manner of drug release from polymeric nanoparticles can be altered owing to the availability of synthetic polymers with high batch-to-batch repeatability and purity (Panyam and Labhasetwar, 2003). Hydrophilic functionalities can be enclosed inside the polymer-based nanoparticles that are synthetic using the double emulsion approach due to the challenge to retain their biological activity in the presence of organic solvents on volatile nature.

Aliphatic polymers that have a tendency to biodegradation, such as polylactide (PLA), polylactide-*co*-glycolide copolymers (PLGA), and poly(-carpolactone), in addition to polymers that are nonbiodegradable such as polyacrylates and poly(methyl methacrylate), are often utilized as synthetic polymers described for drug delivery (Zhang et al., 2013). Polymeric nanoparticles might efficiently shield drug moieties with an unstable nature from deterioration, reducing the likelihood that harmful medications will have side effects.

A medication typically incorporated into drug molecules are usually encapsulated in solid or liquid nanocapsules before being enclosed by a special membrane made of synthetic or organic polymers. Most of the scientists who engage with research are mesmerized by pharmaceuticals related to nanocapsules that are available on the market due to their encapsulation, which shields the encapsulated substance from undesirable issues like breakdown in the fluid base and slows the release of moieties which govern the therapeutic action (Kothamasu et al., 2012). Colon cancer cells may be targeted by resveratrol-loaded lipid-core-nanocapsules (RSV-LNC), which have been developed and characterized recently (Feng, Zhong and Zhan, 2017).

Nanobubbles are spherical and stabilized vesicular structures that contain gas in aqueous solutions with dimensions just under 1,000 nm. However, they are primarily in the region of 100 nm when developed by the technique of hydrodynamic or acoustic cavitation. The vast majority of nanobubbles have a core structure in a shell, in which the core is the area of the nanobubble that contains the chosen gas and the outer shell can have a variety of constituents and topologies. A recent study proves that nanobubbles can be utilized to store O_2 and formulate oxygenated nanobubbles as a treatment strategy for COVID-19 patients who suffer from hypoxia.

These oxygenated nanobubbles can be administered to the bloodstream to overcome the hypoxic states of COVID-19 patients (Afshari et al., 2021).

Nanosponges can be loaded with both hydrophilic, hydrophobic, and lipophilic moieties. They have attracted the interest of experts who engage in pharmaceutical research for drug delivery. These nanosponges are incredibly small, consist low toxicological profile, high porosity, scaffold, and colloidal structures with lots of voids where drug particles could be enclosed. The most often used ingredient in the formation of these nanocarriers is cyclodextrin. Both water and organic solvents are unable to dissolve in these complexes. They have a pH range of 2–11, and have an ability of self-sterilization and being stable up to 300°C. Employing a synthesis approach assisted with ultrasound, Trotta and colleagues developed cyclodextrin nanosponges and investigated their potential as anticancer therapeutics (Prasad et al., 2018).

6.3 CROSS-LINKED NANOGELS

It has been shown that nanogels are soluble in high degrees when employing as drug delivery vehicles. Nanogels are small, round, partially permeable polymer structures with internal voids that can incorporate drug molecules of varied sizes (Vinogradov and Senanayake, 2013). Nanogel expands when exposed to water. Thus, the drug can be introduced straight away, giving the possibility of materializing a rigid, dense nanocarrier which acts like a drug-carrying vehicle by reducing the volume of solvent. Due to its excellent structural qualities, enhanced biocompatibility, and dampness, it has an exceptional status in carrier-based drug delivery systems. Gels provide a vast surface area for bioconjugates and an inner environment for biomolecule incorporation when completing their structure formation. It possesses an effective self-property that facilitates drug release and facilitates the simple removal of any leftover nanogel formulation components (Oh et al., 2008). Core/shell nanogel formulations with N-isopropyl methacrylamide enable controlled release as cancer drugs (Peters et al., 2018).

6.4 DRUG CONJUGATES

Typically, drugs could be chemically bioconjugated or accumulated on the surface of a nanocarrier, either internally or externally. Normally, chemical conjugation occurs on the outermost layers of NPs. There are various methods for conjugating NPs with drug-like responses. When combined into a system of controlled medication release, NPs based on liposomes might be thought of as one of the most promising carriers (DDS). Spherical compartments known as liposomes are produced by suspending phospholipids inside a hydrophobic medium, which is then gradually replaced by a hydrophilic solution. The conjugation is carried out using a variety of chemical techniques and functional groups (Aguilar-Pérez et al., 2020); however ester bonds among a group of carboxylic acids and a group of hydroxyls, which may include the drug or the lipid, correspondingly, are the most popular. To overcome drawbacks such as multidrug resistance, nanoparticles have been conjugated to enhance the pharmacokinetic and pharmacodynamic features of these bulk-carrying structures. Using liposomes as carriers of biomolecules, researchers were able to produce DDS with anticancer potential by conjugating them with microbubbles, specific proteins, or antibodies (Eras et al., 2022).

6.5   ORGANIC NANOPARTICLES FOR DRUG DELIVERY

A variety of organic components are used in the medication delivery methods. Chitosan is capable of performing function at the constrictive epithelial junctions since it has muco-adhesive qualities. In order to provide ongoing medication release systems for different kinds of epithelia, chitosan-based nanoparticles are commonly studied. In the interest of administering the antibiotic ceftazidime to the eye, Silva et al. produced and assessed the effectiveness of a 0.75% w/w isotonic solution of hydroxypropyl methylcellulose (HPMC) containing chitosan/sodium tripolyphosphate/hyaluronic acid nanoparticles (Silva et al., 2017).

Alginate is another organic substance, which is also referred to as a biopolymer, that has been utilized for medication delivery. As contrast to cationic and neutral polymers, such anionic mucoadhesive polymer, which has terminal carboxyl groups, exhibits better mucoadhesive intensity. Xanthan gum is a heteropolysaccharide that comprises a large molecular weight. It has strong bioadhesive qualities and is considered a polyanionic polysaccharide. Xanthan gum is commonly used as a pharmaceutical excipient because it has a low toxicological profile and is a relatively nonirritating polymer material. Cellulose and its derivatives are widely used, mostly to alter the dissolution and gelation of the medicines, which in turn controls their profile for release of active moieties of the medicines (Sun et al., 2019). Repaglinide, an antihyperglycemic drug which is used in diabetic patients, was studied by Elseoud et al. (Elseoud et al., 2018) using nanocrystals of cellulose and nanochitosan for release of the active moieties when administered orally.

Natural biopolymers, which include various saccharides and proteins, are derived from biological sources, including plants, animals, microbes, and seaweed (Balaji et al., 2017; Bassas-Galia et al., 2017). The majority of nanoparticles that have a protein basis may be broken down, metabolized, and easily functionalized for coupling to certain medicines and other targeted ligands. They are often made using a pair of distinct approaches such as insoluble proteins, including zein and gliadin, as well as water-soluble counterparts, including bovine and human serum albumin. In an effort to improve and accelerate their targeting strategy, the protein-based nanoparticles are typically arranged chemically to incorporate targeting ligands that specifically recognize specific cells and tissues (Lohcharoenkal et al., 2014). Similar to monosaccharides, polysaccharides are made up of sugar molecules joined together by O-glycosidic linkages. These polysaccharides can acquire a variety of distinct physical–chemical characteristics due to the nature of their monomers in addition to their biological source.

6.6   INORGANIC NANOPARTICLES FOR DRUG DELIVERY

The inorganic nanoparticles are becoming more and more significant as nanocarriers in drug delivery systems. Endocytosis, a method which enables nanoparticles to enter cells, has been demonstrated to have evidences of the function. The biodistribution is determined by its size and surface characteristics when these nanoparticles have been administered. Hence, nucleic acids could also be delivered into living cells using nanoparticles. Several inorganic nanoparticles have been employed as drug carriers because of the very sophisticated chemical characteristics that nanoparticles now possess. Inorganic nanoparticles like mesoporous silica nanoparticles, calcium phosphate, carbon nanotubes, double hydroxides, gold, silver, iron oxide, quantum dots, magnesium phosphate, and strontium phosphate all have been explored for their ability to carry DNA (Paul and Sharma, 2020).

Considering the recent inorganic nanotherapeutics for drug delivery, Munaweera et al. have synthesized innovative wrinkled structured periodic mesoporous organo-silica (PMO) nanoparticles for the administration of hydrophobic anticancer drugs. These cutting-edge wrinkled PMOs contain pore diameters, hydrophobicity, and surface areas that can be adjusted to facilitating the delivery of hydrophobic drugs. In comparison to mesoporous silica (MS) nanoparticles, the hydrophobic anticancer agent, paclitaxel, was employed as a standard drug, and the PMO demonstrates a better drug-loading efficiency for paclitaxel (Munaweera et al., 2015a). Moreover, Munaweera et al. formulated a new type of platinum drug loaded with holmium in wrinkled mesoporous silica nanoparticles coated with a lipid coating or uncoating. The influence was recognized as an anticancer treatment after *in vitro* platinum drug liberation from both lipids coated and uncoated with chemoradiotherapeutic wrinkled mesoporous silica nanoparticles (Munaweera et al., 2014). In another related study, wrinkle-structured, amine-modified mesoporous silicon (AMS) nanoparticles that release nitric oxide (NO) and cisplatin have been synthesized as an anticancer therapy for treatment of NSCLC (Munaweera et al., 2015b).

6.7 VIRAL NANOPARTICLES FOR DRUG DELIVERY

Viruses are supramolecular entities that have organized architectures and have unique functions and characteristics. Botanical viruses are frequently used in biotechnology, and genetic modification produces particulate debris that resembles viruses. Both provide a material-based method for therapeutic molecule delivery and dispersion. Viruses, especially noninfective viral-like nanoparticles (VLPs), are associated with these desirable traits. Viral nanoparticles (VNPs) are nanostructures produced by mammalian cells, plant cells, and bacteriophage viruses. VNPs are accelerating as nanotherapeutics in drug delivery due to the use and development of VNPs and associated with their genome-free counterparts (Aljabali et al., 2021).

Several active components may be encapsulated in VLPs, which can then be chemically or genetically coupled. VLPs were created using expandable fermentation or molecular farming, and the materials used are both biocompatible and biodegradable. Thus, substantial ongoing research is required to get these medicines to the clinical use (Chung, Cai and Steinmetz, 2020). Figure 6.2 shows schematic illustration of nanocarriers used in drug delivery (Sultana et al., 2022).

6.8 NANOROBOTICS

In contrast to other forms of nanomaterials commonly used in targeted delivery of pharmaceuticals, nanorobots have the potential to deliver drugs to disease areas with

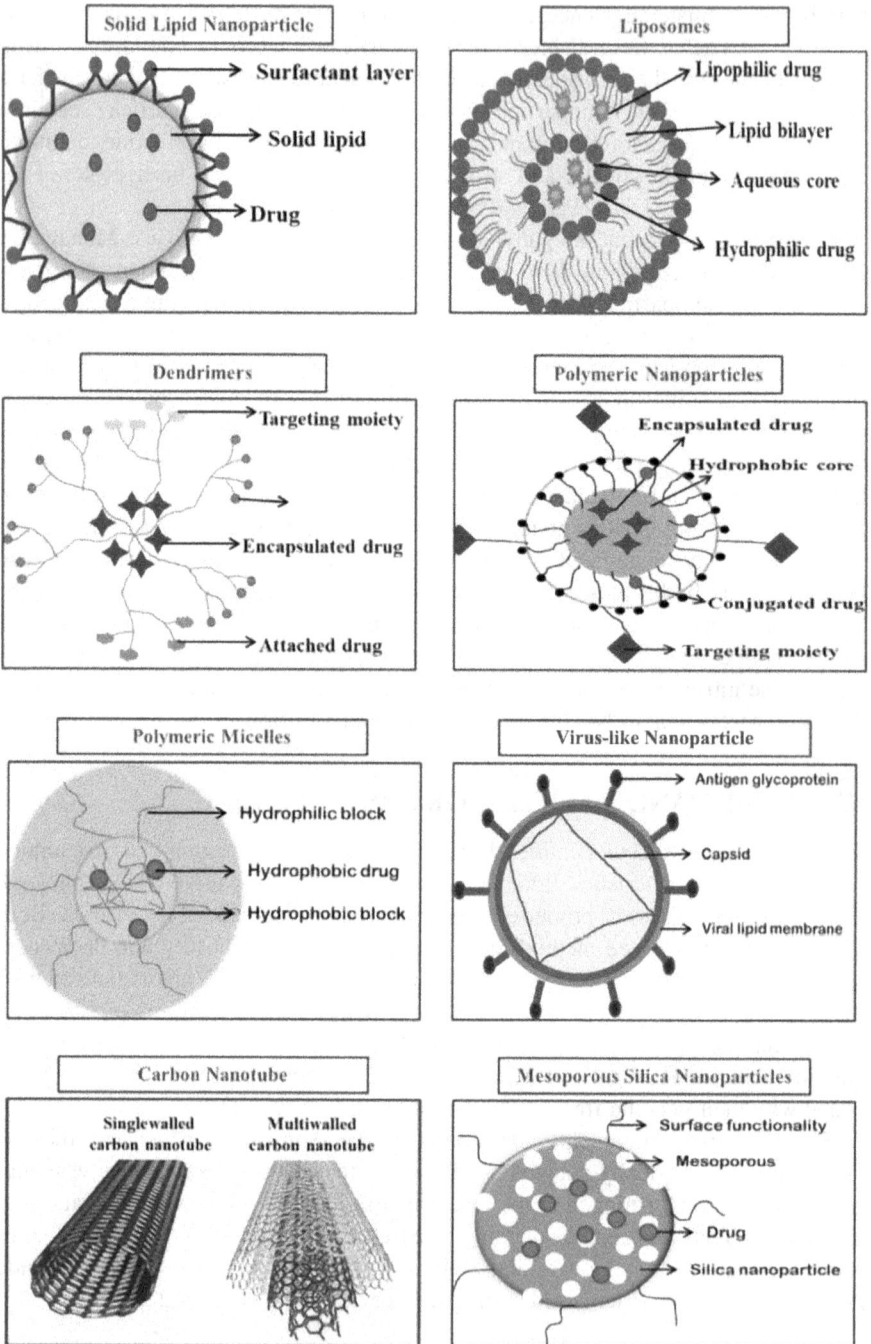

FIGURE 6.2 Schematic illustration of nanocarriers used in drug delivery which includes solid nanoparticles, liposomes, dendrimers, polymeric nanoparticles, polymeric micelles, virus-like nanoparticles, carbon nanotube, and mesoporous silica nanoparticles.

Source: Reproduced with permission from Sultana et al., 2022.

a lot of effectiveness and reduce systemic side effects. The nanorobots for active delivery of various drugs have advanced from test tubes to the cellular level over the last ten years. Several of these tools have even been successfully tried on live animals, which is promising. Furthermore, newly developed transient robots such as Mg/ZnO, Mg/Si, and Zn/Fe Janus particles can disintegrate into their respective environments without causing harm (Luo et al., 2018).

Nanomotors exhibit autonomous self-propulsion through a process known as nanolocomotion, which can be defined as the mechanism that enables a nanoscale object to move forward through an anisotropic energy and is frequently aided by an asymmetric construction. Typically, nanomotors can be used for catalysis, biosensing, and site-specific medicine delivery. The fundamental problems with current micro- and nanomotor platforms, which limit their potential for use in biological applications, appear to be their inability to achieve motion at a non-toxic and neutral pH as well as their lack of biocompatibility (Munaweera et al., 2016).

In this case, Munaweera et al. have developed mesoporous silica nanomotors in gold/palladium-coated magnesium nanoparticles to produce hydrogen gas and perform nanolocomotion simultaneously in a neutral pH environment. The findings of this study, which employed aspirin as a common medication, demonstrate that the built-in nanomotor systems provide acceptable delivery platforms for the preservation of fuel and payload. This concept has high biocompatibility capabilities and can store payloads or fuel wherever needed (Munaweera et al., 2016).

REFERENCES

Afshari, R. et al. (2021) "Review of oxygenation with nanobubbles: Possible treatment for hypoxic COVID-19 patients," *ACS Applied Nano Materials*, 4(11), pp. 11386–11412. doi: 10.1021/acsanm.1c01907.

Aguilar-Pérez, K. M., Avilés-Castrillo, J. I., Medina, D. I., Parra-Saldivar, R. and Iqbal, H. M. N. (2020) "Insight into nanoliposomes as smart nanocarriers for greening the twenty-first century biomedical settings," *Frontiers in Bioengineering and Biotechnology*, 8, p. 1441. doi: 10.3389/fbioe.2020.579536.

Aljabali, A. A. et al. (2021) "The viral capsid as novel nanomaterials for drug delivery," *Future Science OA*, 7(9), p. FSO744. doi: 10.2144/fsoa-2021-0031.

Balaji, A. B. et al. (2017) "Biodegradable and biocompatible polymer composites: Processing, properties and applications," in Shimpi, N. G. (ed.) *Series in composites science and engineering*. Duxford: Woodhead Publishing, pp. 3–32.

Bassas-Galia, M. et al. (2017) "Natural polymers: A source of inspiration," in *Bioresorbable polymers for biomedical applications*. New York: Elsevier, pp. 31–64.

Chung, Y. H., Cai, H. and Steinmetz, N. F. (2020) "Viral nanoparticles for drug delivery, imaging, immunotherapy, and theranostic applications," *Advanced Drug Delivery Reviews*, 156, pp. 214–235. doi: 10.1016/j.addr.2020.06.024.

D'Souza, S. et al. (2002) "Improved tuberculosis DNA vaccines by formulation in cationic lipids," *Infection and Immunity*, 70(7), pp. 3681–3688. doi: 10.1128/IAI.70.7.3681-3688.2002.

Elseoud, W. et al. (2018) "Chitosan nanoparticles/cellulose nanocrystals nanocomposites as a carrier system for the controlled release of repaglinide," *International Journal of Biological Macromolecules*, 111, pp. 604–613.

Eras, A. et al. (2022) "Chemical conjugation in drug delivery systems," *Frontiers in Chemistry*, 10, p. 889083. doi: 10.3389/fchem.2022.889083.

Fang, C.-L., Al-Suwayeh, S. A. and Fang, J.-Y. (2013) "Nanostructured lipid carriers (NLCs) for drug delivery and targeting," *Recent Patents on Nanotechnology*, 7(1), pp. 41–55. doi: 10.2174/187221013804484827.

Feng, M., Zhong, L. X. and Zhan, Z. Y. (2017) "Enhanced antitumor efficacy of resveratrol-loaded nanocapsules in colon cancer cells: Physicochemical and biological characterization," *European Review for Medical and. Pharmacological Science*, 21, pp. 375–382.

Gao, F. et al. (2011) "Nanoemulsion improves the oral absorption of candesartan cilexetil in rats: Performance and mechanism," *Journal of Controlled Release: Official Journal of the Controlled Release Society*, 149(2), pp. 168–174. doi: 10.1016/j.jconrel.2010.10.013.

Gröschel, A. H. et al. (2012) "Precise hierarchical self-assembly of multicompartment micelles," *Nature Communications*, 3(1), p. 710. doi: 10.1038/ncomms1707.

Kothamasu, P. et al. (2012) "Nanocapsules: The weapons for novel drug delivery systems," *Bioimpacts*, 2(2), pp. 71–81. doi: 10.5681/bi.2012.011.

Lohcharoenkal, W. et al. (2014) "Protein nanopar-ticles as drug delivery carriers for cancer therapy," *BioMed Research International*, 2014.

Luo, M. et al. (2018) "Micro-/nanorobots at work in active drug delivery," *Advanced Functional Materials*, 28(25), p. 1706100. doi: 10.1002/adfm.201706100.

Manikkath, J. et al. (2017) "Influence of peptide dendrimers and sonophoresis on the transdermal delivery of ketoprofen," *International Journal of Pharmaceutics*, 521(1–2), pp. 110–119. doi: 10.1016/j.ijpharm.2017.02.002.

Munaweera, I. et al. (2014) "Chemoradiotherapeutic wrinkled mesoporous silica nanoparticles for use in cancer therapy," *APL Materials*, 2(11), p. 113315. doi: 10.1063/1.4899118.

Munaweera, I. et al. (2015a) "Novel wrinkled periodic mesoporous organosilica nanoparticles for hydrophobic anticancer drug delivery," *Journal of Porous Materials*, 22(1), pp. 1–10. doi: 10.1007/s10934-014-9897-1.

Munaweera, I. et al. (2016) "Chemically powered nanomotor as a delivery vehicle for biologically relevant payloads," *Journal of Nanoscience and Nanotechnology*, 16(9), pp. 9063–9071. doi: 10.1166/jnn.2016.12904.

Munaweera, I., Shi, Y., Koneru, B., Patel, A. et al. (2015b) "Nitric oxide- and cisplatin-releasing silica nanoparticles for use against non-small cell lung cancer," *Journal of Inorganic Biochemistry*, 153, pp. 23–31. doi: 10.1016/j.jinorgbio.2015.09.002.

Oh, J. K., Drumright, R., Siegwart, D. J. and Matyjaszewski, K. (2008) "The development of microgels/nanogels for drug delivery applications," *Progress in Polymer Science*, 33, p. 448e477.

Panyam, J. and Labhasetwar, V. (2003) "Biodegradable nanoparticles for drug and gene delivery to cells and tissue, Adv," *Advance Drug Delivery Reviews*, 55, pp. 329–347.

Patra, J. K. et al. (2018) "Nano based drug delivery systems: Recent developments and future prospects," *Journal of Nanobiotechnology*, 16(1), p. 71. doi: 10.1186/s12951-018-0392-8.

Patri, A. K., Majoros, I. J. and Baker, J. R. (2002) "Dendritic polymer macromolecular carriers for drug delivery," *Current Opinion in Chemical Biology*, 6(4), pp. 466–471. doi: 10.1016/s1367-5931(02)00347-2.

Paul, W. and Sharma, C. P. (2020) "Inorganic nanoparticles for targeted drug delivery," In Chandra P. Sharma (Ed.), *Biointegration of medical implant materials*. Boca Raton, FL: Elsevier, pp. 333–373.

Peters, J. T., Hutchinson, S. S., Lizana, N., Verma, I. and Peppas, N. A. (2018) "Synthesis and characterization of poly(N-isopropyl methacrylamide) core/shell nanogels for controlled release of chemotherapeutics," *Chemical Engineering Journal*, 340, p. 58e65.

Prasad, M. et al. (2018) "Nanotherapeutics: An insight into healthcare and multi-dimensional applications in medical sector of the modern world," *Biomedecine & Pharmacotherapie [Biomedicine & Pharmacotherapy]*, 97, pp. 1521–1537. doi: 10.1016/j.biopha.2017.11.026.

Rana, V. and Sharma, R. (2019) "Recent advances in development of nano drug delivery," In Shyam S. Mohapatra, Shivendu Ranjan, Nandita Dasgupta, Raghvendra Kumar Mishra and Sabu Thomas (Eds.), *Applications of targeted nano drugs and delivery systems.* Amsterdam: Elsevier, pp. 93–131.

Shazly, G. A. (2017) "Ciprofloxacin controlled-solid lipid nanoparticles: Characterization, in vitro release, and antibacterial activity assessment," *BioMed Research International*, 2017, p. 2120734. doi: 10.1155/2017/2120734.

Shidhaye, S. S., Vaidya, R. and Sutar, S. (2008) "Solid lipid nanoparticles and nanostructured lipid carriers-innovative generations of solid lipid carriers," *Current Drug Delivery*, 5, pp. 324–331.

Silva, M. M., Calado, R., Marto, J., Bettencourt, A., Almeida, A. J. and Gonçalves, L. (2017) "Chitosan nanoparticles as a mucoadhesive drug delivery system for ocular administration," *Marine Drugs*, 15, p. 370.

Simion, V. et al. (2016) "P-selectin targeted dexamethasone-loaded lipid nanoemulsions: A novel therapy to reduce vascular inflammation," *Mediators of Inflammation*, 2016, p. 1625149. doi: 10.1155/2016/1625149.

Souto, E. B. and Muller, R. H. (eds.) (2007) *Nanoparticulate drug delivery systems, 166 Informa Healthcare.* New York and London: CRC Press. doi: 10.1201/9781420008449.

Sultana, A. et al. (2022) "Nano-based drug delivery systems: Conventional drug delivery routes, recent developments and future prospects," *Medicine in Drug Discovery*, 15(100134), p. 100134. doi: 10.1016/j.medidd.2022.100134.

Sun, B. et al. (2019) "Applications of cellulose-based materials in sustained drug delivery systems," *Current Medicinal Chemistry*, 26(14), pp. 2485–2501. doi: 10.2174/0929867 324666170705143308.

Vinogradov, S. V. and Senanayake, T. (2013) "Nanogeledrug conjugates: A step towards increasing the chemotherapeutic efficacy," *Nanomedicine*, 8, p. 1229e1232.

Zauner, W., Farrow, N. A. and Haines, A. M. (2001) "In vitro uptake of polystyrene microspheres: Effect of particle size, cell line and cell density," *Journal of Controlled Release: Official Journal of the Controlled Release Society*, 71(1), pp. 39–51. doi: 10.1016/s0168-3659(00)00358-8.

Zhang, Z. et al. (2013) "Polymeric nanoparticles-based topical delivery systems for the treatment of dermatological diseases: Polymeric nanoparticles-based topical delivery systems," *Wiley Interdisciplinary Reviews: Nanomedicine and Nanobiotechnology*, 5(3), pp. 205–218. doi: 10.1002/wnan.1211.

7 Nanotherapeutics in Surgery

INTRODUCTION

The definition of surgery allows addressing physiologically and technologically surgical management of certain injuries, deformations, and ailments. From just being "no more science than butchery," surgical procedures has grown into an extremely renowned science as well as artistry. However, delicate microsurgeons may encounter concerns when operating tissues at the nanoscale due to the lack of knowledge in nanotechnological advancements. In conventional surgery that is also called an open surgery, the internal organs that need surgical intervention may be exposed due to the cutting of healthy tissues. Hence, there has been a shift in favor of minimally invasive techniques over the last 20 years. Minimally invasive nanosurgery has several advantages, including less tissue damage and thus less scarring, fewer side effects and comorbidities, less postoperative discomfort, and faster recovery. Nowadays, the prime motivator is to reduce the invasiveness of surgery. One might envision a surgeon becoming able to alter and monitor individual cells by developing novel tools on the nanoscale. Nanotechnology has recently been used to improve surgical tools. Thus, using these nanotherapeutics-based surgical tools, the internal and external factors of the patient and the surrounding environment are crucially regulated (Shrikant, 2013).

7.1 NANOSURGICAL TOOLS

The nanosurgical tools are categorized depending on their invasive limits and levels. Nanotherapeutics-based surgical tools have progressed from nano-scalpel blades and nanotweezers to sophisticated techniques such as femtosecond lasers, surgical nanorobots, and so on. When it comes to surgical treatments, diamond-coated nanomaterials made of hard metal can significantly improve the effectiveness of surgical blades. The minimal physical adherence to substances or biological membranes, as well as chemical and biological inertness of diamond nanolayers, are significant advantages of this technique. Moreover, diamond possesses a relatively low friction coefficient, which lowers the required piercing force. The development of new manufacturing has enabled the production of surgical blades with cutting-edge diameters ranging from 5 nm to 1 μm. The diamond scalpels with sharp edges that are only a few atoms thick (about 3 nm) have been developed for use in ophthalmology, neurosurgery, and minimally invasive surgery.

Both crystalline and polycrystalline materials have been employed in the fabrication of surgical blades used for ophthalmic surgeries with edge radii ranging from 5 to 500 nm (Shrikant, 2013). The surgical blades are made either crystalline or polycrystalline silicon by assembling them and cutting tunnels into the silicon wafers. Every necessary angle may be produced with this technique, and the final blade has a sharp edge that is comparable to a blade with a diamond edge. These blades can

 DOI: 10.1201/9781003442202-8

be utilized in a variety of difficult surgical procedures, including cataract surgery. Nevertheless, these blades have a tendency to bend when they come into contact with tissues, which causes surgeons to apply greater power when cutting, raising the risk of tissue injury. Trephines with nanostructured carbon coatings have been designed to produce cutting edges with greater stability and diamond-like character-istics (Lingenfelder et al., 2005; Shrikant, 2013).

Femtosecond lasers are additionally being employed to cut single actin stress fibers and chromosomes in cells to analyze the morphology changes in the cell over time. Furthermore, they have used to maintain cell growth and division while remov-ing mitochondria from living cells. It demonstrates how specific organelles can be removed using lasers for nanosurgical procedures without compromising long-term survival (Juhasz et al., 1999). As demonstrated in nerve cells (Yanik et al., 2004), ultrashort pulse laser is capable of performing exceedingly accurate surgery and slicing nanosized cellular components. Conventional lasers often first preheat the desired location before cutting it, although this causes a risk of tissue injury. The benefit of "nanoscissors" is that they can serve cell organelles despite of damaging the heathy tissue around them. The method makes use of a succession of low-energy near-infrared laser pulses that last for a few femtoseconds (0–15 femtoseconds). The less energy and brief laser pulse may greatly limit mechanical impacts, such as propagation of plasma and shock waves, accumulation of the heat, and prolonged thermal injury to the external environment of the tissue with comparison to other laser-surgery approaches (Colombelli, Grill and Stelzer, 2004). The femtosecond laser axotomy method could be used to investigate the processes that influence nerve cell growth and regeneration. Femtosecond laser devices are also used in dermato-logical plastic surgeries (Kumru et al., 2005) and ophthalmic surgery for corneal refractive surgery. Figure 7.1 shows the process of capsulotomy by femtosecond laser in the left eye of a human (Yu, Zhang and Zhu, 2020).

A potent method for noninvasive handling of tiny sized objects in micro- or nanoscale, such as individual living cells, cellular components, organs, and microbes for employment of biological molecules in nanoscale is the single-gradient optical trap. They are also known as optical tweezers. Whenever a consistent wave laser beam collides with them, forces resulting from the motion of the light on its own can accurately relocate items by guiding the laser beam. Surgical instruments called nanotweezers may be employed to capture and transport individual biological mate-rials inside the cells. Carbon nanotubes, for example, were attached to electrode ter-minals to create these nanotweezers. Following that, the nanotubes are manipulated using electric forces to gain the ability of bending inward and capture the compo-nents. The first nanotweezers had a diameter of 50 nm and began working at 8.5 V (Kim and Lieber, 1999). It is possible to use nanotweezers to operate on individual cells. Mechanical operations of DNA molecules were accomplished using silicon nanotweezers, including an initial tip distance of 20 nm. The method was used to investigate the viscoelastic behavior of DNA bundles, yielding static results with a resolution greater than 0.2 nm (Yamahata et al., 2008).

An automatic device which acts autonomously within the human body can be referred to nanorobots in surgery. They act as on-site surgeons within the human body and most of the times they have been programmed for surgical procedures by

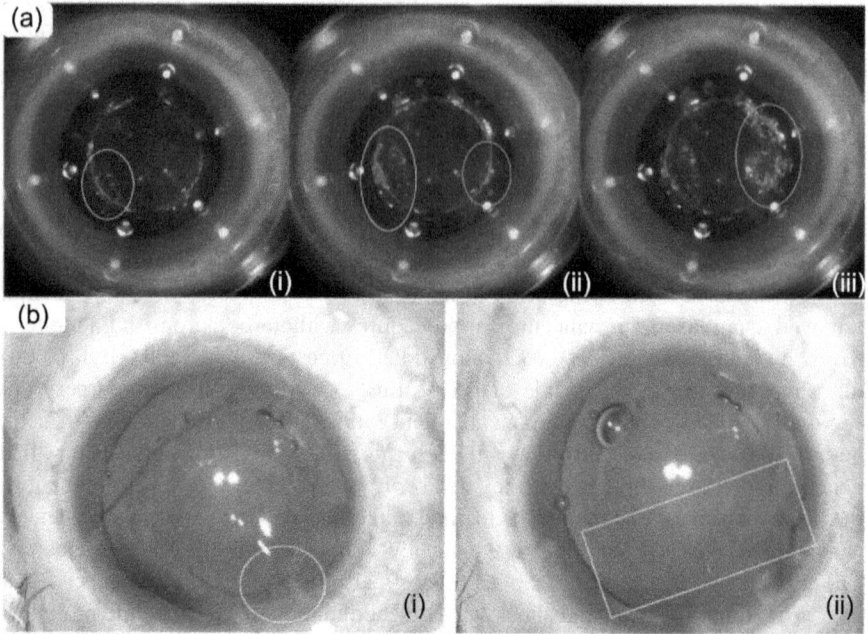

FIGURE 7.1   (a) The process of capsulotomy by femtosecond laser in the left eye (from [i] to [iii]). The circles indicate the big bubble's formation at two o'clock (from [i] to [ii]), while the other circles indicate the big bubble's formation at nine to ten o'clock (from [ii] to [iii]). (b) The photographs of the left eye during the surgery (from [i] to [ii])—(i) the circle shows the rupture of the ICL; (ii) the rectangle shows the incomplete area of femtosecond laser-assisted capsulotomy.

Source: Reproduced with permission from Yu, Zhang, and Zhu, 2020.

a human surgeon. An on-board computer might conduct a number of tasks, including screening and diagnostic tools, reveal pathogenic states, and eradicate or repair the abrasion by nanomanipulation, all the while staying in touch with the directing surgeon through ultrasound signals that are coded. Nanorobots would be performing delicate intracellular surgery far beyond the scope of what the human hand is capable of. Scavengers for atherosclerotic plaque are an example of how nanorobots can be used in surgical procedures. Stents used to place in interior arteries will be replaced by minimally invasive nanorobots, allowing for laparoscopic renovations. The use of nanoparticles during surgery already makes malignancies visible, allowing physicians to entirely eradicate them or perhaps even visibly examine for metastases throughout the body (Manjunath and Kishore, 2014).

Research is being carried out on nanorobots to employ in retinal surgery as well as artificial flagella that are developed to emulate natural bacteria in morphology and their motion style. Nanorobot aims to challenge the fundamental paradigm of contemporary medicine by employing in-body sensors that look for and eradicate microbes before the patient experiences any infective effects (Poorva Manjunath,

2014). Dendrites of a single neuron have been entirely severed using a fast oscillating (100 Hz) micropipette with a 1 μm tip diameter, all without compromising cell survival. Roundworm neurons were axotomized using femtosecond laser surgery, and the axons later functionally recovered (Manjunath and Kishore, 2014).

7.2   SUTURE NEEDLES AND SUTURES

Surgical needles and suture needles that are made of nanoscale stainless steel crystals are already available on the market as nanosurgical items. Suture needles with high ductility, durability, and resistance to corrosion are excellent to be utilized in cosmetic and ocular surgery (Wilkinson, 2004). Needles are constructed of stainless steel, and through the use of thermal aging processes, nanosized particles with a size range of 1–10 nm that are quasi-nanocrystals obtain the aforementioned properties. Silver nanocoating over silk sutures is an innovative strategy for preventing surgical infections.

Nanoneedles made of silicon that are coupled toward an atomic force microscope have the potential to distribute chemicals into the nuclei of biological systems as well as being utilized to perform cell surgery. Such nanoneedles are 200–300 nm in diameter and 6–8 μm in length. Nanoneedles were shown to pierce through the cellular layers rather than impact the plasma membrane or nucleus. Cell manipulation requires the least amount of cell deformation possible even though unintended mechanical reactions could affect the outcome of the manipulation. Different molecules, including DNA, proteins, or drugs, can be mounted onto a nanoneedle by altering its surface using conventional immobilization methods (Shrikant, 2013).

Nanoneedle-based atomic force microscopy is indeed a sort of microscopy that involves contacting and indenting the cell using an extremely slender nanoneedle to investigate certain characteristics. The probe is then scanned throughout the specimen to be operated to gain information about its own surface. Such surgical procedures could be used to prepare healthy cells for functional cell transplantation to a patient by inducing differentiation using stem cells (Shrikant, 2013). Figure 7.2 shows porous silicon nanoneedles that are used in nanosurgeries (Chiappini et al., 2015).

Surgical sutures that are developed with advanced sophisticated technologies are fabricated using cutting-edge technologies. They have adequate mechanical capabilities and the ability to elute drugs. For the treatment of postoperative complications and pain management, electrospinning drug-eluting sutures either with or without bupivacaine have been designed. Antibiotic-eluting sutures minimize the likelihood of infection while achieving appreciable healing properties. Multifilament suture components pose a greater danger of infection. During eye surgery, absorbable antibiotic-eluting sutures containing poly(L-lactide), PEG, and levofloxacin are utilized successfully (Kashiwabuchi et al., 2017). Additionally, there are surgical sutures treating infections at the surgical site (SSI) that are wrapped using curcumin-loaded gold nanoparticles (Sunitha et al., 2017). Heparin-immobilized nanofiber is employed as a suture application that are employed in cardiovascular compartments for cardiovascular diseases (Mariappan, 2019).

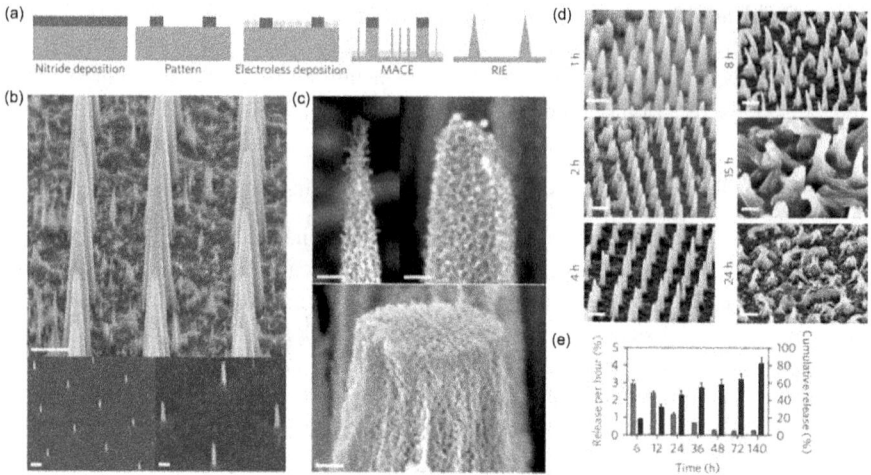

FIGURE 7.2 Porous silicon nanoneedles. (a) Schematic of the nanoneedle synthesis combining conventional microfabrication and metal-assisted chemical etch (MACE). RIE, Reactive ion etching. (b and c) SEM micrographs showing the morphology of porous silicon nanoneedles fabricated according to the process outlined in part (a). (b) Ordered nanoneedle arrays with pitches of 2 μm, 10 μm, and 20 μm, respectively. Scale bars: 2 μm. (c) High-resolution SEM micrographs of nanoneedle tips showing the nanoneedles' porous structure and the tunability of tip diameter from <100 nm to >400 nm. Scale bars: 200 nm. (d) Time course of nanoneedles incubated in cell-culture medium at 37°C. Progressive biodegradation of the needles appears, with loss of structural integrity between 8 hours and 15 hours. Complete degradation occurs at 72 hours. Scale bars: 2 μm. (e) ICP-AES quantification of Si released in solution. The bars represent the rate of silicon release per hour and the cumulative release of silicon, respectively, at each timepoint, expressed as a percentage of total silicon released. Error bars represent the S.D. of 3–6 replicates.

Source: Reproduced with permission from Chiappini et al., 2015.

7.3 NANOFABRICATED DRAINS

Catheters are tiny tubes that are introduced into the cavities or entries within the human body in order to deliver medicine, discharge, or maintain the debris free channel. The development of thrombus upon the outside surfaces of catheters is a major concern of their problems. In order to improve the durability and adaptability of catheters utilized in minimally invasive surgery and lessen their thrombogenic impact, nanomaterials, such as carbon nanotubes, were effectively incorporated. The nucleation mechanism of carbon nanotubes has presumably improved electrostatic characteristics as well as dense surface topology, which are attributed to the antithrombotic characteristic. Silver nanoparticles may additionally be employed to wrap catheters to offer them antibacterial characteristics and inhibit the development of surface biofilm (Roe et al., 2008).

Recently, nanofabricated drains have been used for the management of glaucoma. The gradual deterioration of vision in glaucoma is brought on by the chronically high intraocular pressure, which also causes irreversible destruction of the optic nerve. In a recent investigation, the researchers have reported on an entirely novel concept for treating glaucoma that uses a nano-drainage apparatus made with MEMS and nano-fabrication technology. This entails restoring the trabecular meshwork, which serves as the pathological drainage conduit for water-based fluid outflow. The synthetic drainage implant will lower intraocular pressure and prevent the growth of glaucoma by improving fluid outflow (Pan, Brown and Ziaie, 2006).

7.4 MINIMAL INVASIVE SURGERIES

Chemotherapy and surgery are common examples of conventional treatment methods that have serious adverse reactions and extreme pain. The development of nanotherapeutics and minimally invasive treatments (MITs) has provided an inspiration for those suffering from serious disorders. Particularly, minimally invasive nanomedicines (MINs) that merge the benefits of nanotherapeutics and MITs are capable of successfully targeting malignant cells, tissues, anatomical structures, and organs to increase drug bioavailability, reduce adverse effects, and accomplish pain-free therapies with a tiny incision or without incision, thus obtaining excellent therapeutic benefits.

Moreover, nanoelectromechanical systems (NEMS) and microelectromechanical systems (MEMS) technologies have been recognized as a significant advancement in nanosurgery. Instruments produced at the nano- and microscales are referred to as NEMS and MEMS accordingly. Actuators, nanobeams, biosensors in nanoscale, pumps for various biological activities, resonators, and nanomotors are a few of the sophisticated, miniature electrical and mechanical components that comprise such systems. The ability of NEMS and MEMS to assess mechanical physiological factors, including pressure differences in cranial areas, pulsatility of cerebral spinal fluid (CSF) fluid, weight stress, and strain, is particularly intriguing to the field of neurosurgery (Mattei and Rehman, 2015).

Scientists have already designed arrays that employed microelectrodes and nanowires that can monitor potentials of electrical field while also allowing the assessment of such crucial mechanical characteristics. Many approaches, including the biopolymers included in these products, are being explored to address the consequences of these nanosurgical tools (Mattei and Rehman, 2015).

Advances in NEMS technology is also being exploited as a way of mechanical manipulation at the cellular as well as molecular level, in addition to their prospective function in physiological screening. In almost an *in vivo* mouse model, it has been shown that a newly established nanoknife can chop particular axons upon peripheral nerves (Jourabchi et al., 2014). The potential uses of this technique in several subdisciplines of neurosurgery are promising. For instance, it would be an intriguing instrument for epilepsy surgery, in which the potential to precisely and selectively disassociate particular white matter bundles could result in both a marked merits in surgical outcomes and a significant decrease in the percentages of morbidity related to present surgical techniques (Mattei and Rehman, 2015).

Furthermore, noninvasive method of employing high-frequency alternating magnetic fields for the noninvasive treatment of prosthetic joint infections have been demonstrated recently. It has revealed that this innovative noninvasive treatment is capable of eradicating the biofilms through the generation of heat (Chopra et al., 2017).

7.5 OPTICAL NANOSURGERIES

In optical nanosurgery, optical tweezers, also referred to as single-beam gradient force traps, are an effective tool with intensely concentrated laser beams. In addition to individual living cells or compartments encircled by cells, viruses, microbes, and micrometer-sized materials in the range of piconewtons, are employed for nonintrusive handling (Ashkin, Dziedzic and Yamane, 1987; Ashkin and Dziedzic, 1987). They are perfect for manipulating biological systems and structures at the nanoscale, such as DNA. By introducing an integrated heat shock-responsive gene encoding in nematodes, near-infrared continuous wave laser light using optical tweezers induces stress (Leitz et al., 2002). Tracking their motion allows monitoring of drug metabolism as well as dissemination. Dye-coated cells illuminate when stimulated by light beam of a specific wavelength.

Human corneas have been sliced and reshaped using femtosecond lasers that address vision impairment. The endothelial tissues upon that surface of the cornea had their injuries removed using a femtosecond laser (Juhasz et al., 1999). Moreover, ophthalmic nanosurgery observation is done using "Nano cameras," while nanosurgical tools are controlled with computers (Afarid, Mahmoodi and Baghban, 2022).

7.6 NANOTHERAPEUTICS IN WOUND HEALING

Millions of individuals experience slow wound healing, which raises mortality percentages and related costs globally. The absence of a cellular environment suitable for cell migration, cellular proliferation, and the process of angiogenesis; microbial infection; and unpredictable and persistent inflammation seem to be the three main consequences linked to wounds. Regrettably, these fundamental issues have not been fully resolved by current therapeutic approaches, and as a result, their level of medical success is insufficient. Significant outcomes have been achieved throughout time by incorporating the amazing capabilities of nanomaterials into wound healing. Nanomaterials can activate a variety of cellular and molecular mechanisms that promote the microsetting of wound and may even shift the setting from nonhealing toward healing via antibacterial, anti-inflammatory, antifungal, and angiogenic activities.

There is a research and knowledge gap for both the clear information regarding mechanisms and post–wound adaptations. The majority of the literature concentrates on the advancement of hemostasis, anti-infective activity, immunological regulation, and cell proliferation. Due to their unusual physicochemical and biological characteristics, nanoparticles (NPs) with highly specialized surface areas also indicated potential use in wound dressings for the sustained delivery and liberation of therapeutic medicines. Moreover, NPs for wound healing have the ability to absorb radiation and light and convert it into thermal impulses or reactive oxygen species ROS, which finally causes the bacterial growth in the wounds to terminate. Moreover, NPs may cooperate to fabricate a keen dressing for wound management that is dependent on endogenous stimuli, including pH, chemicals, temperature, enzymes, and toxic materials released by the bacterium, to cure microbial infections. Latest researches on laboratory rats using topical AuNPs to treat cutaneal lesions have shown enhanced healing, as evidenced by increased re-epithelialization, granulation tissue development, deposition of extra cellular matrix, and collagen fiber density (Kushwaha, Goswami and Kim, 2022).

The ability of AuNPs to treat wounds was considerably improved when they were combined with polymeric materials or stem cells. The free radical scavenging capacity of AuNP was multiplied by chitosan–AuNP conjugation, which also increased biocompatibility (Kushwaha, Goswami and Kim, 2022). Compared to using conventional chitosan and a Tegaderm dressing alone, an experiment on a laboratory rat surgical wound model showed that chitosan–AuNPs dramatically improved hemostasis, development of epithelia along with a great healing efficiency, and wound closure (Kushwaha, Goswami and Kim, 2022). In a different study on rats, wounds caused by burns were treated using AuNPs that had been coupled with human cryopreserved fibroblasts. The wounds displayed a rapid rate of healing, less amount of inflammation, and more collagen deposition (Rajendran et al., 2018).

Electrospun nanofiber membranes are an emerging dressing type for postoperative wound healing as well as other lesions. To gain antimicrobial activity within the wounds, these membranes can be reinforced with a variety of nanoparticles and nanocomposites. They can be employed to accelerate tissue proliferation and cell regeneration in wounds, as well as drain the exudates of the wounds by acting as an absorbent due to their high porosity. These electrospun membranes minimize the painful procedures of wound management as a new hope for surgical dressings (Liu et al., 2021). Figure 7.3 shows an electrospun membrane which is fabricated and tested for wound healing (Liu et al., 2021).

Many researchers have chosen to combine the two types of fibers due to the advantages of easy deterioration and great biocompatibility of natural polymers along with the controllability and dependable mechanical durability of synthetic polymers (Zhu et al., 2019). In order to create a coaxial electrospun core-sheath nanofiber film with the antibiotic minocycline as well as herbal extracts that serves as a multifunctional scaffold to aid in the healing of secondary burns, Ramalingam et al. (Ramalingam et al., 2021) reported employing PCL/gelatin as a polymer vehicle. The core-sheath construction keeps the biologically active chemicals released consistently. It additionally exhibits potent antibacterial activity and also encourages epithelial cell proliferation and diffusion. The skin of pig with a second-degree burn injury can be used as a model to demonstrate how collagen tissue has grown in this condition.

Furthermore, the ability to add a range of biologically active substances to create functionalized materials is another significant benefit of electrospinning to fabricate nanofiber membranes for wound dressings. Recently, antibiotics, herbal extracts, and phytochemical substances like curcumin, inorganic NPs (AgNP, ZnO, TiO_2, AuNP), organic materials (honey, essential oils, chitosan), as well as growth factors are all frequently utilized active substances for enhancing the wound healing. Yang et al.

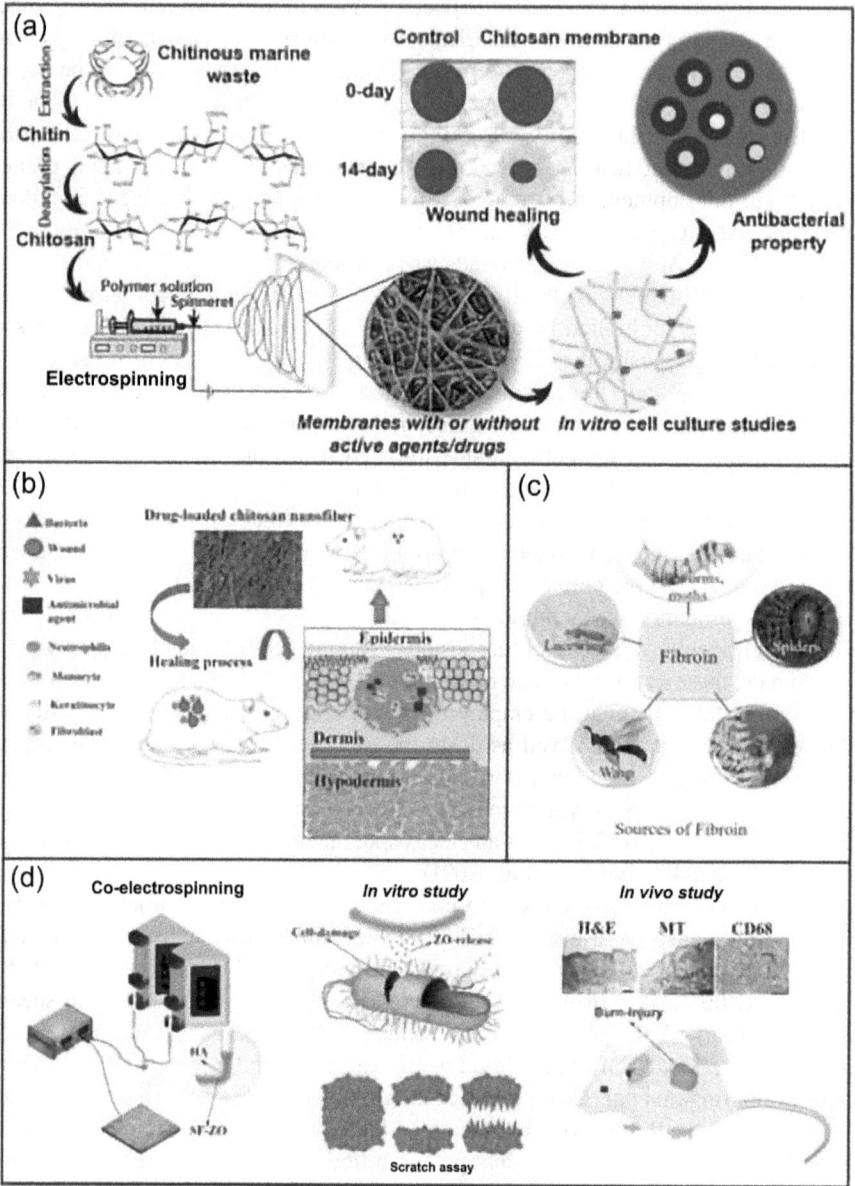

FIGURE 7.3 (a) Chitosan extracted from natural sources and developed into electrospun fiber membranes and its application in wound healing. (b) A schematic diagram of the wound healing process of a drug-loaded chitosan dressing. (c) The sources of fibroin. (d) Preparation and *in vitro* and *in vivo* study of HA/SF-ZO nanofiber by coaxial electrospinning.

Source: Reproduced with permission from Liu et al., 2021.

produced Janus nanofibers with ciprofloxacin and AgNP as the polymer framework using side by side the electrospinning method and investigated the impacts on the healing of wounds. The antibacterial action offers a fresh perspective for creating novel antibacterial dressings for wounds (Yang et al., 2020). On the basis of PCL and gelatin, Jafari et al. developed a bilayer nanofiber framework. Amoxicillin is present in the top level, and n-ZnO is present at the bottom surface to hasten wound healing. Amoxicillin released over time, according to an *in vitro* test (Jafari et al., 2020).

REFERENCES

Afarid, M., Mahmoodi, S. and Baghban, R. (2022) "Recent achievements in nano-based technologies for ocular disease diagnosis and treatment, review and update," *Journal of Nanobiotechnology*, 20(1), p. 361. doi: 10.1186/s12951-022-01567-7.

Ashkin, A. and Dziedzic, J. M. (1987) "Optical trapping and manipulation of viruses and bacteria," *Science (New York, N.Y.)*, 235(4795), pp. 1517–1520. doi: 10.1126/science.3547653.

Ashkin, A., Dziedzic, J. M. and Yamane, T. (1987) "Optical trapping and manipulation of single cells using infrared laser beams," *Nature*, 330(6150), pp. 769–771. doi: 10.1038/330769a0.

Chiappini, C. et al. (2015) "Biodegradable silicon nanoneedles delivering nucleic acids intracellularly induce localized in vivo neovascularization," *Nature Materials*, 14(5), pp. 532–539. doi: 10.1038/nmat4249.

Chopra, R. et al. (2017) "Employing high-frequency alternating magnetic fields for the non-invasive treatment of prosthetic joint infections," *Scientific Reports*, 7(1), p. 7520. doi: 10.1038/s41598-017-07321-6.

Colombelli, J., Grill, S. W. and Stelzer, E. H. K. (2004) "Ultraviolet diffraction limited nanosurgery of live biological tissues," *The Review of Scientific Instruments*, 75(2), pp. 472–478. doi: 10.1063/1.1641163.

Jafari, A. et al. (2020) "Bioactive antibacterial bilayer PCL/gelatin nanofibrous scaffold promotes full-thickness wound healing," *International Journal of Pharmaceutics*, 583(119413), p. 119413. doi: 10.1016/j.ijpharm.2020.119413.

Jourabchi, N. et al. (2014) "Irreversible electroporation (NanoKnife) in cancer treatment," *Gastrointestinal Intervention*, 3(1), pp. 8–18. doi: 10.1016/j.gii.2014.02.002.

Juhasz, T. et al. (1999) "Corneal refractive surgery with femtosecond lasers," *IEEE Journal of Selected Topics in Quantum Electronics: A Publication of the IEEE Lasers and Electro-Optics Society*, 5(4), pp. 902–910. doi: 10.1109/2944.796309.

Kashiwabuchi, F. et al. (2017) "Development of absorbable, antibiotic-eluting sutures for ophthalmic surgery," *Translational Vision Science & Technology*, 6(1), p. 1. doi: 10.1167/tvst.6.1.1.

Kim, P. and Lieber, C. M. (1999) "Nanotube nanotweezers," *Science (New York, N.Y.)*, 286(5447), pp. 2148–2150. doi: 10.1126/science.286.5447.2148.

Kumru, S. S. et al. (2005) "ED50 study of femtosecond terawatt laser pulses on porcine skin," *Lasers in Surgery and Medicine*, 37(1), pp. 59–63. doi: 10.1002/lsm.20195.

Kushwaha, A., Goswami, L. and Kim, B. S. (2022) "Nanomaterial-based therapy for wound healing," *Nanomaterials (Basel, Switzerland)*, 12(4), p. 618. doi: 10.3390/nano12040618.

Leitz, G. et al. (2002) "Stress response in Caenorhabditis elegans caused by optical tweezers: Wavelength, power, and time dependence," *Biophysical Journal*, 82(4), pp. 2224–2231. doi: 10.1016/s0006-3495(02)75568-9.

Lingenfelder, C. et al. (2005) "Can the cutting performance of trephines still be improved? Application of nanotechnology for manufacturing trephines with diamond-like cutting edges," *Klinische Monatsblätter für Augenheilkunde*, 222(9), pp. 709–716.

Liu, X. et al. (2021) "Electrospun medicated nanofibers for wound healing: Review," *Membranes*, 11(10), p. 770. doi: 10.3390/membranes11100770.

Manjunath, A. and Kishore, V. (2014) "The promising future in medicine: Nanorobots," *Biomedical Science and Engineering*, 2(2), pp. 42–47. doi: 10.12691/bse-2-2-3.

Mariappan, N. (2019) "Current trends in nanotechnology applications in surgical specialties and orthopedic surgery," *Biomedical & Pharmacology Journal*, 12(3), pp. 1095–1127. doi: 10.13005/bpj/1739.

Mattei, T. A. and Rehman, A. A. (2015) "'Extremely minimally invasive': Recent advances in nanotechnology research and future applications in neurosurgery," *Neurosurgical Review*, 38(1), pp. 27–37; discussion 37. doi: 10.1007/s10143-014-0566-2.

Pan, T., Brown, J. D. and Ziaie, B. (2006) "An artificial nano-drainage implant (ANDI) for glaucoma treatment," *Conference Proceedings: . . . Annual International Conference of the IEEE Engineering in Medicine and Biology Society: IEEE Engineering in Medicine and Biology Society, Conference*, pp. 3174–3177. doi: 10.1109/IEMBS.2006.260147.

Poorva Manjunath, V. (2014) "The promising future in medicine: Nanorobots," *Biomedical Science and Engineering*, 2(2), pp. 42–47. doi: 10.12691/bse-2-2-3.

Rajendran, N. K. et al. (2018) "A review on nanoparticle based treatment for wound healing," *Journal of Drug Delivery Science and Technology*, 44, pp. 421–430. doi: 10.1016/j.jddst.2018.01.009.

Ramalingam, R. et al. (2021) "Core—shell structured antimicrobial nanofiber dressings containing herbal extract and antibiotics combination for the prevention of biofilms and promotion of cutaneous wound healing," *ACS Applied Materials & Interfaces*, 13(21), pp. 24356–24369. doi: 10.1021/acsami.0c20642.

Roe, D. et al. (2008) "Antimicrobial surface functionalization of plastic catheters by silver nanoparticles," *The Journal of Antimicrobial Chemotherapy*, 61(4), pp. 869–876. doi: 10.1093/jac/dkn034.

Shrikant, M. (2013) "Nanotechnology for surgeons," *The Indian Journal of Surgery*, 75(6), pp. 485–492. doi: 10.1007/s12262-012-0726-y.

Sunitha, S. et al. (2017) "Fabrication of surgical sutures coated with curcumin loaded gold nanoparticles," *Pharmaceutica Analytica Acta*, 8(1). doi: 10.4172/2153-2435.1000529.

Wilkinson, J. M. (2004) "Micro- and nanotechnology: Fabrication processes for metals," *Medical Device Technology*, 15, pp. 21–23.

Yamahata, C. et al. (2008) "Silicon nanotweezers with subnanometer resolution for the micromanipulation of biomolecules," *Journal of Microelectromechanical Systems: A Joint IEEE and ASME Publication on Microstructures, Microactuators, Microsensors, and Microsystems*, 17(3), pp. 623–631. doi: 10.1109/jmems.2008.922080.

Yang, J. et al. (2020) "Electrospun Janus nanofibers loaded with a drug and inorganic nanoparticles as an effective antibacterial wound dressing," *Materials Science & Engineering. C, Materials for Biological Applications*, 111(110805), p. 110805. doi: 10.1016/j.msec.2020.110805.

Yanik, M. F. et al. (2004) "Neurosurgery: Functional regeneration after laser axotomy," *Nature*, 432(7019), p. 822. doi: 10.1038/432822a.

Yu, Y., Zhang, C. and Zhu, Y. (2020) "Femtosecond laser assisted cataract surgery in a cataract patient with a '0 vaulted' ICL: A case report," *BMC Ophthalmology*, 20(1), p. 179. doi: 10.1186/s12886-020-01440-x.

Zhu, Z. et al. (2019) "Tazarotene released from aligned electrospun membrane facilitates cutaneous wound healing by promoting angiogenesis," *ACS Applied Materials & Interfaces*, 11(39), pp. 36141–36153. doi: 10.1021/acsami.9b13271.

8 Nanotherapeutics in Gene Therapy

INTRODUCTION

Gene therapy is employed to manage a monogenic hereditary as well as acquired disorder by introducing therapeutic genes via either integrative or nonintegrative vectors. Integrative vectors are secured and modified viral carriers that allow the delivery of a therapeutic transgene toward the DNA of the target cell. The therapeutic transgene is just not persistently expressed in the specific target cell while using nonintegrative vector models. The transgenes that will be expressed and also the delivering vectors which will be employed will determine how well the gene therapy works. Gene therapy can be categorized in accordance with the selected delivery vector. Vector materials can be viral (integrative or nonintegrative) or nonviral, as was previously mentioned. Typically, viral vectors serve as integrative vectors where adeno-associated viruses, gamma retroviruses, foamy viruses, and lentiviruses can be showed as exemplifications. Adenoviruses, herpesviruses, poxviruses, and vaccinia viruses are examples of viruses that can be utilized as nonviral vectors. Nonviral vectors, typically relied on lipid molecules, polymers that have a cationic nature, as well as nanocarriers can be helpful when significant or sustained transgene expression is not required as the goal is to stimulate an immune response against the malignancies. Viral vectors are particularly helpful when significant and prolonged expression is necessary even though they offer greater consistency and higher degrees of transgene expression, although they are nonintegrative (Prosen et al., 2013; Liu and Zhang, 2011).

There are two crucial elements that are necessary for effective gene therapy. They consist of both *in vitro* and *in vivo* gene delivery that is effective and secure. The efficiency of the transduction, viral density when utilizing viral gene therapy, and the efficiency of transfection while employing nucleic acids are needed to accomplish this objective. The efficient use of imaging techniques that are noninvasive is extremely important for detecting manipulated cells or modifying materials. It will really make it possible to monitor the gene delivery and their expression (Do et al., 2019).

The utilization of magnetic nanoparticles to transfer genetic materials, nucleic acids, and viral vectors has been reported by numerous research groups in recent years, sparking the development of novel techniques known as magnetofection. Employing superparamagnetic nanoparticles in the viral and nonviral techniques is described as magnetofection to enhance gene transport in the magnetic field that exists. Figure 8.1 shows a schematic illustration of the magnetofection by using magnetic nanoparticles in gene therapy (Jinturkar, Rathi and Misra, 2011).

Tiny ferromagnetic as well as ferrimagnetic NPs exhibit superparamagnetism. The magnetism of these nanoparticles may spontaneously reverse the direction when temperature influences them if their dimensions are sufficiently small. The Néel relaxation time is the

DOI: 10.1201/9781003442202-9

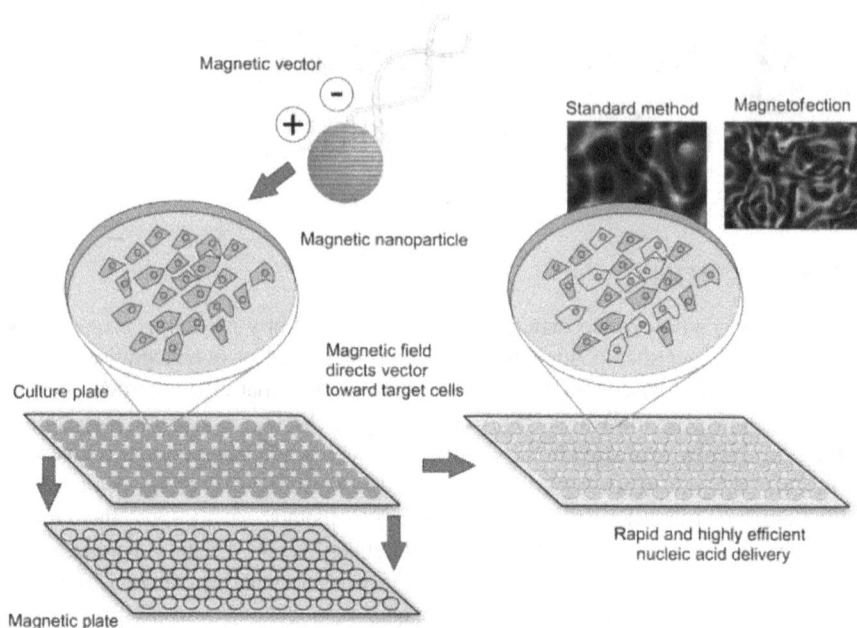

FIGURE 8.1   Magnetofection technique in cell culture.

Source: Reproduced with permission from Jinturkar, Rathi and Misra, 2011.

interval among two flips (Deissler et al., 2013). The term "superparamagnetic state" refers to nanoparticles that appear to have zero average magnetization when their measured magnetization duration is substantially longer when compared with the Néel relaxation time and when there is also no evident external field of magnetism (Deissler et al., 2013).

Superparamagnetism of magnetic substances that exhibit dimensions in the nanoscale seems to be a notion which explains that nanoparticles could be comprised of magnetic substances with appropriate small particle sizes. Moreover, they might exhibit superparamagnetic characteristics. Superparamagnetic nanoparticles can be coated with a suitable coating to formulate a ferrofluid, which can then be disseminated inside an aqueous solution that can be remained consistent. These ferrofluids may be employed in both *in vitro* and *in vivo* biomedical applications, especially in gene therapies (Enriquez-Navas and Garcia-Martin, 2012).

In a recent study, Gal-PEI-SPIO nanomaterials were developed, and siRNA-encapsulated Gal-PEI-SPIO properties were examined. The results exhibited that the particles transport therapeutic siRNA to the liver cancer in a targeted manner by virtue of the iron oxide nucleus that has been altered by galactose (Gal) and polyethylenimine (PEI), which serve as shells (Yang et al., 2018). Another related study has been demonstrated by the safe and efficient magnetofection of both cells and tumors in laboratory mice using surface-modified superparamagnetic iron oxide nanoparticles (SPIONs) combined with polyacrylic acid (PAA) and polyethylenimine (PEI). In comparison to commercially accessible SPIONs, SPIONs-PAA-PEI had a higher transfection efficiency when used in magnetofect cells alongside plasmid

DNA encoding reporter genes. A strong anticancer impact was seen after magnetofection of murine mammary adenocarcinoma containing plasmid DNA encoding IL-12 employing SPIONs-PAA-PEI. This technique could be improved for cancer immuno-gene therapy (Prijic et al., 2012).

8.1 VIRAL MAGNETOFECTION

Viral vectors, which can be categorized as integrative and nonintegrative vectors, constitute one of the most popular methods for delivering genes during gene and cellular treatment strategies. The application of nonintegrative viral vectors as delivery systems for gene therapy has several benefits. The potential of insertional mutagenesis is decreased as well as the therapeutic gene is expressed shortly as a result of their inability to integrate into the genomic materials of the host cells. This is enormously beneficial in circumstances that demand for quick action, like suicide therapy or even the commencement of cascade events. Whenever long-term effort is required, for instance, in the management of long-term illnesses, it might be a drawback. Adenovirus (Ad), herpes simplex virus (HSV), and vaccinia virus are the most prevalent types of nonintegrative viral vectors (VV). Nonintegrative vectors are essential for immediate gene expression. Undesirable consequences and side effects will be mitigated by the insufficient integration. Integrative vectors, which, on the other hand, are perfect where long-term expression is required.

The integrative type of viral vectors is well-suited for usage as gene therapy and gene delivery systems due to their numerous strengths. The expression of the therapeutic gene for a long term is ensured by their capacity to integrate into the genomes of the host cells. This is enormously beneficial when treating chronic illnesses is necessary. Nevertheless, insertional mutagenesis and other dangers are connected with the utilization of integrative viral vectors. Adeno-associated virus, lentivirus, and retrovirus are the most prevalent integrative viral vectors (AAV) (Crespo-Barreda et al., 2016).

In a recent study, researchers have revealed how to successfully conquer transduction impedance in skeletal muscle cells by designing recombinant adenoviral vectors using suitable iron oxide MNPs into magneto-adenovectors (RAd-MNP) and then subjecting them to a gradient magnetic field. While contrasted with transduction alongside naked virus, the expression of green fluorescent protein and insulin-like growth factor 1 substantially rose after magnetofection using RAd-MNPs complexes in C_2C_{12} myotubes *in vitro* and mouse skeletal muscle *in vivo* (Pereyra et al., 2016).

Tresilwised et al. investigated at a trio core–shell-type IO magnetic NPs with different surface coatings, particle dimensions, and magnetic characteristics to determine if they could boost the adenovirus Ad520's oncolytic potency and keep it stable against the impacts of serum as well as a neutralizing antibody. It was discovered that physical and chemical properties of magnetic NPs play a crucial role in determining the characteristics that control the oncolytic productivities associated with their complexes with Ad520. Even though a neutralizing antibody or excessive serum concentration throughout infection experienced a strong inhibitory effect on the ingestion or oncolytic productivity of the naked virus, an individual particle kind was found to confer significant protection toward both inhibitory aspects while boosting the oncolytic productivity of the internalized virus. Following intratumoral injection through the complex with Ad520 along with magnetic field impact, this particle category, which has a silica coating as well as adsorbed polyethylenimine and exhibits a significant magnetic moment with elevated saturation magnetization, mediates a 50% reduction in tumor growth rate compared to control, whereas Ad520 alone is ineffective (Tresilwised et al., 2012).

8.2 NONVIRAL MAGNETOFECTION

Even though viral vectors exhibit a higher transfection efficiency, they might have a greater immunogenicity and require complicated formulations (Mukherjee and Thrasher, 2013). In the laboratory conditions, nonviral vectors are developed from biocompatible starting materials. They exhibit poor cytotoxicity as well as diminished immunogenic activities compared to viral vectors, and their exterior chemical environment can be infinitely customizable, which may be advantageous for large-scale production (Yin et al., 2014).

The exterior interfaces of nanoparticles are designed and synthesized with polymers that are cationic in nature to enhance the nucleic acid association, making them promising agents for gene delivery. These are extremely viable options to viral vectors; however, before they can be used in clinical settings, more *in vivo* research is required. Lin et al. were among the innovators who used magnetofection for *in vitro* applications by employing nanoscale magnets (Lin et al., 2008). There are several different types of magnetic nanoparticles that are cationic in their nature that can bind nucleotypic substances to their surfaces. With this technique, the impact of an external magnetic field concentrates the magnetic nanoparticles mostly in target cells (EMF). As internalization often occurs through endocytosis or pinocytosis, the structural features of the membrane are retained. Compared to other mechanical transfection techniques, this has an added benefit. Additional benefits include the short incubation period necessary for attaining efficiency of high transfection and the low dose of the vector required to obtain the saturation yield. Furthermore, magnetic nanoparticle-transfected cells may be employed to pinpoint the targeted area *in vivo* by applying an EMF (Hen et al., 2012).

On the other hand, organic or inorganic materials are also employed in this strategy. They are made to attach and shield DNA or RNA, achieving great efficacy, sustained gene expression, and low toxicological effects all at once. Polymers, dendrimers, cationic liposomes, and other organic vectors can be exemplified in this category. Due to the unique characteristics of their nanoarchitecture, these nanomaterials have a better capacity to transport genetic materials.

Silica, iron oxide, carbon nanotubes (CNTs), and gold nanoparticles (GNPs) are a few examples of inorganic materials that are employed in gene therapy. Inorganic nanovectors offer a straightforward, manageable, and scalable synthesis procedures. They also have excellent dispersion, a high capacity for cargo loadings, low immunogenic reactions, and low cytotoxic effects. The inorganic nanovectors might bind to DNA and RNA by electro or chemical reactions. These interactions enable the inorganic nanomaterial as well as the nucleotidic sequence that combines into a complex. The complex boosts transfection effectiveness and safeguards genetic material against enzymatic deterioration. Even though endocytosis seems to be the primary pathway by which nanovectors enter cells, some components, including antibodies, may be linked to the surfaces of nanomaterials to facilitate interactions with compounds on cell surfaces. Gene transfection seems to be more precise and successful when receptor mediation is present (Sunshine, Bishop and Green, 2011). Figure 8.2 shows some exemplifications of different nanoparticle types that are used in gene therapy.

There are various factors that have to be taken into account in every situation, including the ratio of nanoparticles to nucleotidic substance, the coverage of the surface charge, or the hydrophobic nature of the material. The endosomal exodus is the most important aspect for a successful transfection. As aforementioned, it is believed that the "proton sponge" plays a significant part in this phenomenon. It is crucial to enhance the properties of the surface of the nanoparticles for this technique with cationic polymers like PEI or poly-L-Lysine (PLL) (Benjaminsen et al., 2013).

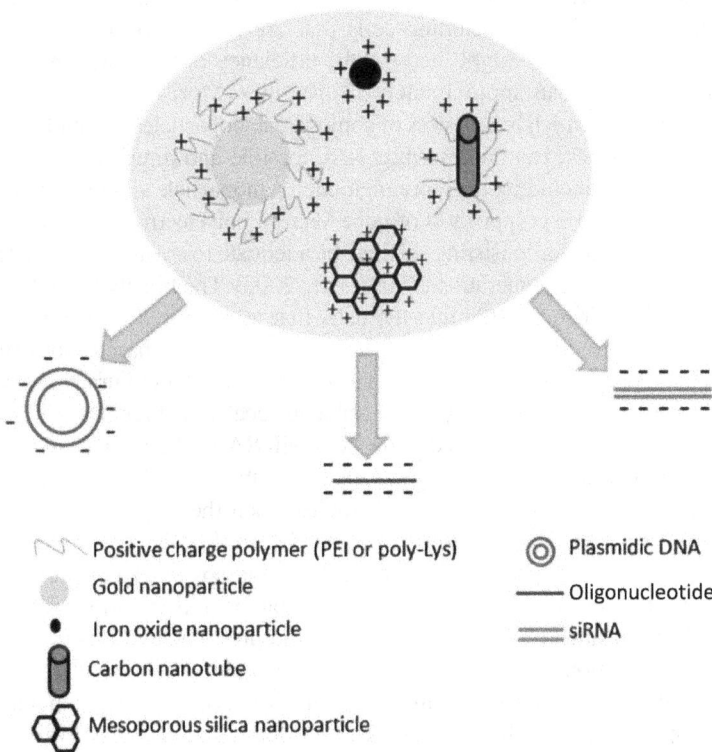

Positive charge polymer (PEI or poly-Lys)   Plasmidic DNA

Gold nanoparticle   Oligonucleotide

Iron oxide nanoparticle   siRNA

Carbon nanotube

Mesoporous silica nanoparticle

FIGURE 8.2 Examples of inorganic nanoparticles. There are many types of inorganic nanoparticles. In this figure, we show several examples of them. In general, they act as nucleic acid vectors for *in vitro* or *in vivo* transfections.

Source: Reproduced with permission from Crespo-Barreda et al., 2016.

8.3   EMERGING NANOTHERAPEUTICS AND APPLICATIONS IN GENE THERAPY

As aforementioned, magnetic nanoparticles-based viral and nonviral magnetofection is an emerging technique that is used to make the gene therapies fruitful. These techniques have overcome several bottlenecks that are arisen with conventional approaches of gene therapy. It is evident with a number of successful researches based on nanotherapeutics associated with viral and nonviral magnetofection approaches in gene therapies.

Many researchers have utilized the potent biotin–streptavidin interaction inside the context of viruses. Novel hybrid envelope proteins with a biotin motif are able to create retroviral and lentiviral vectors (Hughes et al., 2001; Kaikkonen et al., 2009; Weber et al., 2009). A persistent complex that is capable of being separated emerges from the coupling of this novel protein to the streptavidin nanoparticles. The transduction efficiency of adenoviruses and retroviruses can be improved by magnetofection, according to several research (Bhattarai et al., 2008; Kamei et al., 2009). Specifically, when paired with magnetite nanoparticles, transduction of lentiviral vectors accelerates significantly under the influence of magnetic fields (Haim, Steiner and Panet, 2005). Including cells that are receptor-positive and receptor-negative, magnetofection might increase the efficiency of transduction of the paramyxovirus measles virus approximately 30–70 times (Morishita et al., 2005).

Bioconjugation, which is a process of conjugate nanoparticles and biological materials, including genes, can be described as a possible and direct correlation among the two substances including the aforementioned nanoparticle and the respective biological substance. The proper ratio of gene vectors polyelectrolyte-coated magnetic nanoparticles in a media consisting salt may be adequate to create their relationship by salt-induced colloid agglomeration (Plank et al., 2003). The freshly formulated "magnetic vectors" are incorporated into the cells that are cultured on magnetic culture plates after a brief incubation period. Such plates could be purchased commercially or they can be manufactured in laboratory settings with regular culture plates and powerful Nd-Fe-B magnets. Currently, it is feasible to accelerate direct DNA transfection, the uptake of viruses by cells, and delivery of siRNA in the vicinity of a magnetic field owing to commercially accessible magnetic substances. In other instances, the virus enters into the cell by a variety of routes when the magnetic field is present, permitting nonpermissive cells to be infected. Figure 8.3 shows various functional magnetite nanoparticles that are employed in gene therapy (Ito and Kamihira, 2011).

Magnetic resonance imaging (MRI) of the biological distribution of baculovirus *in vivo* offers an intriguing demonstration of the utilization of magnetic nanoparticles for the creation of a persistent nanobioconjugate when considering the gene therapy (Räty et al., 2006). Commercial nanoparticulate superparamagnetic iron oxide nanoparticles were the materials used in this research. This covalent method required functionalizing both the viral capsid and the nanoparticle. This virus displayed a strong affinity for biotinylated substances because it was coupled to avidin proteins (Räty et al., 2006).

In order to transduce HepG2 cell lines, these investigators used baculoviruses, which are efficient vectors for gene transfer in vertebrate cells (Airenne et al., 2000).

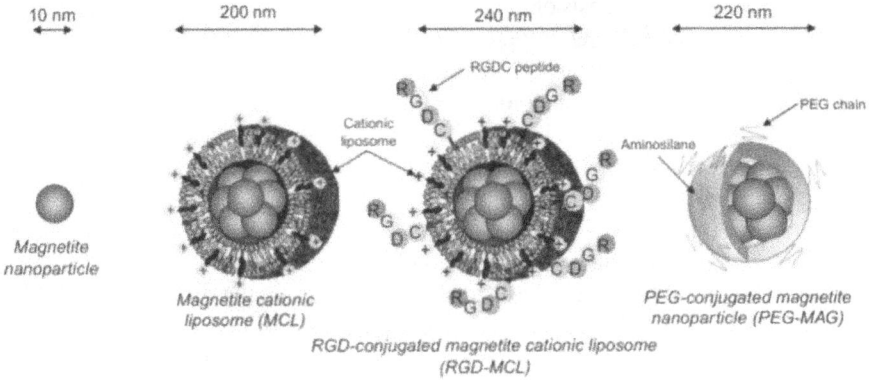

FIGURE 8.3 Functional magnetite nanoparticles.

Source: Reproduced with permission from Ito and Kamihira, 2011.

Characterization of the interaction among the virus and the respective nanoparticles was done using atomic force microscopy (Sinha Ray, 2013). The outcomes demonstrated that, on average, one to two virions per nanoparticle of the expected dimension were attached to the surface of the virus. Along with virions, superparamagnetic iron oxide nanoparticles of 42–67 nm were found.

A recent publication that employed a similar procedure (Huh et al., 2007) used an adenovirus and hybridization of magnetic nanoparticle to formulate one bioconjugate also with twin functionalities of aim MRI and gene delivery. As magnetic nanoparticles, the researchers used a combination of manganese and magnetism-engineered iron oxide (MnMEIO). Although the addition of manganese may increase toxicological effects, MnMEIO is especially appealing due to its exceptional magnetization in high mass value of 110 (emu/g of magnetic atoms) and remarkable magnetic resonance contrast properties (Huh et al., 2007.

Superparamagnetic nanoparticles have been used in gene theranostics investigations, according to several researchers (Bhattarai et al., 2008; Jin and Ye, 2007; Chorny et al., 2009). Ionic interaction among the virus and the respective nanoparticle should be employed as the second phase in the production and purifying of nanobioconjugates as applications in gene theranostics. While it continues to undergo development, this sophisticated and adaptable strategy has several benefits.

Gold nanoparticles (AuNP) have indeed been utilized for gene transfer and imaging. Even though this technique has not been extensively explored in MRI, mostly because the nanoparticles require a second alteration to be operative. AuNPs are a proven nanomaterials used in the technique for medication and gene delivery which was studied by various researchers recently (Cho et al., 2006; Conde, de La Fuente and Baptista, 2010; Ghosh et al., 2008). A fascinating publication by Kamei et al. (Kamei et al., 2009) demonstrated an excellent explanation of how gene therapy is promoted with nanotherapeutics and also how gold nanoparticles help to enhance the potential of various imaging techniques. This publication was halfway among both magnetofection and synthesis of nanobioconjugate. The technique provides a base of magnetic iron oxide (g-Fe_2O_3 or Fe_3O_4) containing tiny gold nanoparticles anchored on it (hydrodynamic diameter of 240 nm).

Additional AuNP-based methods rely on the direct attachment of DNA or RNA toward the interface and their initiation by light to liberate them. This technique has been employed using 780 nm nanorods attached to thiolated DNA and nanorods encapsulated with phosphatidylcholine for such an ionic contact with DNA (Takahashi, Niidome and Yamada, 2005).

Mesoporous silica nanoparticles (MSN) have been researched as siRNA delivery vehicles. For instance, to boost the positive charge on the nanoparticle surface, Hom et al. treated MSNs with PEI. Contrasting the cytotoxicological effects of their PEI–MSNs to certain other transfection agents such as Lipofectamine 2000 and PEI/siRNA complexes, they demonstrated that with less toxicity profiles. Moreover, their PEI–MSNs had a significant impact on the capacity to silence EGFP, Akt, and K-ras (Hom et al., 2010). Zhu et al. who employed PLLNPSNs to attach and shield c-myc antisense oligonucleotides got similar outcomes. In HNE1 and HeLa cell lines, they discovered a considerable downregulation of c-myc mRNA (Zhu et al., 2004).

Graphene oxide as well as carbon nanotubes (CNT) represent intriguing prospects for use in biomedical applications, including scaffolds and implantable devices. Carbon atoms are grouped in compressed atomic rings to form CNTs. They can indeed be arranged as either single-walled carbon nanotubes (SWNTs) or multiple concentric sheets that are rolled up to forming cylinders (MWNTs). A total of 107 CNTs can be functionalized to make them more soluble and to make nucleic acid binding easier (DNA, siRNA, etc.). The most noteworthy accomplishment with binding nucleic acids was already achieved with MWNTs, where Siu et al. had been capable of binding siRNA to SWNTs for managing the treatments for melanoma, displaying a decline in the significant tumor development in a time interval of 25 days. All these types of CNTs were utilized to attach nucleic acids (Siu et al., 2014).

Quantum dots (QDs) can be described as semiconductor nanoparticles capable of being utilized as markers for bioimaging photoluminescence. These QDs are crystalline nanoparticles within 2 and 10 nm. The electronic characteristics of these nanomaterials fall in the range of discrete molecules as well as bulk semiconductors. Due to the liberation of cadmium into the cellular environments or organs, the fundamental issue with QD utilization in biomedical applications concerns their toxicity. However, their surface modification and functionalization may mitigate this issue and also enable the attachment of various biomolecules, especially genes and nucleic acids.

The rupture of the blood–brain barrier (BBB) and the neuroinflammation which arise in many disorders are caused by the matrix-degrading metalloproteinases (MMPs). With the purpose of suppressing the MMP-9 protein and preserving the integrity of the BBB, Bonoiu et al. employed QDs with MMP-9 siRNA. They successfully suppressed about 80% of genes in microvascular endothelial cells of the brain using QD (BMVECs). The capacity of nanoplexes to integrate diagnostic and therapy offered them a significant advantage over all the other therapeutic approaches (Bonoiu et al., 2010).

REFERENCES

Airenne, K. J., Hiltunen, M. O., Turunen, M. P., Turunen, A. M., Laitinen, O. H., Kulomaa, M. S. and Ylä-Herttuala, S. (2000) "Baculovirus-mediated periadventitial gene transfer to rabbit carotid artery," *Gene Therapy*, 7, pp. 1499–1504. [PubMed: 11001370].

Benjaminsen, R. V. et al. (2013) "The possible 'proton sponge' effect of polyethylenimine (PEI) does not include change in lysosomal pH," *Molecular Therapy*, 21(1), pp. 149–157.

Bhattarai, S. R., Kim, S. Y., Jang, K. Y., Lee, K. C., Yi, H. K., Lee, D. Y., Kim, H. Y. and Hwang, P. H. (2008) "Laboratory formulated magnetic nanoparticles for enhancement of viral gene expression in suspension cell line," *Journal of Virological Methods*, 2005–2008.

Bonoiu, A. et al. (2010) "MMP-9 gene silencing by a quantum dot-siRNA nanoplex delivery to maintain the integrity of the blood-brain barrier," *Brain Research*, pp. 142–155.

Cho, S. J., Jarrett, B. R., Louie, A. Y. and Kauzlarich, S. M. (2006) "Gold-coated iron nanoparticles: A novel magnetic resonance agent for T-1 and T-2 weighted imaging," *Nanotechnology*, 17, pp. 640–644.

Chorny, M., Fishbein, I., Alferiev, I. and Levy, R. J. (2009) "Magnetically responsive biodegradable nanoparticles enhance adenoviral gene transfer in cultured smooth muscle and endothelial cells," *Molecular Pharmaceutics*, 6(5), pp. 1380–1387. doi: 10.1021/mp900017m. PMID: 19496618; PMCID: PMC3349935.

Conde, J., de La Fuente, J. M. and Baptista, P. V. (2010) "RNA quantification using gold nanoprobes—Application to cancer diagnostics," *Journal of Nanobiotechnology*, 8, p. 5.

Crespo-Barreda, A. et al. (2016) *Chapter 11—Viral and nonviral vectors for in vivo and ex vivo gene therapies.* Boston: Academic Press.

Deissler, R. J. et al. (2013) "Brownian and Néel relaxation times in magnetic particle dynamics," *2013 International Workshop on Magnetic Particle Imaging (IWMPI)*, IEEE, Berkeley, CA: USA.

Do, M. et al. (2019) "1.26—Cell transfection," in Moo-Young, M. (ed.) *Comprehensive biotechnology.* Oxford: Pergamon.

Enriquez-Navas, P. M. and Garcia-Martin, M. L. (2012) "Chapter 9—Application of inorganic nanoparticles for diagnosis based on MRI," in De La Fuente, J. M. and Grazu, V. (eds.) *Frontiers of nanoscience.* Oxford, UK and Amsterdam, Netherlands: Elsevier.

Ghosh, P. S., Kim, C.-K., Han, G., Forbes, N. S. and Rotello, V. M. (2008) "Efficient gene delivery vectors by tuning the surface charge density of amino acid-functionalized gold nanoparticles," *ACS Nano*, 2, pp. 2213–2218. [PubMed: 19206385].

Haim, H., Steiner, I. and Panet, A. (2005) "Synchronized infection of cell cultures by magnetically controlled virus," *Society*, 79, pp. 622–625.

Hen, Y. et al. (2012) "Development of an MRI-visible nonviral vector for siRNA delivery targeting gastric cancer," *International Journal of Nanomedicine*, 7, pp. 359–368.

Hom, C. et al. (2010) "Mesoporous silica nanoparticles facilitate delivery of siRNA to shutdown signaling pathways in mammalian cells," *Small*, 6(11), pp. 1185–1190. doi: 10.1002/smll.200901966.

Hughes, C., Galea-lauri, J., Farzaneh, F. and Darling, D. (2001) "Streptavidin paramagnetic particles provide a choice of three affinity-based capture and magnetic concentration strategies for retroviral vectors," *Mol. Ther.*, 3, pp. 623–630. [PubMed: 11319925].

Huh, Y.-M., Lee, E.-S., Lee, J.-H., Jun, Y.-w., Kim, P.-H., Yun, C.-O., Kim, J.-H., Suh, J.-S. and Cheon, J. (2007) "Hybrid nanoparticles for magnetic resonance imaging of target-specific viral gene delivery," *Adv. Mater.*, 19, pp. 3109–3112.

Ito, A. and Kamihira, M. (2011) "Tissue engineering using magnetite nanoparticles," *Progress in Molecular Biology and Translational Science*, 104, pp. 355–395. doi: 10.1016/B978-0-12-416020-0.00009-7.

Jin, S. and Ye, K. (2007) "Nanoparticle-mediated drug delivery and gene therapy," *Biomed. Eng.*, pp. 32–41.

Jinturkar, K. A., Rathi, M. N. and Misra, A. (2011) "Gene delivery using physical methods," in Misra, A. (ed.) *Challenges in delivery of therapeutic genomics and proteomics*. London and Burlington, MA, USA: Elsevier, pp. 83–126.

Kaikkonen, M. U., Lesch, H. P., Pikkarainen, J., Räty, J. K., Vuorio, T., Huhtala, T., Taavitsainen, M., Laitinen, T., Tuunanen, P., Gröhn, O., Närvänen, A., Airenne, K. J. and Ylä-Herttuala, S. (2009) (Strept)avidin-displaying lentiviruses as versatile tools for targeting and dual imaging of gene delivery," *Gene Therapy*, 16, pp. 894–904. [PubMed: 19440224].

Kamei, K., Mukai, Y., Kojima, H., Yoshikawa, T., Yoshikawa, M., Kiyohara, G., Yamamoto, T. A., Yoshioka, Y., Okada, N., Seino, S. and Nakagawa, S. (2009) "Direct cell entry of gold/iron-oxide magnetic nanoparticles in adenovirus mediated gene delivery," *Biomaterials*, 30, 1809–1814. [PubMed: 19136151].

Lin, M. M. et al. (2008) "Development of superparamagnetic iron oxide nanoparticles (SPIONS) for translation to clinical applications," *IEEE Transactions on Nanobioscience*, 7(4), pp. 298–305. doi: 10.1109/TNB.2008.2011864.

Liu, C. and Zhang, N. (2011) "Nanoparticles in gene therapy principles, prospects, and challenges," *Progress in Molecular Biology and Translational Science*, 104, pp. 509–562. doi: 10.1016/B978-0-12-416020-0.00013-9. PMID: 22093228.

Morishita, N., Nakagami, H., Morishita, R., Takeda, S., Mishima, F., Terazono, B., Nishijima, S., Kaneda, Y. and Tanaka, N. (2005) "Magnetic nanoparticles with surface modification enhanced gene delivery of HVJ-E vector," *Biochemical and Biophysical Research Communications*, 334, pp. 1121–1126. [PubMed: 16134237].

Mukherjee, S. and Thrasher, A. J. (2013) "Gene therapy for PIDs: Progress, pitfalls and prospects," *Gene*, 525(2), pp. 174–181. doi: 10.1016/j.gene.2013.03.098.

Pereyra, A. S. et al. (2016) "Magnetofection enhances adenoviral vector-based gene delivery in skeletal muscle cells," *Journal of Nanomedicine & Nanotechnology*, 7(2). doi: 10.4172/2157-7439.1000364.

Plank, C., Scherer, F., Schillinger, U., Bergemann, C. and Anton, M. (2003) "Magnetofection: Enhancing and targeting gene delivery with superparamagnetic nanoparticles and magnetic fields," *Journal of Liposome Research*, 13, pp. 29–32. [PubMed: 12725725].

Prijic, S. et al. (2012) "Surface modified magnetic nanoparticles for immuno-gene therapy of murine mammary adenocarcinoma," *Biomaterials*, 33(17), pp. 4379–4391. doi: 10.1016/j.biomaterials.2012.02.061.

Prosen, L. et al. (2013) "Magnetofection: A reproducible method for gene delivery to melanoma cells," *BioMed Research International*, 2013, p. 209452. doi: 10.1155/2013/209452.

Räty, J. K., Liimatainen, T., Wirth, T., Airenne, K. J., Ihalainen, T. O., Huhtala, T., Hamerlynck, E., Vihinen-Ranta, M., Närvänen, A., Ylä-Herttuala, S. and Hakumäki, J. M. (2006) "Magnetic resonance imaging of viral particle biodistribution in vivo," *Gene Therapy*, pp. 1440–1446. [PubMed: 16855615].

Sinha Ray, S. (2013) "Structure and morphology characterization techniques," in *Clay-containing polymer nanocomposites*. Oxford, UK and Amsterdam, The Netherlands: Elsevier, pp. 39–66.

Siu, K. S. et al. (2014) "Non-covalently functionalized single-walled carbon nanotube for topical siRNA delivery into melanoma," *Biomaterials*, 35(10), pp. 3435–3442. doi: 10.1016/j.biomaterials.2013.12.079.

Sunshine, J. C., Bishop, C. J. and Green, J. J. (2011) "Advances in polymeric and inorganic vectors for nonviral nucleic acid delivery," *Therapeutic Delivery*, 2(4), pp. 493–521. doi: 10.4155/tde.11.14.

Takahashi, H., Niidome, Y. and Yamada, S. (2005) "Controlled release of plasmid DNA from gold nanorods induced by pulsed nearinfrared light," *Chemical Communications Journal (Cambridge, England)*, pp. 2247–2249.

Tresilwised, N. et al. (2012) "Effects of nanoparticle coatings on the activity of oncolytic adenovirus-magnetic nanoparticle complexes," *Biomaterials*, 33(1), pp. 256–269. doi: 10.1016/j.biomaterials.2011.09.028.

Weber, W., Lienhart, C., Daoud-El Baba, M., Grass, R. N., Kohler, T., Müller, R., Stark, W. J. and Fussenegger, M. (2009) "Magnet-guided transduction of mammalian cells and mice using engineered magnetic lentiviral particles," *Journal of Biotechnology*, 141, pp. 118–122.

Yang, Z. et al. (2018) "Superparamagnetic iron oxide nanoparticles modified with poly-ethylenimine and galactose for siRNA targeted delivery in hepatocellular carcinoma therapy," *International Journal of Nanomedicine*, 13, pp. 1851–1865. doi: 10.2147/ijn. s155537.

Yin, H. et al. (2014) "Non-viral vectors for gene-based therapy," *Nature Reviews: Genetics*, 15(8), pp. 541–555. doi: 10.1038/nrg3763.

Zhu, S.-G. et al. (2004) "Poly(L-lysine)-modified silica nanoparticles for the delivery of antisense oligonucleotides," *Biotechnology and Applied Biochemistry*, 39(Pt 2), pp. 179–187. doi: 10.1042/BA20030077.

9 Nanotherapeutics in Cancer Therapy

INTRODUCTION

Despite significant technological advances in the field of medicine, there are currently only a few effective cancer treatments available. Metastasis of cancers and recurrence play a significant role in morbidity and mortality, albeit the precise processes are still unclear. Gene mutations are typically thought to be the major cause of cancer. According to the recent census reports, 9.6 million people died due to cancers in 2018 and it estimates 18.1 million of new cases per annum (Sung et al., 2021). The Global Cancer Observatory (GCO) predicts that 30 million people worldwide will die because of cancers annually by 2030 (Sung et al., 2021). Cancer has a high mortality rate, and it also imposes a heavy financial cost on civilization. The economic burden for the families of the patients who suffer from cancers are also considerable. As a result of those impacts, attempts to avert, diagnosis, and treatment strategies for cancers are crucial. Surgical removal of the tumors, chemotherapy, radiation therapies, and biological therapy associated with various drug regimens are frequently employed as anticancer treatments (Xu et al., 2014). Malignant and substantial tumors can be successfully removed with surgery, especially when the cancer remains in its initial stages. Surgery, chemotherapy, and radiotherapy can be combined together to enhance the therapeutic outcome and the quality of the life of patients (Pérez-Herrero and Fernández-Medarde, 2015). Figure 9.1 shows the timeline of nanotherapeutics up to date.

Insufficient specificity, cytotoxic effects, short half-lives, solubility issues, the development of multidrug resistance, as well as the proliferation of stem-like cells are drawbacks with conventional chemotherapy. Nanotherapeutics-based chemotherapy, molecular therapy, targeted therapy, photodynamic therapy (PDT), chemodynamic therapy (CDT), photothermal therapy (PTT), and sonodynamic therapy (SDT) all are employed in anticancer therapy in order to circumvent these drawbacks (Obireddy and Lai, 2021). Furthermore, a significant number of researches have been conducted recently on a range of cancer alternative treatments, including molecular treatment, apoptosis modulation, immunological therapies, therapies regarding signal and responses modification, nucleic acid–associated therapy, and antiangiogenesis therapy (Maeda et al., 2000; Zhao et al., 2022). With the development of nanotechnology, nanotherapeutics reinforced in cancer treatment may lessen the detrimental effects of chemotherapy, and substantial research has been done in this arena.

9.1 EMERGING TYPES OF CANCERS THAT ARE TREATED WITH NANOTHERAPEUTICS

Nanotherapeutics seem to possess the capacity to provide many more important advances in the detection, diagnosis, and treatment therapies of cancer with vast

 DOI: 10.1201/9781003442202-10

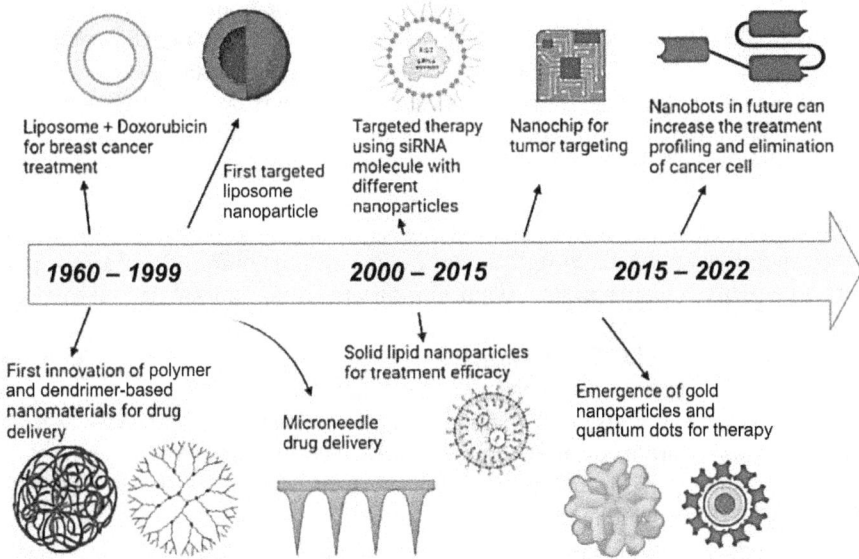

FIGURE 9.1 Timeline of cancer nanotherapeutics.

Source: Reproduced with permission from Nirmala et al., 2023 with permission from the Royal Society of Chemistry.

and specialized research paths earmarked for the future as well as the possibilities of nanotherapeutic-based prevention for cancers. Considering the recent nanotherapeutics-based anticancer researches, Munaweera et al. have synthesized innovative wrinkled structured periodic mesoporous organosilica (PMO) nanoparticles for the administration of hydrophobic anticancer drugs. These cutting-edge wrinkled PMOs contain pore diameters, hydrophobicity, and surface areas that can be adjusted to facilitating the delivery of hydrophobic drugs. In comparison to mesoporous silica (MS) nanoparticles, the hydrophobic anticancer agent, paclitaxel, was employed as a standard drug, and the PMO demonstrates a better drug loading efficiency for paclitaxel (Munaweera et al., 2015a). Moreover, Munaweera et al. formulated a new type of platinum drug loaded with holmium in wrinkled mesoporous silica nanoparticles with a lipid coating or without any coating. The influence was recognized as an anticancer treatment after *in vitro* platinum drug liberation from both lipids coated and uncoated chemoradiotherapeutic wrinkled mesoporous silica nanoparticles (Munaweera et al., 2014a).

Furthermore, it is important to analyze the recent advancements in nanotherapeutics for anticancer therapies according to the anatomical categorization of cancers. Brain cancer is one of the most lethal tumors affecting low- and middle-income economies. It accounts for 9–17% of all cancer cases globally. Glioblastoma multiforme, which accounts for 12–15% including all brain cancers that are observed in adults were reported, is an initial brain tumor that has metastasized. According to Leece et al. 16,050 fatalities and 23,770 incidence of brain cancer were recognized in

2016 (Leece et al., 2017). The anatomical position of the brain and its intracranial location make brain cancer complicated to address. The incapability of the anticancer drug to penetrate the blood–brain barrier (BBB) is the main obstacle and the reason for the low life expectancies for patients with brain cancer (Lin and Kleinberg, 2008).

There are three potential mechanisms for localized medication delivery in anticancer therapy, including passive and active targeting with nanoparticles and nanontheranostic agents. Because the nanomaterials induce the positive accumulation of the drug at the tumor locations, passive targeting seems to be the best way to administer nanopharmaceuticals to intracranial malignant tumors for effective transport across the BBB. Nanomaterials that are administered intravenously (i.v.) take advantage of the increased penetration ability and retention to get close to the tumor cells. Carmustine-loaded PLGA nanoparticles with O_6-benzylguanine preparation were administered intravenously and had a greater beneficial impact than when these two medications were administered separately in a nanoparticle form (Qian et al., 2013). Nanotheranostics are medications and diagnostic agents that are delivered by only one type of nanoparticle for the treatment of brain cancer (Meyers et al., 2013). Employing MRI and polymeric nanomaterials coated with iron oxide nanoparticles, photofrin encapsulation was used in PDT to accumulate surface-decorated malignant tumor vasculature-targeting F3 peptide inside the intracranial tumor. Especially opposed to PDT or photofrin individually, this theranostic improved the rate of survival in the 9L glioma rat model during PDT (Reddy et al., 2006).

For the administration of doxorubicin, that featured a low capacity of drug loading and was difficult to regulate the profile of drug release. Gulati et al. fabricated titanium wires to serve as nanotube clamps or nanocarriers as drug delivering agents. Titanium wires with a 0.75 mm its thickness and a 30 mm in length were anodized using an automated electrochemical process, resulting in arrays of titania nanotubes with a diameter of 170 nm that might load up to 1200 g of the chemotherapy drug doxorubicin. The developed nanoengineered wires demonstrated sustained drug liberation for eight days, were mechanically stable for the loading capacity of doxorubicin, and were proven to be biocompatible (Gulati, Aw and Losic, 2012).

The most common cancer among women worldwide and the second greatest reason of death among them is breast cancer. An incidence of 1.5 million for breast cancer are recorded annually, and the prevalence of this cancer has increased by up to 20% over the last ten years (Torre et al., 2017). Nanotherapeutics, in addition to a combination treatment strategy, aid in overcoming the problems associated with anticancer medication resistance. One of the worst cancers and one that can be challenging to cure if it spreads to other parts of the body is breast cancer. Important anatomical structures and organs like the liver, heart, lung, and bones are susceptible toward its progression and spreading. In the treatment of breast cancer, it is crucial that the nanoformulations be formulated and administered in a way that allows it to adequately reach the cancerous site without causing any adverse reactions.

PLGA nanoparticles containing mannose and abraxane, correspondingly, engage the TAM and EPR in efficient distribution of the anticancer medicines, Paclitaxel and Doxorubicin (Cullis et al., 2017). Parallel to this study, the nanoformulation of CRLX101 (an experimental nanoparticle)–camptothecin combination was evaluated individually or in conjunction with bevacizumab (an antiangiogenic medication) by using a breast cancer–induced laboratory mouse model. This CRLX101 nanoformulation improved susceptibility of cancers to bevacizumab, increased the perfusion of tumors, and lowered hypoxia through effectively inhibiting the hypoxia-inducible factor-1 (Pham et al., 2016).

An incidence of 1.3 million cases of prostate cancer were identified in 2018, indicating that it is the most prevalent cancer afflicting males (Rawla, 2019). The prevalence of prostate-specific antigen (PSA) detection in men is lacking evidence of prostate cancer that has caused age-related incidence (those older than 65) levels of the disease to surge dramatically. A group of scientists have designed silver nanoparticles (100 nm) from an aqueous herbal extract of *Alternanthera sessilis*, and the generated nanoparticles exhibited remarkable action against PC3 prostate cells (Firdhouse and Lalitha, 2013). Corresponding to this, gold nanoparticles (AuNPs) that are bound to glucose with increased toxicity and responsiveness to the DU-145 prostate cancer cell type were developed. Moreover, another research revealed that the nanoparticles in 50 nm in size without a PEGylated surface demonstrated remarkable cellular absorption of AuNPs in the PC3 prostate cell line 344 E. Furthermore, it was established that the docetaxel-encapsulated AuNPs antineoplastic medication exhibited promising outcomes (Arnida and Ghandehari, 2010).

A majority of lung cancers, nearly 85%, are categorized as non-small cell (NSLCC), making it the most common reason for mortality rate of cancers in the United States (NSCLC). In a recent study, holmium-165 (Ho), which can be neutron-activated to generate the holmium-166 radionuclide, as well as a platinum (Pt)-based chemotherapeutic agent have been combined to form a garnet magnetic nanoparticle (HoIG-Pt) in order to obtain selective distribution to tumors utilizing an external magnet (Munaweera et al., 2015b). In another related study, wrinkle-structured, amine-modified mesoporous silicon (AMS) nanoparticles that release nitric oxide (NO) and cisplatin have been synthesized as an anticancer therapy for treatment of NSCLC (Munaweera et al., 2015a).

Another type of most common cancer globally is skin cancer. The most prevalent kinds of cancers found on the skin nowadays are melanoma and nonmelanoma, which have surpassed epidemic proportions. Due to the significant increase in skin cancer cases and the absence of effective drug distribution systems, scientists are conducting more studies to establish skin cancer treatment plans relying on nanotherapeutics (Khan et al., 2022). According to recent research, the investigators have revealed that a bandage made of nonradioactive holmium-165 (165Ho) iron garnet nanoparticles can be placed on a tumor lesion after being neutron-activated to become 166Ho in skin cancers (Munaweera et al., 2014b).

Gastrointestinal (GI) cancers are also a significant type of cancer which affect the anatomical structures and major organs in the GI tract. Gastrointestinal malignancies are aggressive tumors that have a high mortality rate as well as high morbidity. Iron oxide NPs are utilized in colorectal, liver, and gastric cancers in order to detect the specific biomarkers and evaluate the anticancer therapy. QDs are also employed in the same types of cancers, especially for the targeting and imaging of the cancer cells. In colorectal and liver cancers, carbon nanotubes are used for tumor localization. AuNPs are important in photothermal and hyperthermal destruction of tumor and cancer cells. Nanoshells, dendrimers, and polymeric NPs also exhibit same functions toward the cancer cells and tumors (Liang et al., 2022).

The world cancer report of 2020 which is published by the International Agency for Research on Cancer (IARC) of World Health Organization (WHO), colorectal, liver, gastric, and esophageal cancers are ranked third, sixth, fifth, and eighth, respectively, in regard to total cancer morbidity (Liang et al., 2022). Throughout the world, 0.94, 0.83, 0.77, 0.54, and 0.47 million people die from colorectal, liver, gastric, esophageal, and pancreatic cancers, respectively (Liang et al., 2022).

9.2   ANTICANCER MECHANISMS OF NANOMATERIALS

Passive targeting mechanisms, active targeting mechanisms, and mechanisms based on triggered release are the prominent types of targeting used to deliver nanoparticles to tumor tissues.

9.2.1   PASSIVE TARGETING MECHANISMS

Large pores that are located intracellularly, endothelial cells that are interrupted, leaky vasculatures, and high permeability all are evident in tumor cells as a result of the deformed walls of vascular endothelium of tumorous tissues, impaired cell-to-cell connections, and defective lymphatic drainage (Yang et al., 2017). Nanoparticles can concentrate or be accumulated in tumor cells owing to these distinguishing characteristics of tumor cells. The improved permeability and retention phenomenon,

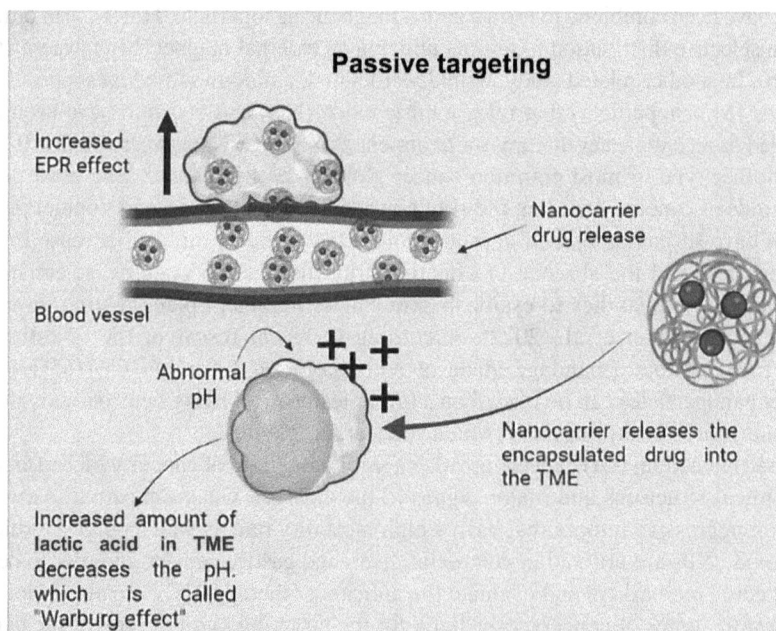

FIGURE 9.2   Passive targeting mechanisms of nanotherapeutics in anticancer therapies.

Source: Reproduced with permission from Nirmala et al., 2023 with permission from the Royal Society of Chemistry.

usually known as EPR, is the mechanism behind passive targeting. This technique prevents damage to the healthy tissues located around the tumor tissue. As a result, the detrimental impacts of chemotherapy are decreased by allowing the cytotoxic medications transported by the nanoparticles to concentrate where they are necessary. Recent research revealed that such medications can be accumulated into tumor tissues using nanoparticles with a size range of 10–100 nm (Danhier, Feron and Préat, 2010).

Other aspects include various kinds of tumor, tumor size, and heterogeneity of tumors that have an impact on the EPR mechanism. This results in variations in the biodistribution of various nanoparticles and a lack of consistency (Shi et al., 2017). Figure 9.2 shows a schematic diagram of passive targeting mechanisms of nanotherapeutics in anticancer therapies.

9.2.2 ACTIVE TARGETING MECHANISMS

This stratagem relies on the alteration of the nanoparticle and its surface by the application of particular ligand conjugation. Such changes enable selective binding to receptors present at the target region. The method distinguishes between cancerous and normal cells based on a specific chemical released on the surfaces of cancerous cells and tumors. The cells are stimulated to take up the nanocarrier and induce

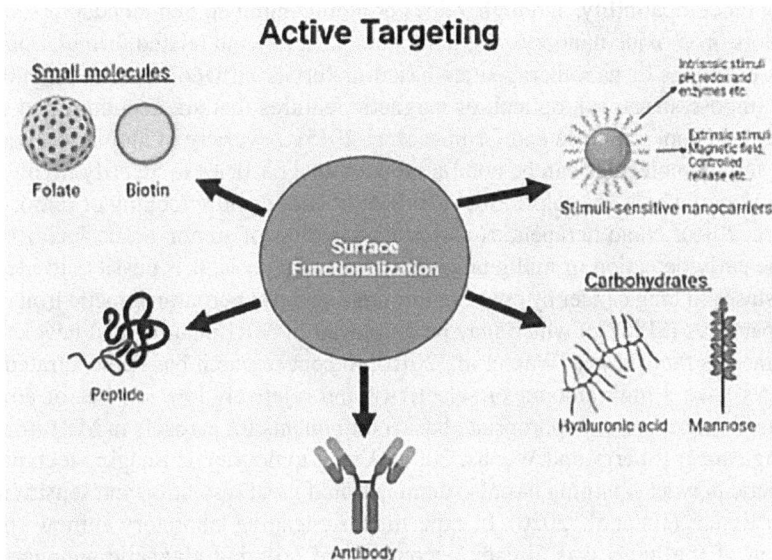

FIGURE 9.3 Active targeting mechanisms of nanotherapeutics in anticancer therapies.

Source: Reproduced with permission from Nirmala et al., 2023. Furthermore, active targeting facilitates the distribution of particles like proteins and nucleic acids that are unable to pass through cellular membranes on their own (Sykes et al., 2014). Besides, it reduces the multidrug resistance (MDR) because proteins like P-glycoprotein (P-gp), which promote resistance are unable to expel drug or the conjugate of drug and polymer nanoparticles that invaded the cell through endocytosis. Tumor cells tend to display one or more surface molecular structures and behaviors, providing locations for active targeting (Blagosklonny, 2003).

the cell death when the altered ligands upon this nanoparticle surface attach to these particular receptors. The absorption of mononuclear phagocyte system (MPS) is reduced as a result of this mechanism, lengthening the duration that blood circulates. Figure 9.3 shows a schematic diagram of active targeting mechanisms of nanotherapeutics in anticancer therapies.

9.2.3 MECHANISMS BASED ON STIMULI RESPONSIVE RELEASE

Both internal and external triggers can cause nanocarriers to modify. Target tissues may experience a variety of internal triggers, including pH, ionic strength, redox potential, and stress—similar to how diverse external stimuli such as magnetic fields, electric fields, light, ultrasound and temperature can cause the medication to be released (Cai et al., 2008).

9.3 NANOTHERAPEUTICS FOR EARLY CANCER DETECTION

Many types of nanoparticles are recently employed for molecular imaging as a result of the recent surge in interest in the utilization of nanotherapeutics in detection and diagnosis of cancer and monitoring. They have become more popular in recent cancer research and detection of cancers because of their perks, including tiny size, strong biocompatibility, and high values of atomic number. Semiconductors, quantum dots, iron oxide nanocrystals, gold nanoparticles, and related formulations are a few examples of nanotherapeutics-based materials utilized in cancer treatment. They impose structural, optical, or magnetic features that are uncommon in other molecules (Popescu, Fufă and Grumezescu, 2015). A variety of antitumor medications and biomolecules can be combined with nanoparticles to identify highly specific tumors, which are helpful for early identification and screening of tumor cells (Singh, 2019). Nanotherapeutics-assisted screening of tumor tissue has allowed for the early detection of malignancy in cancer diagnosis. It is possible to identify metastases in lung cancer by creating immunological superparamagnetic iron oxide nanoparticles (SPIONs) which may be employed in MRI imaging and have cancer cell lines as their target (Wan et al., 2016). Recent research has demonstrated that SPIONs have a high amount of selectivity and relatively low number of adverse effects, rendering them appropriate basic components for aerosols in MRI imaging of lung cancer (Sherry and Woods, 2008). Using tomographic imaging techniques, magnetic powder scanning has also demonstrated great resolution and sensitivity to tumor tissues (Jin et al., 2020). In experiments engaging laboratory animals, nebulization of the lungs was already accomplished utilizing magnetic nanoparticles (MNPs) that target the epidermal growth factor receptor (EGFR) protein, a protein that is frequently found in individuals with non-small cell lung cancer (NSCLC). On the basis of amphiphilic dendritic molecules that are self-assembled, *in vitro* investigations employing nanosystem for positron emission tomography (PET) were additionally established. These dendritic molecules organize on their own to form regular supramolecular nanoparticles with hundreds of PET indicating units on the exterior surface. The dendritic nanoscale system successfully aggregates in tumors by utilizing dendritic multivalence as well as the increased penetration and retention (EPR) impact. Moreover, it results in exceptionally sensitive and specific monitoring of diverse malignancies while lowering treatment toxicities (Garrigue et al., 2018).

According to recent studies, cancer detection at the cellular, tissue, and molecular stages can be validated by nanotechnology (Garrigue et al., 2018). This is facilitated by the capability of nanotechnology in its implementations to investigate the surroundings of the tumor. For example, the pH sensitivity to fluorescent nanoprobes is able to identify fibroblast-triggered protein-A on the cellular membranes of tumor-associated fibroblasts (Ji et al., 2013). Nanotechnology-related spatial and temporal approaches, such as nanoshells, near-infrared quantum dots, and colloidal gold nanoparticles, could enable identifying precisely the living cells and observing dynamic biological events in tumor environment.

Cancer biomarkers are biochemical characteristics whose appearance indicates the presence or stage of a tumor. These indicators are employed to study the cellular mechanisms, track or detect changes in cancer cells, and also the outcomes may eventually assist in comprehending malignancies. Proteins, amino acids, protein fragments, or DNA all can be used as biomarkers. Investigations are possible on tumor biomarkers, which are signs of a tumor to confirm the existence of particular malignancies. Nanoparticles interact with carrier proteins by virtue of their surface properties, including electric charge or active biomolecules. Mesoporous silica particles, hydrogel nanoparticles, and carbon nanotubes presently possess these properties (Geho et al., 2005).

Enhancing the sensitivity of mass spectrometry is another technique for improving screening with nanocarriers. The distinctive optical as well as thermal characteristics of carbon nanotubes improve the ability of the analyte to transmit energy, leading to its absorption and ionization, and obviating the interference of native matrix ions (Najam-ul-Haq et al., 2007). Using nanotechnology to create lab-on-chip microfluidic devices which may be utilized for screening of immunological features and functions or to research the characteristics of tumor cells is another strategy. For instance, the lab-on-a-chip for excellent performance of multimodal protein identification by utilizing quantum dots has been investigated. It consists of cadmium selenide (CdSe) nucleus with a shell made of zinc sulfide (ZnS) and connected to antibodies. These antibodies are attached to carcinoembryonic antigen, cancer antigen 125, and Her-2/Neu (Jokerst et al., 2009). This device exhibits potentialities as a device for anticancer therapies.

9.4 NANOCARRIERS FOR TARGETED CANCER THERAPY

The effectiveness of immunotherapy as an anticancer treatment has the capability to be greatly enhanced by nanomaterials. Vaccines used for cancers and tumor microenvironment (TME) regulation are two components of cancer immunotherapy. Cancer vaccines are designed to deliver cancer antigen to DCs and stimulate a strong effector T-cell response; meanwhile TME manipulation seeks to increase the capacity of cytotoxic T cells for the death of cancer cells. Additionally, certain cells can uptake nanoparticles that have been preloaded with targeted ligands (Melero et al., 2014). It is noteworthy that recent research revealed the creation of a D-enantiomeric supermolecule nanoparticle, which demonstrated p53-dependent antiproliferative effect and improved immunity in cell. The ability of nanoparticles to transport tumor antigens will aid immunotherapy, and owing to their unique properties, they can also control the immune reactions (Yan et al., 2020). It ought to be noted that the PC7A nanoparticles stimulated the mechanism for the modulator of interferon genes, which helped the antitumor immunotherapy work effectively (Luo et al., 2017).

Liposomes, porous silica nanoparticles, micelles, nanoemulsions, polymeric nanomaterials, dendrimers, carbon nanotubes, carbon nanomaterials, extracellular vesicles, monoclonal antibodies (mAb) nanoparticles, quantum dots, metallic nanoparticles, organic and inorganic nanoparticles, lipid-based nanomaterials, nanogels, nanocapsules, and DNA nanococoons are some of the major nanocarriers that play a crucial role in drug and gene delivery treatments related to anticancer therapies (Oon and Chan, 1990).

9.5 NANOTHERAPEUTICS FOR CANCER RADIOTHERAPY

An essential component of anticancer treatment is radiotherapy. The advancement of the area was fueled by discoveries in physics, chemistry, engineering, and biology. The continuing incorporation of innovations from other sectors will be essential for the development of radiation oncology. Nanotherapeutics is a recent branch of science that has the potential to influence radiation oncology. Materials with unique features with the dimensions in nanoscale, including superparamagnetism, increased penetration, and retention effect are quite well-adapted to be employed in radiation oncology. According to Barcellos-Hoff et al., radiotherapy constitutes one of the most popular and efficient cancer treatment techniques (Barcellos-Hoff et al., 2005). Currently, 60% cancer victims undergo radiotherapy as part of their anticancer therapies (Schaue and McBride, 2015) that is delivered via a variety of modalities, such as brachytherapy (internal radioactive source) and exterior beam (photons, protons, and electrons).

In order to increase the antitumor effectiveness of radioisotopes or radiosensitizers, nanomaterials can be employed to enhance their distribution and accumulation. Recent research on the impact of radiotherapy on microenvironments of cancerous tumors has also sparked curiosity about alternative radiotherapy adjuvant therapy, particularly those that combine radiotherapy and immunotherapy. Radiation therapy increases the exposure to and expression of tumor antigens that prompts the activation of cytokines and the mobilization of immune cells.

It is commonly known that radioisotopes (radionuclides) are used in clinical settings. DNA single-strand breaks are brought about by radioactive isotopes, which release energy out from nucleus and produce ionized atoms as well as free radicals. Beta-emitters, including ^{186}Re, ^{188}Re, ^{166}Ho, ^{89}Sr, ^{32}P, and ^{90}Y, as well as alpha-emitters, including ^{225}Ac, ^{211}At, and ^{213}Bi, are radioisotopes used in clinical oncology (Hamoudeh et al., 2008).

Nevertheless, radioisotopes can circumvent these biological removal processes by packing or combining the nanocarriers. For instance, while the physiological half-life of ^{89}Sr is 50.5 days, its plasma clearance takes on average 47 hours. Given their distinctive pharmacokinetic features and the enhanced adverse effects, nanostructures like liposomes, dendrimers, micelles, or polymeric complexes are often larger than 10 nm, which significantly reduces the renal clearance and extends their half-life in systemic environment (Kim, Rutka and Chan, 2010).

The transport of radiosensitizers toward the intended location of tumor can be impacted by nanotherapeutics. For instance, wortmannin inhibits phosphatidylinositol 3′-kinases and kinases linked to phosphatidylinositol 3′-kinases, including DNA-dependent protein kinases. Preclinical outcomes have demonstrated its potency as a radiosensitizer. However, due to solubility issues, instability, and high toxicological effects, its clinical applicability is constrained. These issues were resolved by creating wortmannin with nanoparticles, which has an PLGA polymer center and a DSPE-PEG lipid exterior. The nanoradiosensitizer was shown to be more efficacious than 5-FU, and its MTD was many times higher than that of wortmannin in laboratory mice with KB cell xenografts (Karve et al., 2012). Nanoradiosensitizers proved its ability to destroy hypoxic tumor cells when combined with tirapazamine due to their synergistic effects (Liu et al., 2015). Research is being done on the possibility of additional inorganic nanoparticles, such as Y_2O_3 and $ZnFe_2O_3$, in radiotherapy (Meidanchi et al., 2015).

Negative consequences of radiological therapies may be reduced by reducing the dispersion of radiosensitizers or radioisotopes in healthy tissues and by limiting the discharge of these radiotherapeutic compounds (Win and Feng, 2005). Adverse effects of radiation therapy are frequently brought on by unanticipated damage to healthy tissue. In numerous physiological areas, including the epidermis, lungs, and heart, nanoparticles have been demonstrated to have decreased penetration into regular vasculature and capillaries (Eblan and Wang, 2013). As a result, longer exposure to the substances caused by the regulated and continuous liberation of nanomaterials into the tissue has been associated with beneficial effects and greater tolerance for healthy tissue. This was proven through the clinical application of Doxil with different nanoparticles, which significantly decreased the cardiotoxicity of doxorubicin while maintaining its antitumor activity (Barenholz, 2012).

REFERENCES

Arnida, M. A., & Ghandehari, H. (2010) "Cellular uptake and toxicity of gold nanoparticles in prostate cancer cells: A comparative study of rods and spheres," *Journal of Applied Toxicology*, 30, pp. 212–217. https://doi.org/10.1002/jat.1486.

Barcellos-Hoff, M. H., Park, C. and Wright, E. G. (2005) "Radiation and the microenvironment— tumorigenesis and therapy," *Nat. Rev. Cancer*, 5(11), pp. 867–875. doi: 10.1038/nrc1735.

Barenholz, Y. (2012) "Doxil(R)—the first FDA-approved nano-drug: Lessons learned," *J. Control Release*, 160(2), pp. 117–134. doi: 10.1016/j.jconrel.2012.03.020.

Blagosklonny, M. V. (2003) "Targeting cancer cells by exploiting their resistance," *Trends in Molecular Medicine*, 9, pp. 307–312. https://doi.org/10.1016/S1471-4914(03)00111-4.

Cai, W., Gao, T., Hong, H. and Sun, J. (2008) "Applications of gold nanoparticles in cancer nanotechnology," *Nanotechnology, Science and Applications*, 1, pp. 17–32. https://doi.org/10.2147/NSA. S3788.

Cullis, J., Siolas, D., Avanzi, A. et al. (2017) "Macropinocytosis of nab-paclitaxel drives macrophage activation in pancreatic cancer," *Cancer Immunology Research*, 5, pp. 182–190. https://doi.org/10.1158/2326-6066.CIR-16-0125.

Danhier, F., Feron, O. and Préat, V. (2010) "To exploit the tumor microenvironment: Passive and active tumor targeting of nanocarriers for anti-cancer drug delivery," *Journal of Controlled Release*, 148, pp. 135–146. https://doi.org/10.1016/j.jconrel.2010.08.027.

Eblan, M. J. and Wang, A. Z. (2013) "Improving chemoradiotherapy with nanoparticle therapeutics," *Transl. Cancer Res.*, 2(4), pp. 320–329. doi: 10.3978/j.issn.2218-676X. 2013.08.04.

Firdhouse, M. J. and Lalitha, P. (2013) "Biosynthesis of silver nanoparticles using the extract of alternanthera sessilis-antiproliferative effect against prostate cancer cells," *Cancer Nanotechnology*, 4, pp. 137–143. https://doi.org/10.1007/s12645-013-0045-4.

Garrigue, P. et al. (2018) "Self-assembling supramolecular dendrimer nanosystem for PET imaging of tumors," *Proceedings of the National Academy of Sciences of the United States of America*, 115(45), pp. 11454–11459. doi: 10.1073/pnas.1812938115.

Geho, D. H. et al. (2005) "Nanoparticles: Potential biomarker harvesters," *Current Opinion in Chemical Biology*, 15, pp. 56–61.

Gulati, K., Aw, M. S. and Losic, D. (2012) "Nanoengineered drug-releasing Ti wires as an alternative for local delivery of chemotherapeutics in the brain," *International Journal of Nanomedicine*, 7, pp. 2069–2076. https://doi.org/10.2147/IJN.S29917.

Hamoudeh, M., Kamleh, M. A., Diab, R. and Fessi, H. (2008) "Radionuclides delivery systems for nuclear imaging and radiotherapy of cancer," *Adv. Drug Deliv. Rev.*, 60(12), 1329–1346. doi: 10.1016/j.addr.2008.04.013.

Ji, T. et al. (2013) "Tumor fibroblast specific activation of a hybrid ferritin nanocage-based optical probe for tumor microenvironment imaging," *Small*, 9(14), pp. 2427–2431. doi: 10.1002/smll.201300600.

Jin, C. et al. (2020) "Application of nanotechnology in cancer diagnosis and therapy—A mini-review," *International Journal of Medical Sciences*, 17(18), pp. 2964–2973. doi: 10.7150/ijms.49801.

Jokerst, J. V. et al. (2009) "Nano-bio-chips for high performance multiplexed protein detection: Determinations of cancer biomarkers in serum and saliva using quantum dot bioconjugate labels," *Biosensors & Bioelectronics*, 24(12), pp. 3622–3629. doi: 10.1016/j. bios.2009.05.026.

Karve, S., Werner, M. E., Sukumar, R., Cummings, N. D., Copp, J. A., Wang, E. C. and Wang, A. Z. (2012) "Revival of the abandoned therapeutic wortmannin by nanoparticle drug delivery," *Proc. Natl. Acad. Sci. USA*, 109(21), 8230–8235. doi: 10.1073/ pnas.1120508109.

Khan, N. H. et al. (2022) "Skin cancer biology and barriers to treatment: Recent applications of polymeric micro/nanostructures," *Journal of Advanced Research*, 36, pp. 223–247. doi: 10.1016/j.jare.2021.06.014.

Kim, B. Y., Rutka, J. T. and Chan, W. C. (2010) "Nanomedicine," *N. Engl. J. Med.*, 363(25), pp. 2434–2443. doi: 10.1056/NEJMra0912273.

Leece, R. et al. (2017) "Global incidence of malignant brain and other central nervous system tumors by histology, 2003–2007," *Neuro-Oncology*, 19(11), pp. 1553–1564. doi: 10.1093/neuonc/nox091.

Liang, M. et al. (2022) "Nanotechnology in diagnosis and therapy of gastrointestinal cancer," *World Journal of Clinical Cases*, 10(16), pp. 5146–5155. doi: 10.12998/wjcc.v10. i16.5146.

Lin, S. H. and Kleinberg, L. R. (2008) "Carmustine wafers: Localized delivery of chemotherapeutic agents in CNS malignancies," *Expert Review of Anticancer Therapy*, 8(3), pp. 343–359. doi: 10.1586/14737140.8.3.343.

Liu, Y., Liu, Y., Bu, W., Xiao, Q., Sun, Y., Zhao, K. and Shi, J. (2015) "Radiation-/hypoxia-induced solid tumor metastasis and regrowth inhibited by hypoxia-specific upconversion nanoradiosensitizer," *Biomaterials*, 49, pp. 1–8. doi: 10.1016/j.biomaterials.2015.01.028.

Luo, M. et al. (2017) "A STING-activating nanovaccine for cancer immunotherapy," *Nature Nanotechnology*, 12(7), pp. 648–654. doi: 10.1038/nnano.2017.52.

Maeda, H. et al. (2000) "Tumor vascular permeability and the EPR effect in macromolecular therapeutics: A review," *Journal of Controlled Release: Official Journal of the Controlled Release Society*, 65(1–2), pp. 271–284. doi: 10.1016/s0168-3659(99)00248-5.

Meidanchi, A., Akhavan, O., Khoei, S., Shokri, A. A., Hajikarimi, Z. and Khansari, N. (2015) "ZnFe$_2$O$_4$ nanoparticles as radiosensitizers in radiotherapy of human prostate cancer cells," *Mater. Sci. Eng. C. Mater. Biol. Appl.*, 46, pp. 394–399. doi: 10.1016/j.msec.2014.10.062.

Melero, I. et al. (2014) "Therapeutic vaccines for cancer: An overview of clinical trials," *Nature Reviews: Clinical Oncology*, 11(9), pp. 509–524. doi: 10.1038/nrclinonc.2014.111.

Meyers, J. D., Doane, T., Burda, C. and Basilion, J. P. (2013) "Nanoparticles for imaging and treating brain cancer," *Nanomedicine (Lond)*, 8, pp. 123–143. https://doi.org/10.2217/nnm.12.185.

Munaweera, I. et al. (2014a) "Chemoradiotherapeutic wrinkled mesoporous silica nanoparticles for use in cancer therapy," *APL Materials*, 2(11), p. 113315. doi: 10.1063/1.4899118.

Munaweera, I. et al. (2014b) "Radiotherapeutic bandage based on electrospun polyacrylonitrile containing holmium-166 iron garnet nanoparticles for the treatment of skin cancer," *ACS Applied Materials & Interfaces*, 6(24), pp. 22250–22256. doi: 10.1021/am506045k.

Munaweera, I. et al. (2015a) "Novel wrinkled periodic mesoporous organosilica nanoparticles for hydrophobic anticancer drug delivery," *Journal of Porous Materials*, 22(1), pp. 1–10. doi: 10.1007/s10934-014-9897-1.

Munaweera, I., Shi, Y., Koneru, B., Saez, R. et al. (2015b) "Chemoradiotherapeutic magnetic nanoparticles for targeted treatment of nonsmall cell lung cancer," *Molecular Pharmaceutics*, 12(10), pp. 3588–3596. doi: 10.1021/acs.molpharmaceut.5b00304.

Najam-ul-Haq, M. et al. (2007) "Role of carbon nano-materials in the analysis of biological materials by laser desorption/ionization-mass spectrometry," *Journal of Biochemical and Biophysical Methods*, 70(2), pp. 319–328. doi: 10.1016/j.jbbm.2006.11.004.

Nirmala, M. J. et al. (2023) "Cancer nanomedicine: A review of nano-therapeutics and challenges ahead," *RSC Advances*, 13(13), pp. 8606–8629. doi: 10.1039/d2ra07863e.

Obireddy, S. R. and Lai, W.-F. (2021) "Preparation and characterization of 2-hydroxyethyl starch microparticles for co-delivery of multiple bioactive agents," *Drug Delivery*, 28(1), pp. 1562–1568. doi: 10.1080/10717544.2021.1955043.

Oon, C. J. and Chan, S. H. (1990) "Frontiers in oncology," *Annals of the Academy of Medicine, Singapore*, 19(2), p. 131.

Pérez-Herrero, E. and Fernández-Medarde, A. (2015) "Advanced targeted therapies in cancer: Drug nanocarriers, the future of chemotherapy," *European Journal of Pharmaceutics and Biopharmaceutics: Official Journal of Arbeitsgemeinschaft für Pharmazeutische Verfahrenstechnik e.V*, 93, pp. 52–79. doi: 10.1016/j.ejpb.2015.03.018.

Pham, E., Yin, M., Peters, C. G. et al. (2016) "Preclinical efficacy of bevacizumab with CRLX101, an investigational nanoparticle—drug conjugate, in treatment of metastatic triple-negative breast cancer," *Cancer Research*, 76, pp. 4493–4503. https://doi.org/10.1158/0008-5472.CAN-15-3435.

Popescu, R. C., Fufă, M. O. M. and Grumezescu, A. M. (2015) "Metal-based nanosystems for diagnosis," *Revue roumaine de morphologie et embryologie [Romanian Journal of Morphology and Embryology]*, 56(2 Suppl), pp. 635–649.

Qian, L., Zheng, J., Wang, K. et al. (2013) Cationic core—shell nanoparticles with carmustine contained within O6-benzylguanine shell for glioma therapy. *Biomaterials*, 34, pp. 8968–8978. https://doi.org/10.1016/j.biomaterials.2013.07.097.

Rawla, P. (2019) "Epidemiology of prostate cancer," *World Journal of Oncology*, 10(2), pp. 63–89. doi: 10.14740/wjon1191.

Reddy, G. R., Bhojani, M. S., McConville, P. et al. (2006) "Vascular targeted nanoparticles for imaging and treatment of brain tumors," *Clinical Cancer Research*, 12, pp. 6677–6686. https://doi. org/10.1158/1078-0432.CCR-06-0946.

Schaue, D. and McBride, W. H. (2015) "Opportunities and challenges of radiotherapy for treating cancer," *Nat. Rev. Clin. Oncol.*, 12(9), 527–540. doi: 10.1038/nrclinonc.2015.120.

Sherry, A. D. and Woods, M. (2008) "Chemical exchange saturation transfer contrast agents for magnetic resonance imaging," *Annual Review of Biomedical Engineering*, 10(1), pp. 391–411. doi: 10.1146/annurev.bioeng.9.060906.151929.

Shi, J., Kantoff, P. W., Wooster, R. and Farokhzad, O. C. (2017) "Cancer nanomedicine: Progress, challenges and opportunities," *Nature Reviews Cancer*, 17, 20–37. https://doi. org/10.1038/nrc. 2016.108.

Singh, R. (2019) "Nanotechnology based therapeutic application in cancer diagnosis and therapy," *Biotech*, 9(3).

Sung, H. et al. (2021) "Global cancer statistics 2020: GLOBOCAN estimates of incidence and mortality worldwide for 36 cancers in 185 countries," *CA: A Cancer Journal for Clinicians*, 71(3), pp. 209–249. doi: 10.3322/caac.21660.

Sykes, E. A., Chen, J., Zheng, G. and Chan, W. C. W. (2014) "Investigating the impact of nanoparticle size on active and passive tumor targeting efficiency," *ACS Nano*, 8, pp. 5696–5706. https://doi.org/10.1021/nn500299p.

Torre, L. A., Islami, F., Siegel, R. L. et al. (2017) "Global cancer in women: Burden and trends," *Cancer Epidemiology, Biomarkers and Prevention*, 26, pp. 444–457. https:// doi.org/10.1158/1055-9965.EPI-16-0858.

Wan, X. et al. (2016) "The preliminary study of immune superparamagnetic iron oxide nanoparticles for the detection of lung cancer in magnetic resonance imaging," *Carbohydrate Research*, 419, pp. 33–40. doi: 10.1016/j.carres.2015.11.003.

Win, K. Y. and Feng, S. S. (2005) "Effects of particle size and surface coating on cellular uptake of polymeric nanoparticles for oral delivery of anticancer drugs," *Biomaterials*, 26(15), 2713–2722. doi: 10.1016/j.biomaterials.2004.07.050.

Xu, J.-J. et al. (2014) "Functional nanoprobes for ultrasensitive detection of biomolecules: An update," *Chemical Society Reviews*, 43(5), pp. 1601–1611. doi: 10.1039/c3cs60277j.

Yan, J. et al. (2020) "Chiral protein supraparticles for tumor suppression and synergistic immunotherapy: An enabling strategy for bioactive supramolecular chirality construction," *Nano Letters*, 20(8), pp. 5844–5852. doi: 10.1021/acs.nanolett.0c01757.

Yang, C., Chan, K. K., Lin, W.-J. et al. (2017) "Biodegradable nanocarriers for small interfering ribonucleic acid (siRNA) co-delivery strategy increase the chemosensitivity of pancreatic cancer cells to gemcitabine," *Nano Research*, 10, pp. 3049–3067. https://doi. org/10.1007/s12274-017-1521-7.

Zhao, T. et al. (2022) "Reactive oxygen species-based nanomaterials for the treatment of myocardial ischemia reperfusion injuries," *Bioactive Materials*, 7, pp. 47–72. doi: 10.1016/j. bioactmat.2021.06.006.

10 Nanotherapeutics in Inflammatory Diseases

INTRODUCTION

Inflammation that can be described as a defense mechanism occurs naturally in the human body. It is essential for defending tissues from injury and infection by promoting tissue repair. It boosts the responsive reactions of immune cells and blood supply to injured areas. Hence, inflammation is crucial to the recovery process and required for sustaining human life. However, it can develop inadvertently in the human body, leading to chronic inflammatory illnesses or persisting even after the initial trigger of inflammation has subsided (Goldstein, Snyderman and Gallin, 1992; Medzhitov, 2008).

Inflammation can be divided into two categories according to the duration that it lasts: acute inflammation, which lasts just a short time, such as in allergic reactions. Other category is chronic inflammation, which lasts for several months or even years. Chronic inflammation can be described as a serious illness that can seriously harm the organ or tissue that is afflicted. According to WHO, chronic diseases constitute a danger to human wellness since they claim the lives of three individuals of every five individuals globally (Jogpal et al., 2022). Chronic inflammatory illnesses have grown in incidence and prevalence during the past few decades, particularly in Westernized nations (Jogpal et al., 2022).

Nanotherapeutics are a novel kind of drug distribution system which might enhance therapeutic bioavailability and improve pharmacokinetics and pharmacodynamics (PKPD) of the drugs. These features are enhanced with their significant capacity of drug-loading and potential for targeted selectivity for specific cells and tissues. Phytochemical substances are also identified as promising therapeutic agents for inflammatory diseases. However, they have a great difficulty crossing the blood–brain barrier (BBB), endothelial lining of blood vessels, GI tract, and mucosal layer due to their size and polarity. They are tending to enzymatically digest in the GI tract. Nanoparticles or nanocrystals are used as emerging agents to encapsulate or conjugate these compounds in order to increase their organic potency because of their stability against enzymes in the GI tract, rapid absorption capacity, and dissemination (Jogpal et al., 2022). Moreover, nanoparticles are a key component in the management therapies of many inflammatory diseases, including arthritis, gastritis, nephritis, hepatitis, ulcerative colitis, Alzheimer's disease, atherosclerosis, allergic reactions (asthma, eczema), and autoimmune disorders. Recently, there are numerous medications that are commercially available which can manage inflammations. The aim of contemporary research is on using nanotherapeutics to relieve severe illnesses both *in vitro* and *in vivo*. Most investigations on the application of nanotherapeutics to inflammation have produced a number of extremely positive and encouraging results (Brusini, Varna and Couvreur, 2020).

DOI: 10.1201/9781003442202-11

10.1 PROGRESS OF INFLAMMATORY DISEASES

As mentioned above, inflammation can be categorized depending on the possibility of being brought on by an exogenous chemical or by an endogenous deviant response. According to the duration it lasts, inflammation can either be acute or chronic (Xiao, 2017). Symptoms and signs of subacute inflammation can last between two and six weeks, while symptoms and signs of acute inflammation frequently last for several weeks. The body produces twice as many leukocytes within the region of the injured tissue during an acute inflammatory response. The immunological cells that are engaged in inflammatory responses include eosinophils, mononuclear cells such as monocytes and macrophages, neutrophils, serum proteins, cell receptors, including stimulation of Toll-like receptors, interferon-gamma (IFN-g), granulocytes–monocyte colony-stimulating factor (GM-CSF), and cells that liberate cytokines and biomarkers in inflammatory reactions such as macrophages (Cronkite and Strutt, 2018). Leukocytes, which belong to the category of white blood cells, are attracted to the region to assist in the removal of debris (Shi et al., 2012). The goal of the inflammation is to compensate for the harm and start the recovery pathway. Moreover, this is preceded by a variety of steps that persist to engage the immune system until the lesion or infection restores to equilibrium (Schauss, 2013). When the patient experiences none of the aforementioned symptoms or indicators, the inflammation is said to be a "silent inflammation."

Chronic inflammation can be described as an inflammation at a lower level that is characterized as persistent inflammation. It can last a lifespan or only a few months. This type of infection manifests as persistent fatigue, mouth ulcers, joint pain, discomfort in the stomach, redness, rash, and fever. On the contrary, a prolonged duration of the toxic by-products or pathogen being perceptible is the primary reason for persistent infection. Defense mechanisms are occasionally difficult to manage, causing harm to the vasculature, neurological system, musculoskeletal system, and other vital organs (Pahwa, Goyal and Jialal, 2022). It causes bowel disease, malignancy, sepsis, asthmatic conditions, obesity, diabetes, cardiac diseases, neurological diseases, and certain publications have documented Crohn's disease and rheumatoid polyarthritis (Molinaro et al., 2016). The condition is connected with an array of several conditions, including autoimmune disorders (Abdulkhaleq et al., 2018).

The ongoing generation of inflammatory cytokines, such as IFN-g, IL series of cytokines, as well as the generation of reactive oxygen species (ROS), which is the reason for oxidative stress including metabolic stress (hypoxia), represent the most potential culprits (Schauss, 2013). IL-1, IL-6, and TNF are examples of pro-inflammatory cytokines that have an impact on the pathophysiological basis of pain. Interleukin (IL-6) plays a crucial role inside the neural activity to microglia by activation of astrocytes, neurological damage, and the control of a neuropeptides in a neuronal phase. Two significant receptors on the cell surface called TNFR1 and TNFR2 govern the activation of the NF-B, inflammation, protein kinases activated by stress (SAPKs), and apoptotic cascades. Another inflammatory cytokine is TNF that is essential for innate and adaptive immunity, pro-inflammatory traits, proliferation and differentiation of cells, and inflammatory and neuropathic hyperalgesia (Tanaka, Narazaki and Kishimoto, 2014). The pathophysiological basis of inflammation can be understood by the proteins released by specific cells throughout

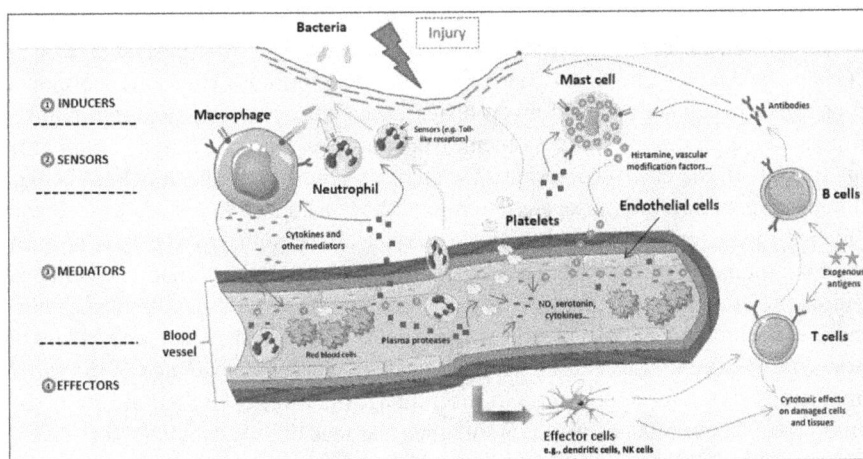

FIGURE 10.1 Schematic representation of the inflammatory response. Briefly, inducer signals (1) (e.g., wound, pathogens) trigger sensors (2) on inflammatory cells present in the damaged area, which start to induce the production and release of multiple mediators (3). Mediators, including plasma proteases, chemokines, cytokines, and vascular modification factors, lead in turn to vascular modifications, recruitment of blood platelets, and other inflammatory cells such as phagocytic leukocytes (e.g., neutrophils) and act on effector cells (4) and tissues to resolve inflammation. Adaptive immunity is also implicated in inflammation response, lymphocytes B and T are able to recognize and respond to antigens presented by antigen-presenting cells such as dendritic cells. Adaptive mechanisms may function either by direct cytotoxic effects or by secretion of antibodies interacting with elements of the innate inflammatory response (complement proteins, phagocytic cells, etc.).

Source: Reproduced with permission from Brusini, Varna and Couvreur, 2020.

inflammation (Zarrin et al., 2021). The aforementioned mechanisms and cellular components that play an important role in the inflammatory diseases are the therapeutic targets for developing nanotherapeutic formulations. Figure 10.1 shows the schematic representation of the inflammatory responses.

10.2 APPROACHES OF NANOTHERAPEUTICS IN INFLAMMATORY DISEASES

Immunological organs, immunological cells, and immunological chemicals are the building blocks of immune system. Currently, nanotherapeutic formulations primarily have an impact upon immune system by specifically interacting with a number of immunological cells and molecules. The conceptual basis for nanotherapeutic-based therapy is that nanomaterials can be developed by addressing the molecular and cellular materials that rely on their own characteristics and exert precise regulating activities.

Macrophages, a kingpin in the cellular components of the innate immunity system, are crucial in inflammatory responses. They play distinct functions in nearly every part of biological functions of an organism, including growth, homeostasis, tissue regeneration, and immunity (Wynn, Chawla and Pollard, 2013). They may be present in a variety of tissues and are incredibly diverse and changeable (Locati, Curtale and Mantovani, 2020). Several nanoparticle formulas have been developed to engage with monocytes and macrophages, which are major players in a number of pathogenic processes at the moment. Nanoparticles must be designed with various ligands on the exterior interface Those ligands may be monoclonal antibodies, oligomers, peptides, mannose, etc. Therefore, they can attach to particular receptors which are overexpressed upon the exterior surface of macrophages as well as perform these simultaneous processes. The control of bone marrow stimulation, monocyte migration, and enlistment, as well as the augmentation of vasculature permeability and the modification of polarization are only a few of the impacts of nanoparticles on monocytes/macrophages. Moreover, nanoparticles can take advantage of the inherent characteristics of monocytes and macrophages that improve their ability of targeting specific molecules while avoiding the clearance of the immunological system (Gaspar et al., 2019).

One of the main characteristics of inflammatory illnesses is bone marrow stimulation. Hematopoietic stem cells (HSCs) would multiply during inflammatory circumstances because of increased concentrations of pro-inflammatory cytokines, Toll-like receptors (TLR) agonists, as well as noradrenaline. This excess generation and supply of inflammatory monocytes would aggregate in ulcerations (Heidt et al., 2014; Mendelson and Frenette, 2014). Moreover, techniques to improve nanoparticle deposition in bone marrow were developed. The focusing affinity of bisphosphonates (like alendronate) to hydroxyapatite, the main mineral constituent of bone, can be increased by conjugating them to various varieties of nanoparticles (Ordikhani et al., 2021). Synthetic compounds, such as the anionic amphiphilic N-(3-carboxy-1-oxopropyl)-1,5-dihexadecyl ester of L-glutamic acid, can promote the aggregation of liposomes inside the bone marrow while concurrently inhibiting absorption in the liver (Sou et al., 2007). Furthermore, molecular imaging techniques may be utilized to evaluate the pharmacological impacts that nanoparticles have on the generation of monocytes in the bone marrow. For examples, 18F-3'-fuoro-3'-deoxy-1-thymidine-PET (18F-FLT-PET) can be used to measure the multiplication of bone marrow monocytes and HSCs (Agool et al., 2011).

Nanotherapeutic agents may potentially be developed to regulate the mobilization and engagement of monocytes and macrophages. Monocytes and macrophages can be activated and recruited within the process of chronic inflammation by a wide assortment of chemokines, such as CCL2 (also known as monocyte chemotactic protein 1 or MCP-1) and chemokine C–C motif ligand 7 (CCL7), and receptor molecules, such as angiotensin II (Ang II) receptors (Alaarg et al., 2017) which then concentrate in the location of inflammation (Qi et al., 2019). Inhibiting the migration and recruiting of inflammatory monocytes and macrophages is one way that nanotherapeutic agents designed to target such substances can act as an anti-inflammatory agent (Kratofl, Kubes and Deniset, 2017).

Both local macrophage growth and recruitment of circulating monocytes have been shown to contribute to lesional inflammation (Robbins et al., 2013). Several solutions including nanoparticles are developed to limit the growth of focal macrophages or even to immediately deplete them in order to lessen the consequence of local inflammation. Since many years, clodronate liposomes have served as the preferred drug for depleting macrophages in a number of illness scenarios. In animal models of induced endometriosis, Bacci et al. used clodronate liposomes to deplete macrophages (Bacci et al., 2009).

Macrophage polarization is crucial in the progression of inflammation, particularly in the pathophysiology of several inflammatory disorders. Nanostructured materials with a metallic nature have also been used to control the polarization of macrophages. Gold nanoparticles (AuNP) exhibit anti-inflammatory properties in mice in addition to a number of beneficial biochemical features. Researchers used a laboratory mouse model induced with cecal ligation as well as puncture laboratory animal model of bacterial sepsis to administer AuNP as an additive to antibiotics. According to the outcomes, AuNP may enhance M2 macrophages (CD206+ve in F4/80+ve cells) and diminish M1 macrophages (CD86+ve in F4/80+ve cells) inside the spleens of laboratory mice induced with sepsis. These impacts were further demonstrated by *in vitro* tests (Taratummarat et al., 2018).

Nanomaterials must get through the immune system, traverse the biological barriers in the human body, and then navigate their way to the designated tissues in order to be therapeutically effective [67], which calls for a variety of intricate processes. Nanoporous silicon nanoparticles covered with leukocyte-derived cellular membranes were created by Parodi et al. (Parodi et al., 2013). These hybrid nanoparticles can deliver and discharge their payload throughout an inflamed reconstructed endothelium, escape opsonization and decrease phagocytosis, and interact with endothelial cells via receptor–ligand encounter, all of which suggest a prospects for their use in the treatment of inflammatory diseases and tumors. Monitoring monocytes and macrophages is another method for spotting inflammatory reactions. Iron oxide nanoparticles were produced to mark and detect monocytes in patients with cutaneous inflammation without impairing their viability or functionality (Richards et al., 2012). These particles have been shown to be secure for use in humans.

Another subset of cells in the innate immune system, neutrophils, play an essential part in resistance to external pathogens during acute inflammation despite having a low capacity for biosynthesis (Mantovani et al., 2011). Recent studies have examined using albumin nanoparticles coupled with piceatannol to administer therapeutics to neutrophils for acute lung damage. As inflammation occurs, neutrophils can cling to endothelial layer in the vasculature and penetrate into lesioned area, which is a key factor in a number of inflammatory conditions (Liew and Kubes, 2019). In laboratory mouse models induced with traumatic primary spinal cord injury (SCI), treatment with PLG NPs decrease fourfold the overall quantity of neutrophils within the site of injury and reduce threefold the scar ring of fibrosis, suggesting the development of a prodegenerative extracellular matrix that endorses regeneration and improved recovery in their function (Park et al., 2019).

The development of inflammatory ailments is significantly influenced by the generation of neutrophils, which is a significant component of the acute immune response. The capacity to preferentially target and deplete active neutrophils has been described for one form of pH-responsive albumin nanomaterials coupled with doxorubicin (DOX) (Zhang et al., 2019). Neutrophils are additionally employed as carriers to distribute therapeutic substances, much like the hitchhiking techniques connected to monocyte or macrophages. Denatured albumin protein nanoparticles (albumin NPs) have been found to be swallowed by neutrophils and may be utilized to distribute therapeutic medicines (Wang et al., 2014).

Nanoparticles with neutrophil membrane coatings take on some characteristics from normal neutrophils. They have the ability to target infected tissue, destroy pathological chemicals, evade immune monitoring, and more. Neutrophil-simulating NPs have been considered as prospective therapeutic portals for the management of

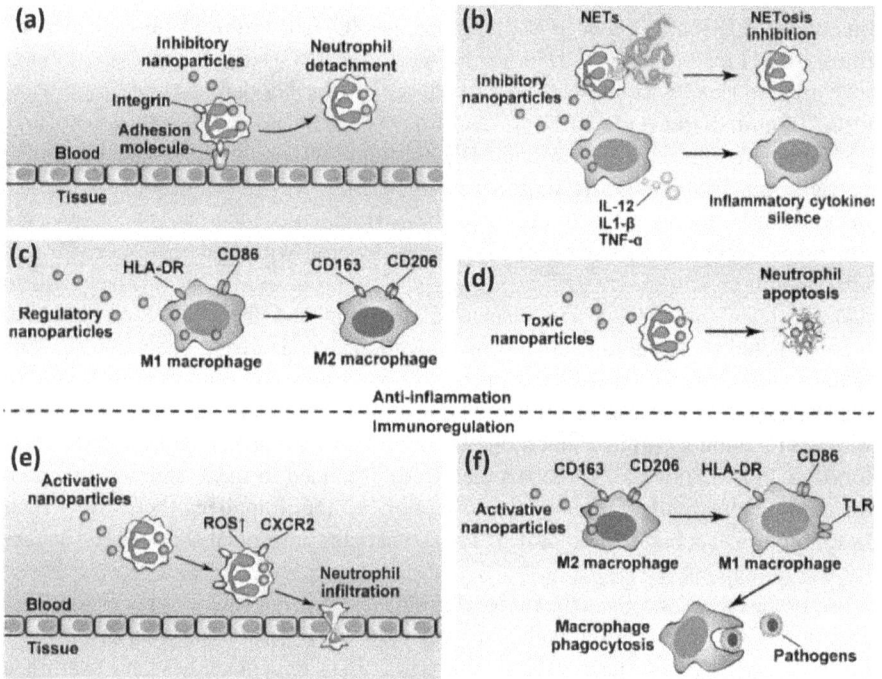

FIGURE 10.2 Targeting neutrophils and macrophages using nanoparticles for immunotherapies in inflammatory disorders. (a) Albumin nanoparticles loaded with piceatannol inhibit the neutrophil adhesion to endothelium, thus blocking neutrophil infiltration. (b) Nanoparticles inhibit the functions of activated neutrophils and macrophages to reduce pro-inflammatory factors and NETs release. (c) Nanoparticles transform macrophages from the pro-inflammatory M1 phenotype (biomarkers of human leukocyte antigen-DR isotype (HLA-DR) and CD86) to anti-inflammatory M2 phenotype (biomarkers of CD163 and CD206). (d) DOX-loaded nanoparticles induce neutrophil apoptosis to induce the resolution of inflammation. (e) Nanoparticles activate neutrophil by upregulating intracellular reactive oxygen species (ROS) level and CXCR2 to restore neutrophil pathogen clearance. (f) Nanoparticles induce the transition of immunosuppressive M2 macrophages to immunoenhancement M1 macrophages to enhance phagocytosis.

Source: Reproduced with permission from Su et al., 2020.

inflammatory disorders (Zhang et al., 2018). Figure 10.2 shows targeting neutrophils and macrophages using nanoparticles for immunotherapies in inflammatory disorders.

Hematopoietic stem cells (HSCs) located in the skeletal system are considered as the prototypes of immune cells. The two types of initially differentiated cells of HSCs are typical lymphoid progenitor (CLP) and myeloid progenitor (CMP) cells. T and B lymphocytes seem to be the primary constituents and primary particle emitters of adaptive immunity, whereas CMP cells represent the progenitors of granulocytes, megakaryocytes, macrophages, erythrocytes, etc. (Orkin and Zon, 2008). An important factor in the pathophysiology of numerous inflammatory illnesses is the autoreactive immune mechanism. Scientists have used poly(lactide-*co*-glycolide) NPs with coated antigen [PLG(Ag)] to address T2-mediated allergic airway inflammation. PLG(Ag) nanoparticles have been readily accepted and efficiently reduced ovalbumin (OVA)-induced T2 reactions and airway inflammation either prophylactically or in a therapeutic manner (Smarr et al., 2016).

Rheumatism and acute inflammation are two examples of inflammatory disorders that can be brought on by autoreactive T cells. In a laboratory mouse model of imiquimod-induced psoriasis, Özcan et al. revealed that gold nanoparticles coupled with MTX had greater anti-inflammatory activity to MTX separately (Özcan et al., 2020). The adaptive immune system is carried out by B lymphocytes, which differentiate to plasma cells and secrete antibodies in response to B cell receptors (BCR) attaching to their corresponding antigens (Yang and Reth, 2016). Another team demonstrated the potential to specifically target and deprive autoreactive B cells for therapeutic strategies in rheumatoid arthritis using poly(DL-lactic-*co* glycolic acid) NPs embellished with synthetic citrullinated peptide as well as complement-activating lytic peptide to significantly decrease the ACPA generation of B cells from peptide seropositive patients with rheumatoid arthritis (Pozsgay et al., 2016).

In addition to the cellular components in the immunological system, cytokines, receptors, enzymes, reactive oxygen species (ROS), and other molecules play crucial roles in the process of inflammation and are now being used as therapeutic targets in disorders that cause inflammation. Moreover, studies have shown that nanoparticles can regulate the concentrations of a variety of cytokines while managing inflammatory disorders. For instance, PLGA nanoparticles loaded with metformin hydrochloride might lower IL-1 and TNF levels (Pereira et al., 2018).

In parallel to the interconnections among nanoparticles and the immune system described above, nanoparticles can further influence immunological responses through interacting with dendritic cells, regulating the activity of natural killer (NK) cells, and other ways.

Many immunomodulatory nanodrugs have already received FDA approval, and more are undergoing preclinical research or clinical trials. In contrast to existing anti-inflammatory substances, which are primarily palliative, nanoparticles are capable of dealing with the infective factors of inflammatory ailments. This is due to their unique properties in their structure, plasticity, and consistency, which give them a tremendous potential to approach and accumulate inside the inflamed tissues (Liu et al., 2022).

REFERENCES

Abdulkhaleq, L. A. et al. (2018) "The crucial roles of inflammatory mediators in inflammation: A review," *Veterinary World*, 11(5), pp. 627–635.

Agool, A. et al. (2011) "Effect of radiotherapy and chemotherapy on bone marrow activity: A 18F-FLT-PET study," *Nuclear Medicine Communications*, 32, pp. 17–22.

Alaarg, A. et al. (2017) "Applying nanomedicine in maladaptive inflammation and angiogenesis," *Advanced Drug Delivery Reviews*, 119, pp. 143–158.

Bacci, M. et al. (2009) "Macrophages are alternatively activated in patients with endometriosis and required for growth and vascularization of lesions in a mouse model of disease," *The American Journal of Pathology*, 175(2), pp. 547–556. doi: 10.2353/ajpath.2009.081011.

Brusini, R., Varna, M. and Couvreur, P. (2020) "Advanced nanomedicines for the treatment of inflammatory diseases," *Advanced Drug Delivery Reviews*, 157, pp. 161–178. doi: 10.1016/j.addr.2020.07.010.

Cronkite, D. A. and Strutt, T. M. (2018) "The regulation of inflammation by innate and adaptive lymphocytes," *J. Immunol. Res.*, 2018, p. 1467538. https://doi.org/10.1155/2018/1467538. PMID: 29992170; PMCID: PMC6016164.

Gaspar, N. et al. (2019) "Active nano-targeting of macrophages," *Current Pharmaceutical Design*, 25(17), pp. 1951–1961. doi: 10.2174/1381612825666190710114108.

Goldstein, I. M., Snyderman, R. and Gallin, J. I. (1992) "Inflammation: Basic principles and clinical correlates". *Annals of Internal Medicine*, 109(6), p. 519. doi: 10.7326/0003-4819-109-6-519_2.

Heidt, T. et al. (2014) "Chronic variable stress activates hematopoietic stem cells," *Nature Medicine*, 20(7), pp. 754–758. doi: 10.1038/nm.3589.

Jogpal, V. et al. (2022) "Advancement of nanomedicines in chronic inflammatory disorders," *Inflammopharmacology*, 30(2), pp. 355–368. doi: 10.1007/s10787-022-00927-x.

Kratofl, R. M., Kubes, P. and Deniset, J. F. (2017) "Monocyte conversion during inflammation and injury," *Arteriosclerosis Thrombosis Vascular Biology*, 37, pp. 35–42.

Liew, P. X. and Kubes, P. (2019) "The neutrophil's role during health and disease," *Physiological Reviews*, 99(2), pp. 1223–1248. doi: 10.1152/physrev.00012.2018.

Liu, J. et al. (2022) "The interaction between nanoparticles and immune system: Application in the treatment of inflammatory diseases," *Journal of Nanobiotechnology*, 20(1), p. 127. doi: 10.1186/s12951-022-01343-7.

Locati, M., Curtale, G. and Mantovani, A. (2020) "Diversity, mechanisms, and significance of macrophage plasticity," *Annual Review of Pathology*, 15.

Mantovani, A. et al. (2011) "Neutrophils in the activation and regulation of innate and adaptive immunity," *Nature Reviews: Immunology*, 11(8), pp. 519–531. doi: 10.1038/nri3024.

Medzhitov, R. (2008) "Origin and physiological roles of inflammation," *Nature*, 454(7203), 428–435. https://doi.org/10.1038/nature0720 1454:428.

Mendelson, A. and Frenette, P. S. (2014) "Hematopoietic stem cell niche maintenance during homeostasis and regeneration," *Nature Medicine*, 20(8), pp. 833–846. doi: 10.1038/nm.3647.

Molinaro, R. et al. (2016) "Vascular inflammation: A novel access route for nanomedicine," *Methodist Debakey Cardiovasc*, 12, pp. 169–174.

Ordikhani, F. et al. (2021) "Targeted nanomedicines for the treatment of bone disease and regeneration," *Medicinal Research Reviews*, 41(3), pp. 1221–1254. doi: 10.1002/med.21759.

Orkin, S. H. and Zon, L. I. (2008) "Hematopoiesis: An evolving paradigm for stem cell biology," *Cell*, 132(4), pp. 631–644. doi: 10.1016/j.cell.2008.01.025.

Özcan, A. et al. (2020) "Nanoparticle-coupled topical methotrexate can normalize immune responses and induce tissue remodeling in psoriasis," *The Journal of Investigative Dermatology*, 140(5), pp. 1003–1014.e8. doi: 10.1016/j.jid.2019.09.018.

Pahwa, R., Goyal, A. and Jialal, I. (2022) *Chronic inflammation*. Tampa, Florida: StatPearls Publishing.

Park, J. et al. (2019) "Intravascular innate immune cells reprogrammed via intravenous nanoparticles to promote functional recovery after spinal cord injury," *Proceedings of the National Academy of Sciences of the United States of America*, 116(30), pp. 14947–14954. doi: 10.1073/pnas.1820276116.

Parodi, A. et al. (2013) "Synthetic nanoparticles functionalized with biomimetic leukocyte membranes possess cell-like functions," *Nature Nanotechnology*, 8(1), pp. 61–68. doi: 10.1038/nnano.2012.212.

Pereira, A. et al. (2018) "Metformin hydrochloride-loaded PLGA nanoparticle in periodontal disease experimental model using diabetic rats," *International Journal of Molecular Sciences*, 19(11), p. 3488. doi: 10.3390/ijms19113488.

Pozsgay, J. et al. (2016) "In vitro eradication of citrullinated protein specific B-lymphocytes of rheumatoid arthritis patients by targeted bifunctional nanoparticles," *Arthritis Research and Therapy*, 18.

Qi, D. et al. (2019) "Hypoxia inducible factor 1α in vascular smooth muscle cells promotes angiotensin II-induced vascular remodeling via activation of CCL7-mediated macrophage recruitment," *Cell Death & Disease*, 10(8), p. 544. doi: 10.1038/s41419-019-1757-0.

Richards, J. M. J. et al. (2012) "In vivo mononuclear cell tracking using superparamagnetic particles of iron oxide: Feasibility and safety in humans," *Circulation: Cardiovascular Imaging*, 5(4), pp. 509–517. doi: 10.1161/CIRCIMAGING.112.972596.

Robbins, C. S. et al. (2013) "Local proliferation dominates lesional macrophage accumulation in atherosclerosis," *Nature Medicine*, 19(9), pp. 1166–1172. doi: 10.1038/nm.3258.

Schauss, A. G. (2013) "Polyphenols and inflammation," in Watson, R. R. and Preedy, V. R. (eds.) *Bioactive food as dietary interventions for arthritis and related inflammatory diseases*. San Diego: Academic Press, pp. 379–392.

Shi, Y. et al. (2012) "How mesenchymal stem cells interact with tissue immune responses," *Trends in Immunology*, 33(3), pp. 136–143. doi: 10.1016/j.it.2011.11.004.

Smarr, C. B. et al. (2016) "Biodegradable antigen-associated PLG nanoparticles tolerize Th2-mediated allergic airway inflammation pre- and postsensitization," *Proceedings of the National Academy of Sciences of the United States of America*, 113(18), pp. 5059–5064. doi: 10.1073/pnas.1505782113.

Sou, K. et al. (2007) "Selective uptake of surface-modified phospholipid vesicles by bone marrow macrophages in vivo," *Biomaterials*, 28, pp. 2655–2666.

Su, Y. et al. (2020) "Neutrophils and macrophages as targets for development of nanotherapeutics in inflammatory diseases," *Pharmaceutics*, 12(12), p. 1222. doi: 10.3390/pharmaceutics12121222.

Tanaka, T., Narazaki, M. and Kishimoto, T. (2014) "IL-6 in inflammation, immunity, and disease," *Cold Spring Harbor Perspectives in Biology*, 6(10), p. a016295. doi: 10.1101/cshperspect.a016295.

Taratummarat, S. et al. (2018) "Gold nanoparticles attenuates bacterial sepsis in cecal ligation and puncture mouse model through the induction of M2 macrophage polarization," *BMC Microbiology*, 18(1), p. 85. doi: 10.1186/s12866-018-1227-3.

Wang, Z. et al. (2014) "Prevention of vascular inflammation by nanoparticle targeting of adherent neutrophils," *Nature Nanotechnology*, 9, pp. 204–210.

Wynn, T. A., Chawla, A. and Pollard, J. W. (2013) "Macrophage biology in development, homeostasis and disease," *Nature*, 496(7446), pp. 445–455. doi: 10.1038/nature12034.

Xiao, T. S. (2017) "Innate immunity and inflammation," *Cellular & Molecular Immunology*, 14(1), pp. 1–3. doi: 10.1038/cmi.2016.45.

Yang, J. and Reth, M. (2016) "Receptor dissociation and B-cell activation," *Current Topics in Microbiology and Immunology*, 393, pp. 27–43. doi: 10.1007/82_2015_482.

Zarrin, A. A., Bao, K., Lupardus, P. and Vucic, D. (2021) "Kinase inhibition in autoimmunity and inflammation," *Nature Reviews Drug Discovery*, 20, 39–63.

Zhang, C. Y. et al. (2019) "Nanoparticle-induced neutrophil apoptosis increases survival in sepsis and alleviates neurological damage in stroke," *Science Advances*, 5(11), p. eaax7964. doi: 10.1126/sciadv.aax7964.

Zhang, Q. et al. (2018) "Neutrophil membrane-coated nanoparticles inhibit synovial inflammation and alleviate joint damage in inflammatory arthritis," *Nature Nanotechnology*, 13, pp. 1182–1190.

11 Nanotherapeutics in Skin Diseases and Cosmetology

INTRODUCTION

The incorporation of active pharmaceutical ingredients (APIs) into medication delivery systems in nanoscale is now being employed to encourage pharmaceutical innovation by designing nanotherapeutics. A variety of dermatological products currently exist on the marketplace for the medical management of wounds to the skin, including atopic dermatitis, carcinoma of the skin, burns on the skin, wound recovery, and shielding from ultraviolet (UV) radiations. These medications demonstrate the effectiveness of nanotherapeutics employed in delivering of APIs across the skin. The development of novel sunscreens with nanoproducts is an exemplification in this case. Consumer safety of these nanomaterials-incorporated products is reportedly enhanced, which reduces the adverse reactions of UV inorganic filtering materials like titanium dioxide (TiO_2) and zinc oxide (ZnO) as well as chemical filters like benzophenone-3 (Barbosa et al., 2019; Osmond-McLeod et al., 2016). Additionally, it is being shown that introducing sunscreen to solid nanomaterials may possess a synergistic impact because nanoparticles can potentially shield sunlight. Various kinds of nanoparticles are being suggested in recent years for incorporating vitamins, antiaging agents, antiwrinkle agents, antioxidants, and sunscreens into skin care formulas (Antonio et al., 2014).

The human skin has multiple layers. The following three methods are proposed for allowing the solvent to pass through the horny epidermal layer: the transfollicle permeation (via hair follicles) as well as sudoriparous hair ducts involved in multiple investigations have demonstrated the existence of transfollicle channel that is a highly important pathway for numerous substances to enter the body; The intercellular permeation of the substances tortuously disperse throughout the horny cells, perpetually residing in the lipid matrices. Finally, the transcellular permeation of the substances move straight across the horny cells into the intercellular lipid matrices (Barry, 2001). The dimensions of the molecules in the medication are also important. Molecules greater than 200–350 Da have an extremely challenging time penetrating intact skin; 400 Da have been considered to represent the maximum molecular size. Whenever the layer of horny cells lacks, the majority of tiny, nonelectrolytic, molecules that are water soluble permeate to the circulatory system approximately a thousand times fast (Cevc et al., 1996).

Researchers aim to remove this hurdle in order to increase substance movement; however, occasionally the follicular pathway can be significant. Skin responds as a mechanically nanoporous barrier that can be breached by numerous, semicircular tunnels or paths from a penetration perspective. According to the majority of reports, the average diameter of these aforementioned hydrophilic "pores" is 0.4–36.0 nm. Different approaches have been suggested to enhance this pathway and alter the molecular design that comprises corneocytes and the numerous intercellular lipid sheets since the majority of passive permeating molecules traverse the skin through those intercellular "microchannels." Nanoparticles are directly involved in this phenomenon (Barry, 2001).

Considering the cosmeceuticals, moisturizing lotions comprising liposomes were the initial cosmetics developed utilizing nanotechnology, and they were introduced four decades ago. Cosmeceuticals, and particularly nanocosmeceuticals, have experienced the fastest increase in the personal care goods sector over the past few decades. The regulated release of active pharmaceutical ingredients (APIs), location-specific targeting, and occlusive qualities with increased hydration are the key benefits of nanocosmeceuticals. Given some of these benefits, clinical trials and regulation of nanocosmeceuticals are essential steps to guaranteeing the safety of the public (Singhal, Khanna and Nasa, 2011).

11.1   THE STRUCTURE OF THE HUMAN SKIN

The architecture of the skin, a multilayered organ made up of epidermis, dermis, and hypodermis, is shown schematically in Figure 11.1. Because it is made up of a stratified, compact epithelium, the epidermis, regarded as the outermost superficial layer, serves as the primary physical–chemical barrier against the penetration of bioactive substances. The epidermis is made up of keratinocytes which are constantly moving from lower to superficial layers. These keratinocytes are attached to one another by desmosomes, adhesive junctions, and tight junctions that prevent chemicals from diffusing into the dermis underneath. The four epidermis layers—the stratum corneum (SC), the stratum granulosum (SG), the stratum spinosum (SS), and the stratum basale (SB)—that run from the outermost layer downward to the underlying basement membrane (BM) are various phases of keratin maturation (Salvioni et al., 2021).

This has been described as a "brick and mortar" structure laden with desmosomes, in which nonaligned corneocytes (displacement 15–30%) are dispersed in a lipidic matrix. The SC constitutes a nonaligned "brick-and-mortar" architecture made up of enucleated deceased cells (corneocytes) that are enveloped by a lipidic matrix. The surface of the SC is entirely covered in many skin furrows that vary in depth. Although SC that constitutes the lipophilic stratum (approximately 15% water) is responsible for the vast majority of the preventive function governed by the epidermis, the remaining strata, which are combined for convenience into just a single multilayer termed viable epidermis (VE), have a more hydrophilic nature (75% water). Together with the hypodermis, the dermis offers the epidermis trophic as well as structural support. It primarily consists of fibroblasts and a reticulum of elastin and collagen fibers embedded in a proteoglycan-based framework. These more profound layers contain blood vessels (Salvioni et al., 2021).

11.2   THE IMPACT OF THE SIZE OF ACTIVE MOLECULES IN DERMATOLOGICAL AGENTS

Depending on physical and chemical characteristics of various layers of the skin, molecules may penetrate through the epidermal layer in a variety of ways. A 500

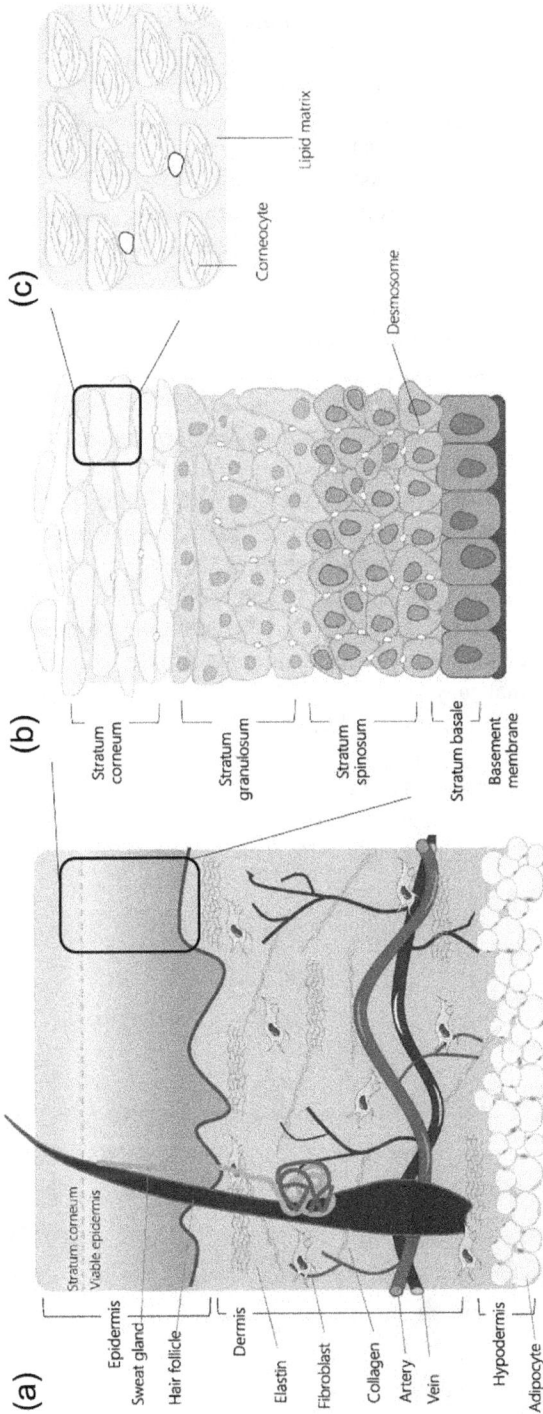

FIGURE 11.1 Schematic representation of the skin. (a) Epidermis and dermis have a thickness of 0.1–0.2 mm and 2.0–5.0 mm, respectively, while the thickness of the hypodermis varies greatly between individuals depending on the anatomical site. (b) Epidermis structure. Viable epidermis (50–150 μm) and the stratum corneum (10–20 μm) differ in hydrophilicity and pH, which ranges between 4.5 and 5.5 on mammalian SC surfaces and approaches neutrality at the SC–SG interface. (c) Stratum corneum composition.

Source: Reproduced with permission from Salvioni et al., 2021.

Da limit has been considered as the molecular weight (MW) threshold permitted for the penetration into the skin of compounds (Bos and Meinardi, 2000). The scientific arena differs on the matter of NP penetration for a minimum of a pair of factors: first, the toxicological consequences associated with nanotechnology, and second, the requirement to reveal the function of nanomaterials as transporters to improve the penetration regarding the bioactive substance. The SC is each ingredient's initial and most significant barrier, as previously stated. Each of the three paths (transcellular, intercellular, and appendageal route) used to explain the penetration of other compounds has been reported for nanoparticles in skin (Liang et al., 2013). The size of the nanoparticles is crucial in this phenomenon. According to a theoretical examination of the SC framework, nanomaterials that are smaller than 36 nm could potentially be able to infiltrate through aqueous pores with a superficial diameter of 0.4–36 nm, while nanoparticles smaller than 5–7 nm seem more likely to accomplish so through the intercellular lipidic matrices (Baroli, 2010).

In addition, nanoobjects that can be disseminated in perspiration and sebum can accumulate due to the vast follicular spacing (10–210 nm) (Mahmoud et al., 2017). Chemical–physical characteristics of the skin surface can affect the speed with which NPs penetrate (negatively charged NPs may penetrate the epidermis more easily than the positive charged NPs, for example) (Lee et al., 2013) or they can prolong the time that these systems are available in the SC (lipid coating, for example, improves retention in lipid-rich SC) (Jensen, Petersson and Nielsen, 2011). Figure 11.2 shows the potential routes of the penetration of nanomaterials into the skin. There are certain general statements that may be offered to distinguish between insoluble and lipid- or surfactant-based nanoparticles, despite the fact that nanoparticles vary in their capacity to penetrate depending on their dimensions, composition, stability of the colloids, and carrier qualities (Larese Filon et al., 2015). The first category consists of polymeric nanocomplexes which remain bio-persistent following being applied to the human skin and inorganic NPs. The actions of these nanoparticles

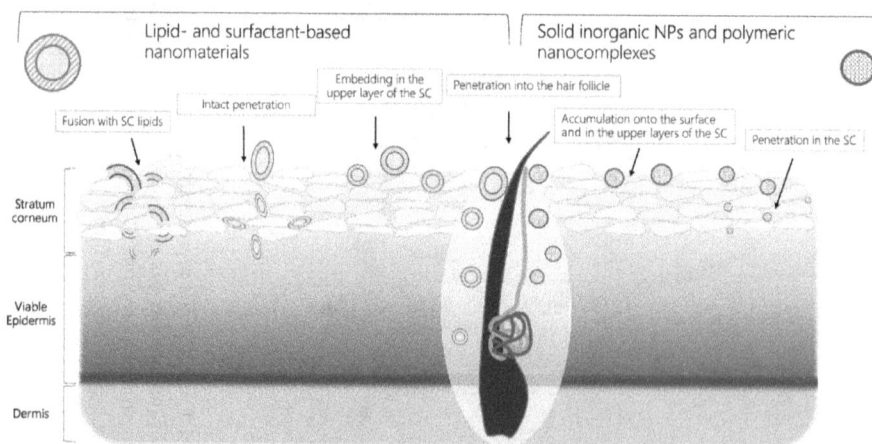

FIGURE 11.2   Potential routes of the penetration of nanomaterials into the skin.

Source: Reproduced with permission from Salvioni et al., 2021.

have been the subject of numerous investigations. Since this experimental design is typically believed to be more trustworthy than alternative laboratory animal models, researchers are concentrating on the findings obtained utilizing human skin herein (Roberts et al., 2017). The information provided indicates that bio-persistent nanoparticles primarily accumulate on the outermost layer of intact skin as well as in the more superficial layers of the SC, considering the small size necessary for penetration. Zinc was identified in the more profound layers of the dermis and epidermis as an outcome of NP dissolution because topically administered ZnO, the type of zinc employed most frequently in sunscreen, exhibited no substantial penetration into normal skin. Additionally, these findings were confirmed on skin with impairment and in occlusive situations (Leite-Silva et al., 2016). Comparable to TiO_2 NPs, another excellent mineral-based sunblock component, SC's initial layers are impermeable to particles 20–100 nm in dimension (Lohani et al., 2014). These nanoparticles are not dispersing throughout the tissues that surround it, despite the fact that they appear to enter the follicular region more deeply (Lekki et al., 2007).

11.3   NANOTHERAPEUTICS AS SUNSCREEN AGENTS

UV radiation is classified as UVA (wavelength = 320–400 nm), UVB (wavelength = 280–320 nm), and UVC (wavelength = 100–280 nm) and accounts for around 10% of the total radiation emissions. The only types of radiation that considerably permeate the atmosphere as well as endanger human health are those featuring the longest wavelengths, such as UVA and UVB. UV filtration systems, which are typically categorized into two categories—inorganic or organic—can be used for photoprotection (D'Orazio et al., 2013).

In the field of cosmetics, the prevention of sunburn and long-exposure consequences (such as skin aging and skin malignancies) depend heavily on a decrease of UV-induced damage to the skin, and the incorporation of filters have become commonplace in daily-use treatments in addition to sunscreens (Burke, 2018). Filter-containing formulas are presently made to provide UVA and UVB protection. Although this type of radiation has higher energy, it plays an important role in the development of cancer: UVA permeates deeper into the epidermal layers, inhibiting immune function and causing precancerous alterations (Burke, 2018). Additionally, UVA upregulates the synthesis of matrix metalloproteinases, which break down collagen and elastin, which is the main cause of skin elasticity decline (Battie et al., 2014). Inorganic filters frequently utilize insoluble TiO_2 and ZnO particles, particularly when they are nanosized in their dimensions (30–150 nm). The utilization of TiO_2 and ZnO-NPs, which reflect just a tiny fraction of the incident light particles and produce a transparent impact, better satisfies consumer expectations than micrometer-sized particles. In addition, as opposed to organic filters, these filters are more environment-friendly, safer, and photostable (Schneider and Lim, 2019).

11.4   NANOTHERAPEUTICS AS ANTIMICROBIAL AGENTS

Because of the emergence of strains that are resistant and toxicities, frequently employed antimicrobic drugs have a limited potency and effectiveness (Singh, Young and Silver, 2017). The antimicrobial activity of several metal-based nanoparticles, including Ag-, Au-, Co-, ZnO-, TiO_2-, and Cu-based nanomaterials, has consequently been explored for a variety of applications (including the textile, nourishment, and cosmetics sectors). Numerous nanoparticles have the inherent capacity to enhance skin well-being, while this is not their primary application. This increases the significance of nanocosmetic products (Niska et al., 2018).

11.5 NANOTHERAPEUTICS FOR ANTISEPSIS

Another important application of nanoparticles is in antisepsis. In addition to providing an instant antibacterial impact due to rapid absorption through the capsule wall, chlorhexidine gluconate transported by nanoparticles (Nanochlorex®) also has a lasting effect owing to persistent liberation from the nucleus of the particle (Roberts et al., 2017). The efficacy of the particles in formulations is equivalent to 60% isopropanol, which renders them a good substitute for alcohol-based hand treatments, which might cause some harm to the skin after prolonged use (Holmes et al., 2020). Because of their photocatalytic activity, other nanoparticles, including bare TiO_2, exhibit antimicrobial characteristics. Uncovered TiO_2 works as a photocatalyst to encourage the peroxidation of the polyunsaturated phospholipid present in the bacterial lipid membrane after being exposed to UV light (Lohani et al., 2014). The most widely utilized antibacterial nanoformulation currently in use is nanosilver, which is employed not only as a bandage for wounds and burns but also as a disinfectant for water and an interior spray. Its antibacterial impact is most likely caused by its mitochondrial toxicity as a result of interactions with oxidative stress-causing moieties of internal membrane protein thiols (Lekki et al., 2007).

11.6 NANOTHERAPEUTICS AS MOISTURIZING AGENTS

To improve skin hydration, moisturizing chemicals are applied. Traditional moisturizing methods use occlusive substances or humectants that trap and preserve water within the skin. Occlusive substances, such as petrolatum, beeswax, and fatty acids, prevent water evaporation by creating a film on the human skin (Kim et al., 2018). For the purpose of providing a sustained liberation of the active component, chitosan was coated onto PLGA NPs that were encasing ceramides. This technique made use of chitosan's adhesiveness and dispersion at an acidic pH. An experimental *in vivo* atopic dermatitis model data revealed that therapy with this formulation promoted skin regeneration with greater efficacy than the commercial medication (Jung et al., 2015).

Unsaturated phospholipid-based liposomes have a tendency to separate after their application to the skin; as a result, their constituent parts might reach deep inside the SC and have a moisturizing impact there. This is a result of both phospholipids' catabolism and internal hygroscopicity. Particularly, the activity of skin phospolipases results in the formation of osmolytes (such as betaine), which inhibit the loss of water by maintaining the number of keratinocytes and boosting the expression of tight junctions (El-Chami et al., 2014).

It was recently suggested that nanocrystals could boost the effectiveness of several kinds of bioactive substances employed in cosmetics in addition to their function as UV filters. Luscious, silky, and soft commodities are often well-received by consumers;

however, plenty of molecules and extracts exhibiting beneficial impacts on skin health are pigmented and insoluble, which limits their effectiveness. Solubility issues of an active ingredient can impact the homogeneity of the product and restrict its absorption in addition to providing it an unpleasant aesthetic. The nanonization of bioactive substances has been suggested as an alternative to these problems; in fact, the vast surface area of nanocrystals enhances penetration kinetics and skin adhesion capability. The usage of nanocrystals for cosmetic purposes has been discussed in a number of publications. For example, flavonoids, ubiquinone, lutein, and resveratrol all are examples of fat-soluble antioxidants that have been the focus of research on bioactive substances (Salvioni et al., 2021).

11.7 NANOTHERAPEUTICS AS RHEOLOGY MODIFIERS OF DERMATOLOGICAL PRODUCTS

Rheology modifiers, frequently referred to as thickening agents, are added to cosmetic compositions to increase viscosity, enhance sensory properties, and give the consumer a sense of quality. It has become quite common to use nanomaterials, primarily clay and silica NPs, as rheology moderators. Additionally, silica NPs are ideal for cosmetic uses due to their chemical inertness. The temporary NP aggregation to create a percolating matrix that has no impact on the product's spreading as it disintegrates under mechanical pressure might be the cause of the thickness impact. In addition to thickening the product, silica nanoparticles give it an opaque appearance and have been researched as skin defenders due to their capacity to absorb and neutralize harmful compounds (Bolzinger, Briançon and Chevalier, 2011).

11.8 NANOTHERAPEUTICS AS ANTIOXIDANTS IN DERMATOLOGY

Retinol, a form of vitamin A, and retinoids, its analogues, are some of the most widely utilized active substances in cosmetics. They are capable to control sebum, boost the generation of extracellular matrix, and support the development, differentiation, and upkeep of epidermal cells, all of which help to lessen wrinkles and acne. Additionally, they are used for managing pigmentation and photoaging diseases due to their capacity to induce cellular turnover, limit melanogenesis, and impede the transfer of melanin into epidermal cells. Antioxidants (AOs) shield DNA from oxidative stress brought on by the presence of ROS. ROS are produced as a result of numerous external or internal triggers. By neutralizing ROS, preventing ROS-producing enzymes, and chelating transition metal particles, AOs are able to achieve this goal. The excessive generation of ROS that UV radiation induces in the skin leads to aging (wrinkles and hyperpigmentation) as well as cancer. Van Tran et al. (Van Tran, Moon and Lee, 2019) recently presented a thorough overview of the difficulties in employing liposomes for the transportation of AOs. Other delivery methods besides liposomes have been used to increase the function of AOs (Sorg et al., 2006).

11.9 NANOTHERAPEUTICS AS ANTIAGING AGENTS

In youthful skin, hyaluronic acid (HA), which is an endogenous glycosaminoglycan, is abundant; nevertheless, as skin ages, its levels inevitably decline. HA is frequently used as an emollient because of its capacity to hold onto water molecules. Furthermore, HA can be employed as an antiwrinkle agent because it is a physiological component of the extracellular matrix of the human skin. Despite these advantageous effects, HA's huge molecular weight (>500 kDa) and high hydrophilicity lead to limited penetration, which severely restricts its potential. In addition to being utilized as a soft-tissue padding, HA may be integrated into a variety of cosmetic products as topical application. In this instance, intradermal microinjection is used to compensate for HA's poor permeability (Bukhari et al., 2018).

11.10 NANOTHERAPEUTICS IN SEBACEOUS GLAND–RELATED DISEASES

A crucial part of the pilosebaceous component is the sebaceous gland. Since the sebaceous duct enters the hair follicle canal, efforts for treating disorders that affect the hair follicle are especially helped by the follicular penetration of externally applied materials. Early studies by Schaefer et al. using adapalene fragments carried by polymerized particles (PLA and PLGA) have demonstrated the usefulness of particle networks for drug delivery for intrafollicular medication delivery and for significantly improved success in addressing sebaceous gland problems like acne in addition to pilose sebaceous disorders (Van Tran, Moon and Lee, 2019).

11.11 NANOTHERAPEUTICS FOR HAIR GROWTH PROBLEMS

Particle delivery networks for medications are demonstrated to be a crucial component in treating hair diseases as they promote the penetration of drugs within hair follicle apertures and serve as a deposition for continuous drug release. Thus, it is thought that nanoparticle-based products are better suited for treating illnesses like androgenic alopecia and alopecia areata than the solutions containing water and alcohol utilized until recently. In contrast to aqueous regulate solutions, particles encapsulating chemicals for hair growth demonstrated 2.0–2.5 times greater permanence inside hair follicle areas. In comparison to a simple solution of the exact same drug, hinokitiol encapsulated in identical particles significantly enhanced the transition of hair follicles during their telogen to anagen phase. Minoxidil's longevity in the hair follicle zone was increased by encapsulating it in polyethylene glycol nanostructures with a size of 40–130 nm (Wu et al., 2015).

11.12 NANOTHERAPEUTICS IN BURN WOUNDS

Burn wound care has been investigated using a wide variety of NPs. These wounds can benefit from the use of nanotherapeutics by having an increased antibacterial action, eliminating bacterial drug resistance, promoting cell proliferation, and reducing the frequency of drug administration. Nanotherapeutics' ability to treat many different kinds and intensities of burns is being examined in a number of animal models. In people who have burn injuries, certain nanotherapeutics have effective therapeutic effects, which renders them ideal candidates for further research into their function in the treatment of these wounds—despite the fact that satisfying therapeutic results have been attained (Huang et al., 2021).

Because of their outstanding antibacterial properties and broad-spectrum antimicrobial actions against a number of microorganisms, AgNPs and Ag ions are remarkable antimicrobial agents in burn wound management. Because of their greater penetration and retention properties, AgNPs in particular exhibit better antibacterial action than ionic silver. As a result, they are frequently employed for the management of burn wounds. Importantly, because Zn has semiconductor characteristics, ZnO-NPs can enhance cell adhesion, proliferation, and migration through GF-mediated routes. Consequently, because ZnO-NPs have antibacterial, anti-inflammatory, and minimal cytotoxicity capabilities, they may also be employed as persistent sources of ionic Zn in the management of burn wounds (Huang et al., 2021).

11.13 NANOTHERAPEUTICS FOR PSORIASIS

An autoimmune etiology underlies the dermatological chronic skin disorder known as psoriasis. It significantly lowers the patients' overall quality of life. Consequently, it served as an intriguing research focus over the years. Anti-inflammatory drugs, immune suppressants, biological treatments, and phototherapy are among the traditional treatment choices. Nanotechnology has potential properties that make it possible to customize a drug carrier for cutaneous targeting, increased efficacy, and reduced side effects. Polymeric, metallic, lipidic, and hybrid nanocarriers integrating various active agents are included in sophisticated systems. Over the years, all of the aforementioned drug delivery system variants have been researched for topical administration on psoriatic plaques. To increase efficiency, security, and adherence for the treatment of psoriasis, researchers are making promising progress toward developing an optimal formula with a practical dosage form. As a result, it will provide patients with a higher quality of life. Figure 11.3 shows psoriatic plaques with healthy normal skin (Fereig et al., 2020).

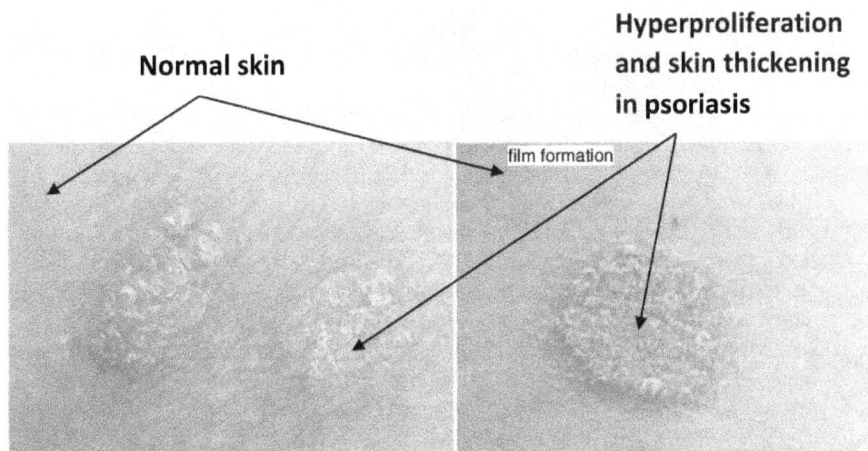

FIGURE 11.3 Psoriatic plaques covered with silvery scales compared to normal skin parts.

Source: Reproduced with permission from Fereig et al., 2020.

11.14   NANOTHERAPEUTICS IN DESIGNING AND CHARACTERIZATION OF NANOPARTICLES IN DERMATOLOGICAL PRODUCTS

A very broad topic is the creation and characterization of NPs in dermatological products. Once the nanoparticles have been synthesized, they need to be incorporated into a vehicle suited for cosmetic usage. In reality, aqueous dispersions of nanoparticles are frequently applied straight to the skin; thus, it is important to mix them in a suitable vehicle. The stability of NPs chemically and physically in skincare products is influenced by both the manner they are delivered and the chemical consistency of the media in which they are disseminated. The proper formulation ensures physical, chemical, and microbial stability and controls the end product's effectiveness and safety. Additionally, the type of cosmetic product, such as a day or night lotion, body lotion, serum products, etc., determines its vehicle of choice. The type and strength of interactions between particles, the dispersion, the emulsifier, and the thickening will determine the physical stability of a cosmeceutical product comprising NPs. Chelating compounds, buffers, and AOs all have been employed to give the finished product chemical stability. Microorganisms cannot grow due to preservatives. In addition to improving the product's organoleptic qualities, dyes and perfumes can also increase customer's appeal. The fundamental benefit of NPs is the fact that they liberate the active substance in the epidermis in significant amounts by releasing it in the outermost strata of the human skin. Cosmetics including liposomes have a strong substantivity that makes them difficult to remove with water. Particularly liposomes can raise the amount of lipids in the SC, which will improve moisturization and lessen skin dryness (Budai et al., 2013).

REFERENCES

Antonio, J. R. et al. (2014) "Nanotechnology in dermatology," *Anais brasileiros de dermatologia*, 89(1), pp. 126–136. doi: 10.1590/abd1806-4841.20142228.

Barbosa, T. C. et al. (2019) "Cytotoxicity and eye irritation profile of a new sunscreen formulation based on benzophenone-3-poly(epsilon-caprolactone) nanocapsules," *Toxics*, 7. doi: 10.3390/toxics7040051.

Baroli, B. (2010) "Penetration of nanoparticles and nanomaterials in the skin: Fiction or reality?," *Journal of Pharmaceutical Sciences*, 99(1), pp. 21–50. doi: 10.1002/jps.21817.

Barry, B. W. (2001) "Novel mechanisms and devices to enable successful transdermal drug delivery," *European Journal of Pharmaceutical Sciences: Official Journal of the European Federation for Pharmaceutical Sciences*, 14(2), pp. 101–114. doi: 10.1016/s0928-0987(01)00167-1.

Battie, C. et al. (2014) "New insights in photoaging, UVA induced damage and skin types," *Experimental Dermatology*, 23, pp. 7–12. doi: 10.1111/exd.12388.

Bolzinger, M.-A., Briançon, S. and Chevalier, Y. (2011) "Nanoparticles through the skin: Managing conflicting results of inorganic and organic particles in cosmetics and pharmaceutics," *Wiley Interdisciplinary Reviews: Nanomedicine and Nanobiotechnology*, 3(5), pp. 463–478. doi: 10.1002/wnan.146.

Bos, J. D. and Meinardi, M. M. (2000) "The 500 Dalton rule for the skin penetration of chemical compounds and drugs," *Experimental Dermatology*, 9(3), pp. 165–169. doi: 10.1034/j.1600-0625.2000.009003165.x.

Budai, L. et al. (2013) "Liposomes for topical use: A physico-chemical comparison of vesicles prepared from egg or soy lecithin," *Scientia Pharmaceutica*, 81(4), pp. 1151–1166. doi: 10.3797/scipharm.1305-11.

Bukhari, S. N. A. et al. (2018) "Hyaluronic acid, a promising skin rejuvenating biomedicine: A review of recent updates and pre-clinical and clinical investigations on cosmetic and nutricosmetic effects," *International Journal of Biological Macromolecules*, 120(Pt B), pp. 1682–1695. doi: 10.1016/j.ijbiomac.2018.09.188.

Burke, K. E. (2018) "Mechanisms of aging and development—A new understanding of environmental damage to the skin and prevention with topical antioxidants," *Mechanisms of Ageing and Development*, 172, pp. 123–130. doi: 10.1016/j.mad.2017.12.003.

Cevc, G. et al. (1996) "The skin: A pathway for systemic treatment with patches and lipid based carriers," *Advanced Drug Delivery Reviews*, 18, pp. 349–378.

D'Orazio, J. et al. (2013) "UV radiation and the skin," *International Journal of Molecular Sciences*, 14(6), pp. 12222–12248. doi: 10.3390/ijms140612222.

El-Chami, C. et al. (2014) "Role of organic osmolytes in water homoeostasis in skin," *Experimental Dermatology*, 23(8), pp. 534–537. doi: 10.1111/exd.12473.

Fereig, S. A. et al. (2020) "Tackling the various classes of nano-therapeutics employed in topical therapy of psoriasis," *Drug Delivery*, 27(1), pp. 662–680. doi: 10.1080/10717544.2020.1754527.

Holmes, A. M. et al. (2020) "Penetration of zinc into human skin after topical application of nano zinc oxide used in commercial sunscreen formulations," *ACS Applied Bio Materials*, 3(6), pp. 3640–3647. doi: 10.1021/acsabm.0c00280.

Huang, R. et al. (2021) "Recent advances in nanotherapeutics for the treatment of burn wounds," *Burns & Trauma*, 9, p. tkab026. doi: 10.1093/burnst/tkab026.

Jensen, L. B., Petersson, K. and Nielsen, H. M. (2011) "In vitro penetration properties of solid lipid nanoparticles in intact and barrier-impaired skin," *European Journal of Pharmaceutics and Biopharmaceutics: Official Journal of Arbeitsgemeinschaft für Pharmazeutische Verfahrenstechnik e.V*, 79(1), pp. 68–75. doi: 10.1016/j.ejpb.2011.05.012.

Jung, S.-M. et al. (2015) "Thermodynamic insights and conceptual design of skin-sensitive chitosan coated ceramide/PLGA nanodrug for regeneration of stratum corneum on atopic dermatitis," *Scientific Reports*, 5(1). doi: 10.1038/srep18089.

Kim, H. et al. (2018) "Seeking better topical delivery technologies of moisturizing agents for enhanced skin moisturization," *Expert Opinion on Drug Delivery*, 15(1), pp. 17–31. doi: 10.1080/17425247.2017.1306054.

Larese Filon, F. et al. (2015) "Nanoparticles skin absorption: New aspects for a safety profile evaluation," *Regulatory Toxicology and Pharmacology: RTP*, 72(2), pp. 310–322. doi: 10.1016/j.yrtph.2015.05.005.

Lee, O. et al. (2013) "Influence of surface charge of gold nanorods on skin penetration," *Skin Research and Technology*, 19(1), pp. e390–e396. doi: 10.1111/j.1600-0846.2012.00656.x.

Leite-Silva, V. R. et al. (2016) "Human skin penetration and local effects of topical nano zinc oxide after occlusion and barrier impairment," *European Journal of Pharmaceutics and Biopharmaceutics: Official Journal of Arbeitsgemeinschaft für Pharmazeutische Verfahrenstechnik e.V*, 104, pp. 140–147. doi: 10.1016/j.ejpb.2016.04.022.

Lekki, J. et al. (2007) "On the follicular pathway of percutaneous uptake of nanoparticles: Ion microscopy and autoradiography studies," *Nuclear Instruments & Methods in Physics Research: Section B, Beam Interactions with Materials and Atoms*, 260(1), pp. 174–177. doi: 10.1016/j.nimb.2007.02.021.

Liang, X. W. et al. (2013) "Penetration of nanoparticles into human skin," *Current Pharmaceutical Design*, 19(35), pp. 6353–6366. doi: 10.2174/1381612811319350011.

Lohani, A. et al. (2014) "Nanotechnology-based cosmeceuticals," *ISRN Dermatology*, 2014, p. 843687. doi: 10.1155/2014/843687.

Mahmoud, N. N. et al. (2017) "Preferential accumulation of gold nanorods into human skin hair follicles: Effect of nanoparticle surface chemistry," *Journal of Colloid and Interface Science*, 503, pp. 95–102. doi: 10.1016/j.jcis.2017.05.011.

Niska, K. et al. (2018) "Metal nanoparticles in dermatology and cosmetology: Interactions with human skin cells," *Chemico-Biological Interactions*, 295, pp. 38–51. doi: 10.1016/j.cbi.2017.06.018.

Osmond-McLeod, M. J. et al. (2016) "Long-term exposure to commercially available sunscreens containing nanoparticles of TiO_2 and ZnO revealed no biological impact in a hairless mouse model," *Particle and Fibre Toxicology*, 13(1), p. 44. doi: 10.1186/s12989-016-0154-4.

Roberts, M. S. et al. (2017) "Topical and cutaneous delivery using nanosystems," *Journal of Controlled Release: Official Journal of the Controlled Release Society*, 247, pp. 86–105. doi: 10.1016/j.jconrel.2016.12.022.

Salvioni, L. et al. (2021) "The emerging role of nanotechnology in skincare," *Advances in Colloid and Interface Science*, 293(102437), p. 102437. doi: 10.1016/j.cis.2021.102437.

Schneider, S. L. and Lim, H. W. (2019) "A review of inorganic UV filters zinc oxide and titanium dioxide," *Photodermatology, Photoimmunology & Photomedicine*, 35(6), pp. 442–446. doi: 10.1111/phpp.12439.

Singh, S. B., Young, K. and Silver, L. L. (2017) "What is an 'ideal' antibiotic? Discovery challenges and path forward," *Biochemical Pharmacology*, 133, pp. 63–73. doi: 10.1016/j.bcp.2017.01.003.

Singhal, M., Khanna, S. and Nasa, A. (2011) "Cosmeceuticals for the skin: An overview," *Asian Journal of Pharmaceutical and Clinical Research*, 4, pp. 1–6.

Sorg, O. et al. (2006) "Retinoids in cosmeceuticals," *Dermatologic Therapy*, 19(5), pp. 289–296. doi: 10.1111/j.1529-8019.2006.00086.x.

Van Tran, V., Moon, J.-Y. and Lee, Y.-C. (2019) "Liposomes for delivery of antioxidants in cosmeceuticals: Challenges and development strategies," *Journal of Controlled Release: Official Journal of the Controlled Release Society*, 300, pp. 114–140. doi: 10.1016/j.jconrel.2019.03.003.

Wu, M.-S. et al. (2015) "Nanodiamonds protect skin from ultraviolet B-induced damage in mice," *Journal of Nanobiotechnology*, 13(1). doi: 10.1186/s12951-015-0094-4.

12 Nanotherapeutics in Orthopedics

INTRODUCTION

One of the most vital organs within the body is bone tissue. It is comprised of approximately 60% of inorganic elements, 30% of organic materials, 10% of tissue cells, along with veins and arteries of the circulatory system. The inorganic elements are referred to as hydroxyapatite (HA) ($Ca_{10}(PO_4)_6(OH)_2$), when the organic framework contains lipids, the protein collagen, along with proteoglycans (Shea and Miller, 2005; Chen et al., 2022). The skeleton has a variety of purposes in the body, including protecting the organs that are located within the structure, supporting the framework of the body, serving as a repository for minerals, and aiding in the generation of blood cells (Florencio-Silva et al., 2015). A healthy structure of bones is continually being digested and reshaped by the highly specific dynamic tissue during lifetime for these purposes.

Bone disorders comprise a wide range of skeletal-related problems, such as abnormalities that significantly impede human mobility and increase mortality. Additionally, there is an imperative necessity for developing novel medicines and drug delivery technologies for secure and efficient therapeutic treatments of a number of most prevalent skeleton diseases, such as osteoarthritis, osteosarcoma, osteoporosis, and metastatic cancer of the bone (Xue X. et al., 2021). Successful achievements are a constant concern in the advancement of medicines for bone malignancies and bone degenerative conditions with the equilibrium between adverse effects of the drug and curative therapy. A targeted delivery approach utilizing nanotechnology has frequently been suggested as a potential tactic to deal with these problems and improve the effectiveness of treatment. In regard to medicine, nanomaterials provide novel opportunities to study illnesses through imaging and diagnostic uses and, increasingly, they serve as delivery systems for medications or therapeutic substances to produce better and safer therapeutic results in orthopedics. Additionally, nanoparticles are transforming tissue engineering in healthcare by offering a fine architecture facilitating regeneration of tissue (Tasker, Sparey-Taylor and Nokes, 2007).

Investigation on bone regeneration possesses a lengthy and varied history. Some of the most popular experimental techniques used to assess growth of the bone tissue are *in vivo* and *in vitro* exposed tests. In the first instance, laboratory rodents are purposely induced bone fractures and deformities to evaluate various treatment options and materials (Luvizuto et al., 2011). The benefit of *in vitro* tests is that they give a more precise understanding of the manner in which a chemical act on cells, cellular components and tissues in an intended organ under certain circumstances. They involve studying the proliferation, morphological features, and intracellular biochemistry of cells linked to bone regeneration by exposing cells that have been cultured to a medication (Qiang et al., 2008) or cultivating cells on a substance (Zhou et al., 2013). Numerous nanomaterials have been invented recently as possible constituents for bone regeneration therapy.

There are several ways to assess whether they are safe and effective as initial components (Zanello et al., 2006) or in the form of composite materials (Hill et al., 2019), even though the majority are employed as composite substances in bone regeneration scaffolds.

The distribution of drugs might represent the most prominent prospect of nanotherapeutics in orthopedics. Nanofabricated interfaces may enable targeted administration of therapeutic enzymes into tumor cells within nanotherapeutics utilized for targeting of bone tumors. Nanocapsules have been found to have a longer-lasting anti-inflammatory impact than other forms of arthritis treatment. The development of wound dressings with nanofibrous membranes is an important milestone in lowering postoperative infections and accelerating recovery. The employing of nanotechnology in orthopedic research, diagnosis, and treatment is relatively young. However, nanotherapeutics has been capable to transform both the science and the practice of orthopedic care in the brief period it has been investigated and used—as a result of the capability of nanotherapeutics for the treatment of the human body in manners that are more accurate, superior for bone formation, and theoretically better, at least in regard to the rate of infection and the need for repeat operations. Hence, many traditional treatments are being substituted (Pokkalath et al., 2021).

Although it is still in the early stages, nanotechnology cannot solve all of the issues facing the discipline of orthopedic surgery. However, it appears that nanotherapeutics is occupying a burgeoning niche in the discipline of orthopedic surgery with additional funding and research (Pokkalath et al., 2021). Figure 12.1 depicts various nanotherapeutic-based approaches in orthopedics methods.

12.1 NANOTHERAPEUTICS IN OSTEOPOROSIS

Decreased density of bones and aberrant bone tissue microscopic structure, which enhance the fragility of bones and fracture susceptibility, are characteristics of osteoporosis (OP). OP can be described as a systemic metabolic bone disorder (Seeman and Delmas, 2006). The aging among people in China is contributing to a spike in osteoporosis cases according to statistics, which also raises medical costs (Wang et al., 2009). The two varieties of OP are primary and secondary. This categorization is based on their etiologies, with primary being the more prevalent type and comprising old age and postmenopause (Li et al., 2021). In the instance of postmenopausal osteoporosis, it is mostly caused by estrogen insufficiency. The decreased bone mass along with elevated conversion osteoporosis that arise from greater bone resorption over bone synthesis is also a major reason on this matter. Estrogen is frequently employed to keep the mineral density of bones intact. However, this treatment is linked to breast swelling and congestion. Moreover, it is linked significantly to higher incidences of malignancies of the breast with hyperplasia of the endometrium (Black and Rosen, 2016). Therefore, the use of bone-targeted treatments for osteoporosis is a significant research topic at present. This is because performing such research can lower the risk of the unwanted effects and enhance treatment outcomes.

The utilization of gene therapy to the treatment of metabolic disorders is still being implemented into practical uses due to the dearth of appropriate targeted methods of delivery to guarantee the safety and effectiveness of the treatment. In order to accomplish the targeted discharge of the osteogenic Plekho1 siRNA, Liang

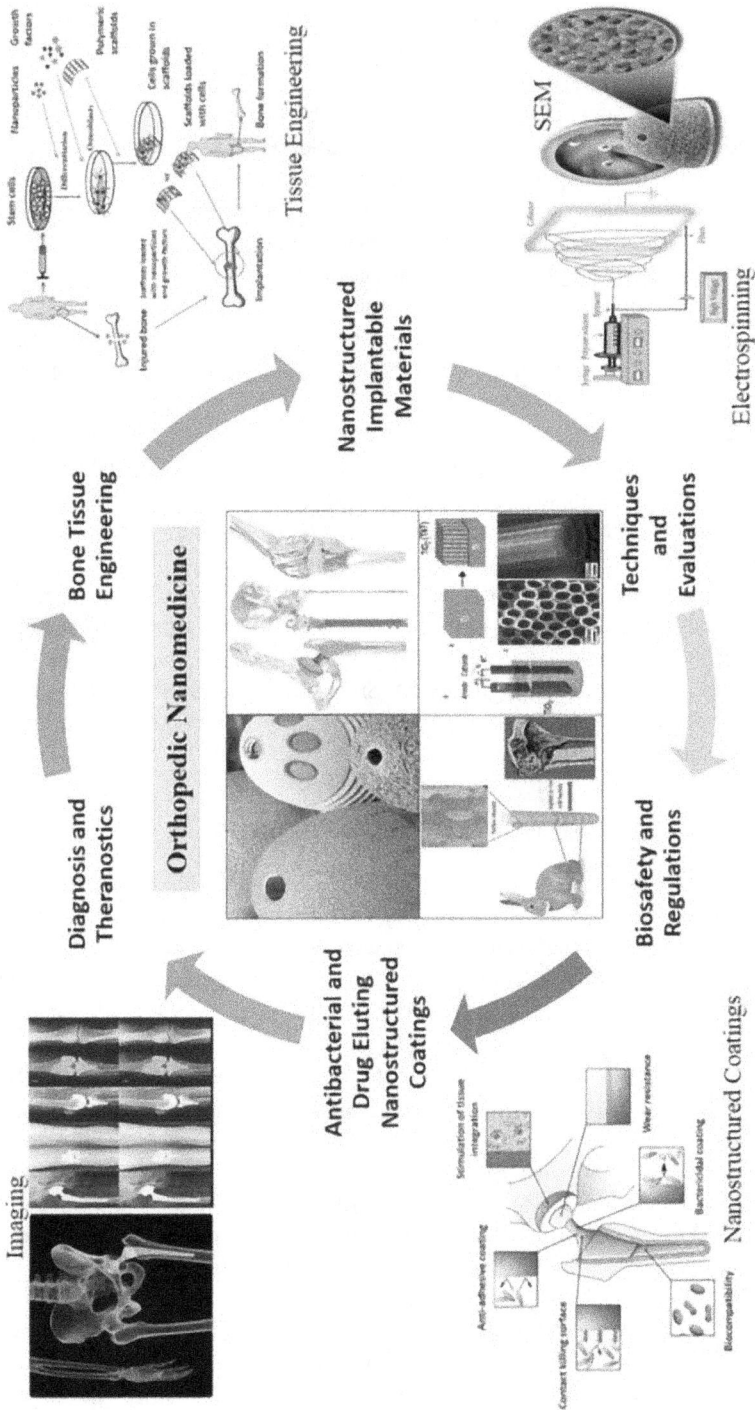

FIGURE 12.1 Nanotherapeutics-based approaches in orthopedics.

Source: Reproduced with permission from Pokkalath et al., 2021.

et al. invented the first aptamer-functionalized liposome nanosystem in 2015. They opted for the osteoblast-specific aptamer CH6 by cell-SELEX, along with the ligand-modified PEGylated liposome, primarily via macropinocytosis. These foster suppressing of the negative regulation of skeletal formation genes in osteoblasts and boost bone formation as demonstrated. Additionally, Cui et al. developed an exosome-loaded Shn3 gene siRNA delivery method called BT-Exo-siShn3. The peptide that is targeting the bone experienced hydrophobic interaction alteration is aimed to enable the exosomes to carry siRNA to osteoblasts. Furthermore, it was tethered to the exosome surface. Suppression of Shn3 genes decreased RANKL expression in osteoblasts, improved osteogenic differentiation, inhibited osteoclast activity, halted OVX-induced reduction in bone mass, and encouraged the development of H-type vessels and mineralization of bones (Cui et al., 2022). The previously described bone-targeting nanomaterials offer an intriguing concept for the investigation of siRNA delivery to cure osteoporosis.

Supplements containing calcium are a therapeutically recommended medication for the first-line treatment of osteoporosis. Although they often require large and repetitive dosages of administration, an absence of targeting results in subpar treatment results. Tao et al. have described a carrier for *in situ* calcium supplementation that target the skeletal structures in the oral region and are responsive to OP microenvironment (water/pH). A bone-targeted medication delivery platform (TMA/Sim) was developed using an amorphous calcium carbonate (ACC) framework as the main structural component, modulated with tetracycline (Tc), capped with monostearin (MS), and preloaded with simvastatin (Sim). Simvastatin might be administered to specific areas of the body in combination with *in situ* supplementation of calcium to produce a potentially effective treatment plan (Tao et al., 2021).

12.2 NANOTHERAPEUTICS IN OSTEOARTHRITIS

Osteoarthritis (OA) is a type of chronic arthropathy that is usually found in elderly patients and is distinguished by osteophytes, subchondral bone sclerosis, localized inflammation, as well as the degenerative breakdown of articular cartilage (Hunter and Bierma-Zeinstra, 2019; Hu et al., 2021). It is mainly triggered by a discrepancy between mechanical and biological processes that results in the normal degeneration and development of articular cartilage, its extracellular matrix, and subchondral bones (Karsdal et al., 2014). Even though there have been a lot of scientific clinical research and laboratory animal investigations, the pathophysiology and development of OA are still not fully understood. Therefore, the primary goals of OA treatment are symptom relief, functional improvement, and process of pathogenesis delaying (McAlindon and Bannuru, 2018). The unique avascular, thick, and occlusive tissue architecture in OA renders drug administration that has become a therapeutic problem (Bijlsma, Berenbaum and Lafeber, 2011). The application of nanoparticles to deliver medications for specific treatments has helped to make a qualitative advancement in improving the penetration of medicines and sustained liberation in OA, relying on the ongoing research and development of traditional pharmaceuticals.

In recognition of the localized characteristics of osteoarthritis in particular joints, intraarticular (IA) injectables are a more efficient method of obtaining therapeutic doses with fewer adverse reactions on the entire joint than systemic delivery. A focused delivery technique may be more efficient since the medicine may be promptly eliminated once it reaches the joint. Mangostemonin (FMN), a medication with exceptionally poor aqueous solubility and limited bioavailability, was used as a therapeutic substance. For the production of cartilage-targeting nanomicrospheres (PCFMN), FMN was PEGylated and then coupled with the cartilage-targeting peptide (CollBP). When FMN was PEGylated, the medication was more soluble in it, and CollBP allowed more drug to accumulate at the joint region. After the therapy, a number of inflammatory reactions–related factors were substantially reduced, which also improved the cartilage damage caused by ACLT and eventually resulted in an effective OA slowing effect (Xiong et al., 2021).

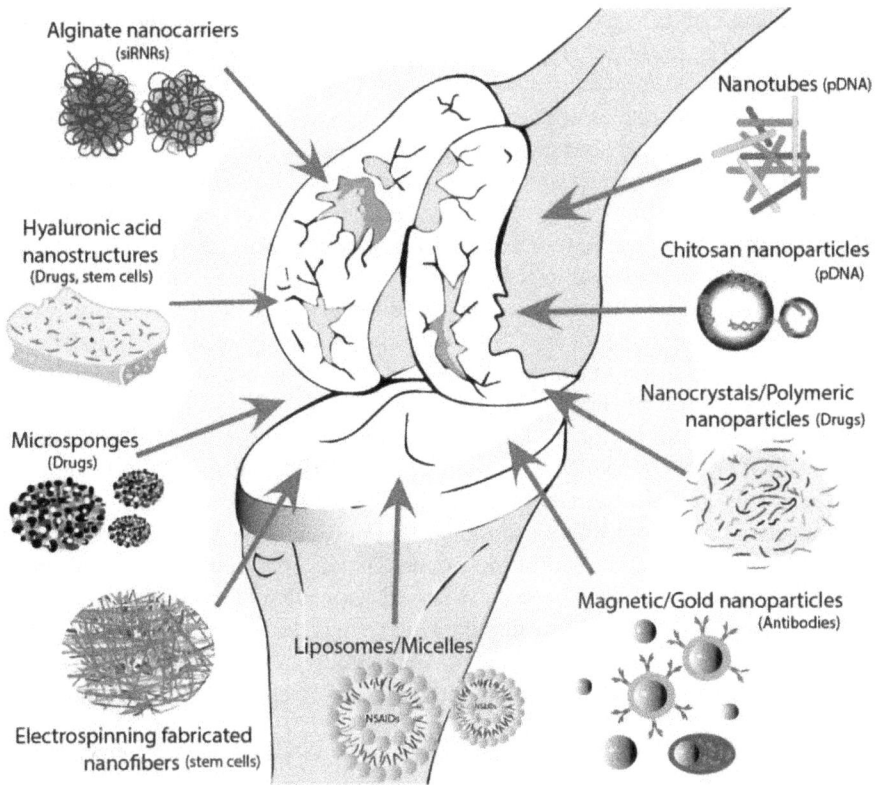

FIGURE 12.2 Nanotubes, magnetic nanoparticles, and other nanotechnology-based drug and gene delivery systems may be used for targeting molecular pathways and pathogenic mechanisms involved in OA development. Nanocomposites are also being explored as potential tools for promoting cartilage repair. Nanotechnology platforms may be combined with cell, gene, and biological therapies for the development of a new generation of future OA therapeutics.

Source: Reproduced with permission from Mohammadinejad et al., 2020.

Figure 12.2 shows various nanotherapeutics-based approaches in the disease management of osteoporosis. A type II collagen-targeting peptide was attached by Xue et al. to a metal organic framework (MOF)-modified mesoporous polydopamine (MPDA) double drug delivery platform (RB@MPMW). Following the near-infrared (NIR) laser stimulated nanoparticles, bilirubin (Br) was liberated for immediate ROS scavenging, enabling the resulting discharge of rapamycin (Rap) increased autophagy initiation and chondrocyte preservation. In the ACLT laboratory rat model, cartilage degradation was effectively postponed by the targeted liberation of both medicines at cartilage locations (Xue et al., 2021).

12.3   NANOTHERAPEUTICS IN OSTEOSARCOMA

The most common basic sarcoma in children and adolescents can be described as osteosarcoma (OS), a malignant skeletal tumor. It poses a major hazard to human health because of its aggressiveness, carcinogenicity, and poor prognosis (Kansara et al., 2014). The present therapeutic paradigm for OS is prior to surgery neoadjuvant chemotherapy, surgical removal of the tumor, and adjuvant chemotherapy, and the overall survival rate after five years of the disorder has increased from 20% to about 60% with medical advancements (Isakoff et al., 2015; Gill and Gorlick, 2021). However, the initial therapy of OS depends on amputation, which harms patients physically and psychologically. However, the current state of clinical practice indicates that the issues with tumor resistance, nontargeted distribution of drugs, high expenses, and adverse reactions of chemotherapy have not fundamentally enhanced the efficacy, particularly for those suffering from metastasis or recurrence (González-Fernández et al., 2017). The creation of personalized drug delivery platforms could prove to be a successful strategy to improve survival rates in the context of precision medicine (Jurek et al., 2017). Two nanoplatforms have been invented by Chen et al. for the specific treatment of osteosarcoma. One example is CDDPHANG/DOX, which refers to cisplatin (CDDP)-cross-linked hyaluronic acid nanogels loaded with DOX. In addition to its anticancer properties, CDDP also functions as a cross-linking substance that prevent early drug release and contribute to drug deposition within the tumor. The second method uses hyaluronic acid nanoparticles that have been cross-linked with calcium carbonate ($CaCO_3$) to administer DOX while also ensuring the long-term stability of those nanoparticles. Both nanoplatforms possess excellent biocompatibility, extended blood circulation times, and sensitivity toward the acidic microenvironment of tumors (Zhang et al., 2018a; Zhang et al., 2018b).

Alendronate (ALN) as well as hyaluronic acid (HA), the ligand from CD44, were coupled in a different study using bisphosphonates as focusing ligands. The modified lipid ALN-HA-SS-L was then attached to liposomes containing the anticancer medication DOX. A substantial growth hindering effect appeared in the *in situ* OS laboratory mouse model, and the survival rate of laboratory mice was developed. *In vitro* experiments confirmed that the receptive liposomes liberated the drug after disassembling in glutathione-comprised cancer cells, demonstrating significant cytotoxicity and an immediate cellular uptake rate toward human OS MG-63 cells

(Feng et al., 2019). In summary, the double-targeting redox-sensitive liposomes treating CD44 and bone were assembled together and it demonstrated a potential for OS.

12.4 NANOTHERAPEUTICS FOR BONE REGENERATION

Scaffolds can be described as mechanical devices that serve as transporters of growth factors or cellular components. The most effective scaffolds are simultaneously biocompatible and biodegradable ensuring they can eventually be replaced with tissue that functions. The extracellular matrix that normally offers support and durability and acts as a lattice enabling cell adhesion, motility, and tissue ingrowth has been imitated by many scaffolds (Frisch, Schaller and Cieply, 2013). Primary biodegradable polymeric substances or ceramics are being researched as scaffolds for tissue engineering of bones. Scaffolds currently contain the popular cell adhesion ligand arginine–glycine–aspartate (RGD), which helps cells adhere more effectively. An ability of a scaffold to replicate the extracellular framework and direct the activity and growth of implanted cells is improved by the incorporation of the RGD ligand, particularly through the development of polymer–RGD peptide hybrid compounds or via the surface modification of premade polymers (Shakesheff, Cannizzaro and Langer, 1998). In terms of bone engineering, this has been demonstrated that adding carbon nanotubes and micro-hydroxyapatite (HA) particles into PLA-based scaffolds to form nanocomposites improves MSC adhesion and osteoprogenitor development (Ciapetti et al., 2012). Additionally, it was discovered that adding a biomimetic HA surface drastically changed the microenvironment of adhering preosteoblasts and encouraged cellular projecting survivability and expansion along irregular surfaces (Chou et al., 2005).

It is therefore not shocking that mimicking apatite nanoparticles could increase the osteogenic ability of progenitor cells given that HA mimics the natural mineral framework of bone. In laboratory rat calvarial imperfections, HA-coated PLGA scaffolds discovered to help with bone regeneration, and more exposition of HA nanoparticles over the scaffold surface were observed to cause rapid bone deposition through local progenitors (Kim et al., 2007). Additionally, it is known that apatite-coated PLGA scaffolds encourage the development of seeded preosteoblasts. Chou et al. discovered that MC3T3-E1 cells grown on 3D apatite-coated PLGA displayed noticeably increased expression amounts for markers of bone development (Chou, Dunn and Wu, 2005). It has recently been demonstrated that protein adsorption layers control the way these cells respond to apatite nanoparticles. The aforementioned protein layers may modify the surface potential or charge or influence phase transformation of the compound calcium phosphate (Tsang et al., 2011).

Regarding bone tissue engineering, designed electrospun thermoplastic polyurethane(TPU)/hydroxyapatite scaffolds is an emerging solution. The researchers assessed the impact of scaffold physical characteristics and osteoblast-like cell functionality on the characteristics and particle dimensions of (micro and nano) HA polymer. Despite the assistance of a carrier polymer, Leszczak et al. (2014) designed an electrospun as natural demineralized matrix of bones (DBM). DBM is referred to as an allograft bone that has the protein building blocks of bone but has had the inorganic material eliminated. These parts include crucial growth factors, including sticky ligands and osteoinductive impulses. Poologasundarampillai et al. (2014) have developed an electrospun of the calcium-incorporated SiO_2 fibers employing sol–gel remedies for bone regeneration in order to generate bioactive three-dimensional scaffolds containing a cotton-wool-like structure (Poologasundarampillai et al., 2014). For the production of Si–O–Si linear chains, tetraethylorthosilicate (TEOS) has been hydrolyzed and condensed beneath acid-catalyzed conditions (Khajavi, Abbasipour and Bahador, 2016).

12.5 NANOTHERAPEUTICS IN ORTHOPEDIC SURGERY

Surgical implantable biomaterials have evolved into crucial elements of orthopedic surgery, partly as a result of their superior osteointegration and stimulation of healthy bone mechanisms when compared to traditional materials (Mazaheri et al., 2015). These critical advancements occur at a crucial moment when the aging population raises the requirement for orthopedic implants. As an example, it is projected that more than 600,000 joint implants are used annually in the United States and that number is rising (Christenson et al., 2007). Orthopedic implants are utilized in an assortment of methods across the human body in various parts; however, nanomaterials added to surgical implants improve their overall functionality and work effectively. Figure 12.3 shows the nanotherapeutic approaches in bone repair in surgeries.

Bone allografts as well as autografts, more traditional ways of treating bone abnormalities, continue to be used frequently. They are thought to make up close to 80% of bone defect procedures (Pd, 2013). Potential risks associated with these methods, particularly for minor abnormalities, include infection, immune system rejection, and protracted repair time frames (Pd, 2013). Nanomaterial implants have reduced many of these hazards, nonetheless they still occasionally fail. Nanomaterial-based implants have not yet been able to restore full capability, and they frequently only last for several decades at most. Complete implant failure is a possibility and can be extremely difficult, necessitating time-consuming and costly re-operations (Christenson et al., 2007).

However, the application of nanotechnology in surgical implants for orthopedics has been demonstrated to be immensely advantageous, enhancing the management of numerous bone abnormalities and orthopedic injuries. Numerous materials have been researched and employed, resulting in the utilization of a wide range of prospective materials, each with their own special qualities and advantages. Gelatin, ceramics that have a bioactive nature, polymers that are biodegradable, and polysaccharides like agarose are a few examples of materials. Since they may encourage cell proliferation and tissue regeneration owing to their physical characteristics and nanoscale capabilities, these nanomaterials can function well inside the human body. In order to replicate the functions of cells, which additionally possess nanometer-scale dimensions and aggregate to create extracellular matrix structures, these nanomaterials must be able to mimic the environment inside of cells. Additionally,

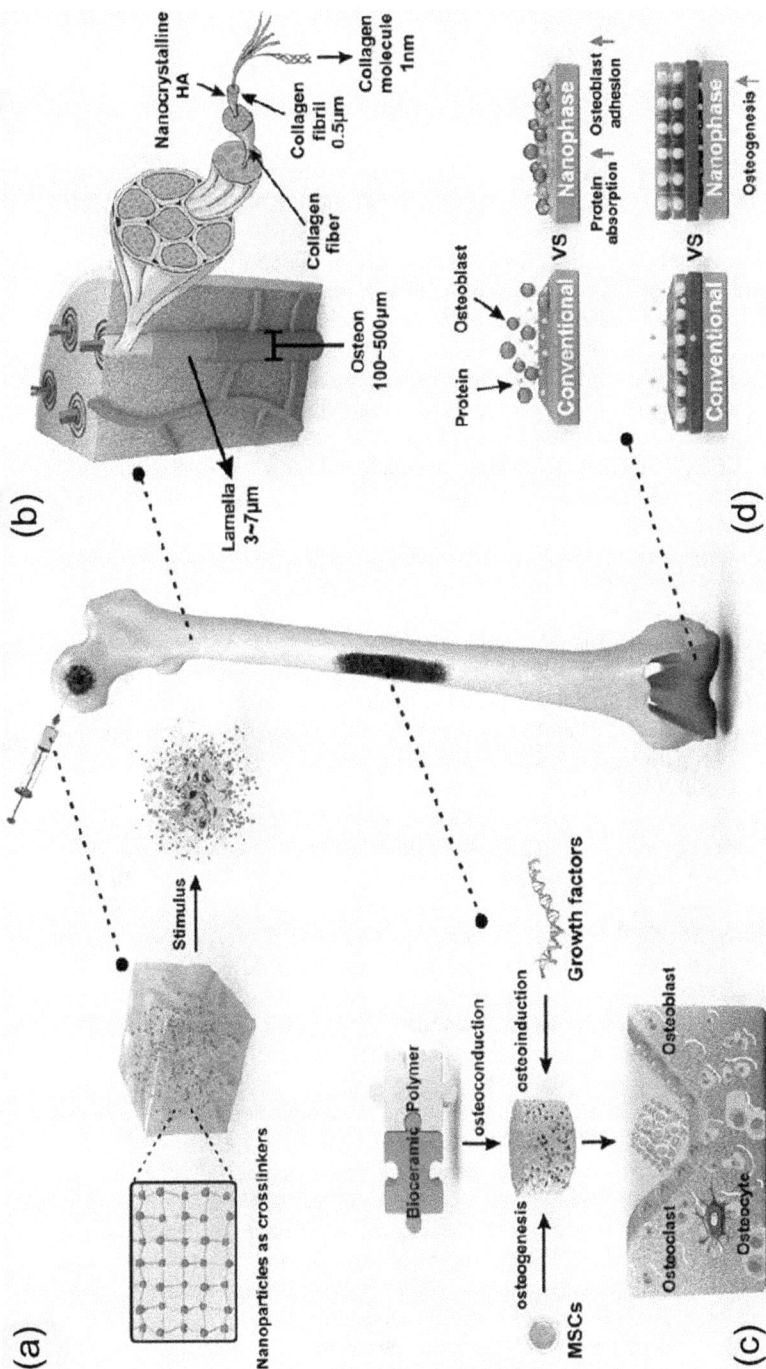

FIGURE 12.3 Nanotechnologies in bone repair. (a) The introduction of nanoparticles can effectively improve the structural properties of the hydrogel network with enhanced mechanical properties, while imparting stimulus responsiveness. (b) The ECM of bone tissues mainly consist of highly ordered collagen nanofibers and nanocrystalline HA. (c) Three essential elements of nanocomposite scaffold-mediated bone regeneration and the cellular composition of bone tissue. (d) Generating nano-surface features on metallic implants through surface modification to enhance the adsorption of proteins as well as adhesion of osteoblasts, thus promoting osteogenesis.

Source: Reproduced with permission from Qiao et al., 2022.

implants made of nanoparticles can create a larger surface area, which promotes a favorable environment for bone formation and lowers infection rates (Garimella and Eltorai, 2017).

REFERENCES

Bijlsma, J. W., Berenbaum, F. and Lafeber, F. P. (2011) "Osteoarthritis: An update with relevance for clinical practice," *Lancet*, 377(9783), pp. 2115–2126. doi: 10.1016/s0140-6736(11)60243-2.

Black, D. M. and Rosen, C. J. (2016) "Clinical practice: Postmenopausal osteoporosis," *N. Engl. J. Med.*, 374(3), pp. 254–262. doi: 10.1056/NEJMcp1513724.

Chen, S. et al. (2022) "The horizon of bone organoid: A perspective on construction and application," *Bioactive Materials*, 18, pp. 15–25. doi: 10.1016/j.bioactmat.2022.01.048.

Chou, Y. F., Dunn, J. C. and Wu, B. M. (2005) "In vitro response of MC3T3-E1 pre-osteoblasts within three-dimensional apatite-coated PLGA scaffolds," *Journal of Biomedical Materials Research Part B Applied Biomaterials*, 75(1), pp. 81–90.

Chou, Y.-F. et al. (2005) "The effect of biomimetic apatite structure on osteoblast viability, proliferation, and gene expression," *Biomaterials*, 26(3), pp. 285–295. doi: 10.1016/j.biomaterials.2004.02.030.

Christenson, E. M. et al. (2007) "Nanobiomaterial applications in orthopedics," *Journal of Orthopaedic Research: Official Publication of the Orthopaedic Research Society*, 25(1), pp. 11–22. doi: 10.1002/jor.20305.

Ciapetti, G. et al. (2012) "Enhancing osteoconduction of PLLA-based nanocomposite scaffolds for bone regeneration using different biomimetic signals to MSCs," *International Journal of Molecular Sciences*, 13(2), pp. 2439–2458. doi: 10.3390/ijms13022439.

Cui, Y., Guo, Y., Kong, L., Shi, J., Liu, P., Li, R. et al. (2022) "A bone-targeted engineered exosome platform delivering siRNA to treat osteoporosis," *Bioactive Materials*, 10, pp. 207–221. doi: 10.1016/j.bioactmat.2021.09.015.

Feng, S., Wu, Z. X., Zhao, Z., Liu, J., Sun, K., Guo, C. et al. (2019) "Engineering of bone- and CD44-dual-targeting redox-sensitive liposomes for the treatment of orthotopic osteosarcoma," *ACS Applied Materials and Interfaces*, 11(7), pp. 7357–7368. doi: 10.1021/acsami.8b18820.

Florencio-Silva, R. et al. (2015) "Biology of bone tissue: Structure, function, and factors that influence bone cells," *BioMed Research International*, 2015, p. 421746. doi: 10.1155/2015/421746.

Frisch, S. M., Schaller, M. and Cieply, B. (2013) "Mechanisms that link the oncogenic epithelial-mesenchymal transition to suppression of anoikis," *Journal of Cell Science*, 126(Pt 1), pp. 21–29. doi: 10.1242/jcs.120907.

Garimella, R. and Eltorai, A. E. M. (2017) "Nanotechnology in orthopedics," *Journal of Orthopaedics*, 14(1), pp. 30–33. doi: 10.1016/j.jor.2016.10.026.

Gill, J. and Gorlick, R. (2021) "Advancing therapy for osteosarcoma," *Nature Reviews Clinical Oncology*, 18(10), 609–624. doi: 10.1038/s41571-021-00519-8.

González-Fernández, Y., Imbuluzqueta, E., Zalacain, M., Mollinedo, F., Patiño-García, A. and Blanco-Prieto, M. J. (2017) "Doxorubicin and edelfosine lipid nanoparticles are effective acting synergistically against drug-resistant osteosarcoma cancer cells," *Cancer Letters*, 388, pp. 262–268. doi: 10.1016/j.canlet.2016.12.012.

Hill, M. J. et al. (2019) "Nanomaterials for bone tissue regeneration: Updates and future perspectives," *Nanomedicine*, 14, pp. 2987–3006.

Hu, Y., Chen, X., Wang, S., Jing, Y. and Su, J. (2021) "Subchondral bone microenvironment in osteoarthritis and pain," *Bone Research*, 9(1), 20. doi: 10.1038/s41413-021-00147-z.

Hunter, D. J. and Bierma-Zeinstra, S. (2019) "Osteoarthritis," *Lancet*, 393(10182), pp. 1745–1759. doi: 10.1016/s0140-6736(19)30417-9.

Isakoff, M. S., Bielack, S. S., Meltzer, P. and Goearchrlick, R. (2015) "Osteosarcoma: Current treatment and a collaborative pathway to success," *J. Clin. Oncol.*, 33(27), pp. 3029–3035. doi: 10.1200/jco.2014.59.4895.

Jurek, P. M., Zabłocki, K., Waśko, U., Mazurek, M. P., Otlewski, J. and Jeleń, F. (2017) "Anti-FGFR1 aptamer-tagged superparamagnetic conjugates for anticancer hyperthermia therapy," *Int. J. Nanomedicine*, 12, pp. 2941–2950. doi: 10.2147/IJN.S125231

Kansara, M., Teng, M. W., Smyth, M. J. and Thomas, D. M. (2014) "Translational biology of osteosarcoma," *Nat. Rev. Cancer*, 14(11), pp. 722–735. doi: 10.1038/nrc3838.

Karsdal, M. A., Bay-Jensen, A. C., Lories, R. J., Abramson, S., Spector, T., Pastoureau, P. et al. (2014) "The coupling of bone and cartilage turnover in osteoarthritis: Opportunities for bone antiresorptives and anabolics as potential treatments?," *Ann. Rheum. Dis.*, 73(2), pp. 336–348. doi: 10.1136/annrheumdis-2013-204111.

Khajavi, R., Abbasipour, M. and Bahador, A. (2016) "Electrospun biodegradable nanofibers scaffolds for bone tissue engineering," *Journal of Applied Polymer Science*, 133(3). doi: 10.1002/app.42883.

Kim, S.-S. et al. (2007) "A poly(lactide-co-glycolide)/hydroxyapatite composite scaffold with enhanced osteoconductivity," *Journal of Biomedical Materials Research. Part A*, 80(1), pp. 206–215. doi: 10.1002/jbm.a.30836.

Leszczak, V. et al. (2014) "Nanostructured biomaterials from electrospun demineralized bone matrix: A survey of processing and crosslinking strategies," *ACS Applied Materials & Interfaces*, 6(12), pp. 9328–9337. doi: 10.1021/am501700e.

Li, M. C. M., Chow, S. K. H., Wong, R. M. Y., Qin, L. and Cheung, W. H. (2021) "The role of osteocytes-specific molecular mechanism in regulation of mechanotransduction—A systematic review," *J. Orthop. Transl.*, 29, pp. 1–9. doi: 10.1016/j.jot.2021.04.005.

Luvizuto, E. R. et al. (2011) "The effect of BMP-2 on the osteoconductive properties of β-tricalcium phosphate in rat calvaria defects," *Biomaterials*, 32(15), pp. 3855–3861. doi: 10.1016/j.biomaterials.2011.01.076.

Mazaheri, M. et al. (2015) "Nanomedicine applications in orthopedic medicine: State of the art," *International Journal of Nanomedicine*, 10, pp. 6039–6053. doi: 10.2147/IJN.S73737.

McAlindon, T. E. and Bannuru, R. R. (2018) "Osteoarthritis in 2017: Latest advances in the management of Knee OA," *Nat. Rev. Rheumatol.*, 14(2), pp. 73–74. doi: 10.1038/nrrheum.2017.219.

Mohammadinejad, R. et al. (2020) "Nanotechnological strategies for osteoarthritis diagnosis, monitoring, clinical management, and regenerative medicine: Recent advances and future opportunities," *Current Rheumatology Reports*, 22(4), p. 12. doi: 10.1007/s11926-020-0884-z.

Pd, P. (2013) "How nanotechnology can really improve the future of orthopedic implants and scaffolds for bone and cartilage defects," *Journal of Nanomedicine & Biotherapeutic Discovery*, 3(2). doi: 10.4172/2155-983x.1000114.

Pokkalath, A. et al. (2021) "Nanomaterials for orthopaedic implants and applications," In Krishnan Anand, Muthupandian Saravanan, Balakumar Chandrasekaran, Suvardhan Kanchi, Sarojini Jeeva Panchu and Quansheng Chen (Eds.), *Handbook on nanobiomaterials for therapeutics and diagnostic applications*. Amsterdam, UK and Cambridge, US: Elsevier, pp. 229–270.

Poologasundarampillai, G. et al. (2014) "Cotton-wool-like bioactive glasses for bone regeneration," *Acta Biomaterialia*, 10(8), pp. 3733–3746. doi: 10.1016/j.actbio.2014.05.020.

Qiang, Y.-W. et al. (2008) "Dkk1-induced inhibition of Wnt signaling in osteoblast differentiation is an underlying mechanism of bone loss in multiple myeloma," *Bone*, 42(4), pp. 669–680. doi: 10.1016/j.bone.2007.12.006.

Qiao, K. et al. (2022) "The advances in nanomedicine for bone and cartilage repair," *Journal of Nanobiotechnology*, 20(1), p. 141. doi: 10.1186/s12951-022-01342-8.

Seeman, E. and Delmas, P. D. (2006) "Bone quality-the material and structural basis of bone strength and fragility," *N. Engl. J. Med.*, 354(21), pp. 2250–2261. doi: 10.1056/NEJMra053077.

Shakesheff, K., Cannizzaro, S. and Langer, R. (1998) "Creating biomimetic micro-environments with synthetic polymer-peptide hybrid molecules," *Journal of Biomaterials Science: Polymer Edition*, 9(5), pp. 507–518. doi: 10.1163/156856298x00596.

Shea, J. E. and Miller, S. C. (2005) "Skeletal function and structure: Implications for tissue-targeted therapeutics," *Advanced Drug Delivery Reviews*, 57(7), pp. 945–957. doi: 10.1016/j.addr.2004.12.017.

Tao, S., Yu, F., Song, Y., Zhou, W., Lv, J., Zhao, R. et al. (2021) "Water/pH dual responsive in situ calcium supplement collaborates simvastatin for osteoblast promotion mediated osteoporosis therapy via oral medication," *J. Control Release*, 329, pp. 121–135. doi: 10.1016/j.jconrel.2020.11.059.

Tasker, L. H., Sparey-Taylor, G. J. and Nokes, L. D. M. (2007) "Applications of nanotechnology in orthopaedics," *Clinical Orthopaedics and Related Research*, 456, pp. 243–249. doi: 10.1097/blo.0b013e31803125f4.

Tsang, E. J. et al. (2011) "Osteoblast interactions within a biomimetic apatite microenvironment," *Annals of Biomedical Engineering*, 39(4), pp. 1186–1200. doi: 10.1007/s10439-010-0245-6.

Wang, Y., Tao, Y., Hyman, M. E., Li, J. and Chen, Y. (2009) "Osteoporosis in China," *Osteoporos. Int.*, 20(10), 1651–1662. doi: 10.1007/s00198-009-0925-y.

Xiong, W., Lan, Q., Liang, X., Zhao, J., Huang, H., Zhan, Y. et al. (2021) "Cartilage-targeting poly(ethylene glycol) (PEG)-formononetin (FMN) nanodrug for the treatment of osteoarthritis," *J. Nanobiotechnol*, 19(1), p. 197. doi: 10.1186/s12951-021-00945-x.

Xue, S., Zhou, X., Sang, W., Wang, C., Lu, H., Xu, Y. et al. (2021a) "Cartilage-targeting peptide-modified dual-drug delivery nanoplatform with NIR laser response for osteoarthritis therapy," *Bioact. Mater.*, 6(8), pp. 2372–2389. doi: 10.1016/j.bioactmat.2021.01.017.

Xue, X. et al. (2021) "Recent advances in design of functional biocompatible hydrogels for bone tissue engineering," *Advanced Functional Materials*, 31(19), p. 2009432. doi: 10.1002/adfm.202009432.

Zanello, L. P. et al. (2006) "Bone cell proliferation on carbon nanotubes," *Nano Letters*, 6(3), pp. 562–567. doi: 10.1021/nl051861e.

Zhang, Y., Cai, L., Li, D., Lao, Y.-H., Liu, D., Li, M. et al. (2018a) "Tumor microenvironment-responsive hyaluronate-calcium carbonate hybrid nanoparticle enables effective chemotherapy for primary and advanced osteosarcomas," *Nano Res.*, 11(9), 4806–4822. doi: 10.1007/s12274-018-2066-0.

Zhang, Y., Wang, F., Li, M., Yu, Z., Qi, R., Ding, J. et al. (2018b) "Self-stabilized hyaluronate nanogel for intracellular codelivery of doxorubicin and cisplatin to osteosarcoma," *Adv. Sci. (Weinh)*, 5(5), p. 1700821. doi: 10.1002/advs.201700821.

Zhou, J. et al. (2013) "Regulation of osteoblast proliferation and differentiation by interrod spacing of Sr-HA nanorods on microporous titania coatings," *ACS Applied Materials & Interfaces*, 5(11), pp. 5358–5365. doi: 10.1021/am401339n.

13 Nanotherapeutics for Global Health Challenges

INTRODUCTION

The term "global health" first emerged in academic writing in the early 1940s (Dunham, 1945). The World Health Organization (WHO) subsequently adopted it as direction and foundational theory (Kickbusch, 1986). It can be concluded that global health is a recently established field of health sciences, emerging from the fields of medicine, public health, and worldwide health with major contributions provided by the WHO. It is based on studies that have been published in the international scientific community and through the experiences in research, instruction, imparting, and practice. They are distinct from the global health initiative because it focuses solely on medical and healthcare challenges with a global effect (Chen et al., 2020). Its primary mission is searching for global remedies for problems with a global health effect; and (Kickbusch, 1999) its ultimate objective is to apply the strength of academic research and science to advance health for all else, increase health equity, and lessen disparities in healthcare (Chen et al., 2020). Therefore, even if global health research studies and practice are able to be carried out locally, global health focuses on populations in every nation and incorporates all sectors outside of the medical and health systems (Beaglehole and Bonita, 2010).

The global health challenges comprise a number of communicable and noncommunicable diseases. Infectious diseases including microbial infections are the kingpins in the category of communicable diseases, and cancers, diabetes, cardiovascular diseases, neurodegenerative diseases, kidney diseases, genetic disorders, etc. are the kingpins in the category of the noncommunicable diseases. Additionally, sanitary issues such as menstruation health, personal hygiene, adult care, and their hygiene are important when taking into account the challenges facing global health. Seven objectives have been set forth by the Grand Challenges in Global Health (GCGH) program in an effort to address the current drawbacks of modern medicine (Singer et al., 2007). The GCGH's improved vaccine program aims to reduce treatment costs, boost therapeutic effectiveness, and provide new methods of drug delivery to completely remove the possibility of reused needles. The therapeutic effectiveness of recently developed pharmacological substances can be directly impacted by a variety of factors, including their scalability, capability to regulate discharge rate, and targeted liberation (Charrois and Allen, 2004; Siepmann et al., 2004). Discovering safer alternatives to therapy is especially important because chemotherapy is currently known to have negative side effects that can last both long and short periods of time (Partridge, Burstein and Winer, 2001). Innovative solutions are required in light of these difficulties in order to enhance treatment for patient successes on an international basis.

DOI: 10.1201/9781003442202-14

Nanotherapeutics may soon be able to help with the resolution of some of the most pressing issues in global health. Numerous studies have previously shown that, as compared to conventional procedures, utilizing nanotechnology may increase therapeutic effectiveness as well as security. Despite the fact that human clinical trials to evaluate the effectiveness and safety of drugs that utilize nanotherapeutics have begun to emerge (Hrkach et al., 2012), there are still numerous issues that need to be resolved before future commercialization, broad adoption, and clinical acceptability can take place. These obstacles encompass the necessity for long-term substance/therapeutic preservation, the accessibility of significant clinical trial financing, social and ethical concerns, potential negative effects on healthcare and ecosystems, regulatory constraints, and an intellectual property framework that is always changing. Fortunately, novel approaches that have received approval from the Food and Drug Administration are paving the way for a wider application of nanotechnology in healthcare. Future collaborative initiatives in nanotherapeutics will have a beneficial effect on society. The prospective of global health appears to be bright as the biomedical research field proceeds to accomplish important strides toward the discipline of nanotherapeutics (Miele, Spinelli and Miele, 2009).

13.1 IMMUNOLOGICAL APPROACHES IN MICROBIAL INFECTIONS

Bacteria, fungi, viruses, and parasites are among the pathogenic organisms causing infectious diseases, which continue to account for a large percentage of hospitalizations and fatalities globally. There are significant hurdles to overcome in the successful management of infectious diseases, despite significant progress made with antibiotic agents (Kaufmann et al., 2018). The continual emergence of novel viruses and bacteria as a result of adaptation and other biological processes further renders it difficult to regulate and prevent infectious diseases. Therefore, in addition to finding novel antiviral drugs and antibiotics for preventing and controlling infection, creative methods must be devised to increase the effectiveness of currently available therapies (Dickey et al., 2017). In fact, vaccination has significantly decreased the number of hospitalizations and mortality rates imposed by infectious diseases, rendering it one of the most simple and cost-effective measures. Unfortunately, there continues to be numerous cases of infectious diseases without vaccines, like *Chlamydia* and tuberculosis infections (Monno et al., 2001). In other instances, the use of vaccinations that contain inactivated or attenuated live pathogenic organisms potentially raises safety concerns, whereas recently produced subunit vaccines typically exhibit poor immunogenicity. As a result, the development of vaccines and novel antibiotics urgently requires breakthrough technology (Pardi et al., 2018). Figure 13.1 shows the global status of infectious diseases (Kirtane et al., 2021).

According to Singh et al. (2017), nanotechnology is a novel approach that can both mitigate the numerous drawbacks of antiviral medications and antibiotics and increase their therapeutic effects. In this regard, a wide range of nanoparticles have been investigated to increase drug dissolution rate/stability, extend circulation period of time, overcome biological obstacles, increase bioavailability, focus on infection locations, and modulate the way drugs release in accordance with biochemical signals associated with pathological alterations in order to enhance therapeutic efficacy

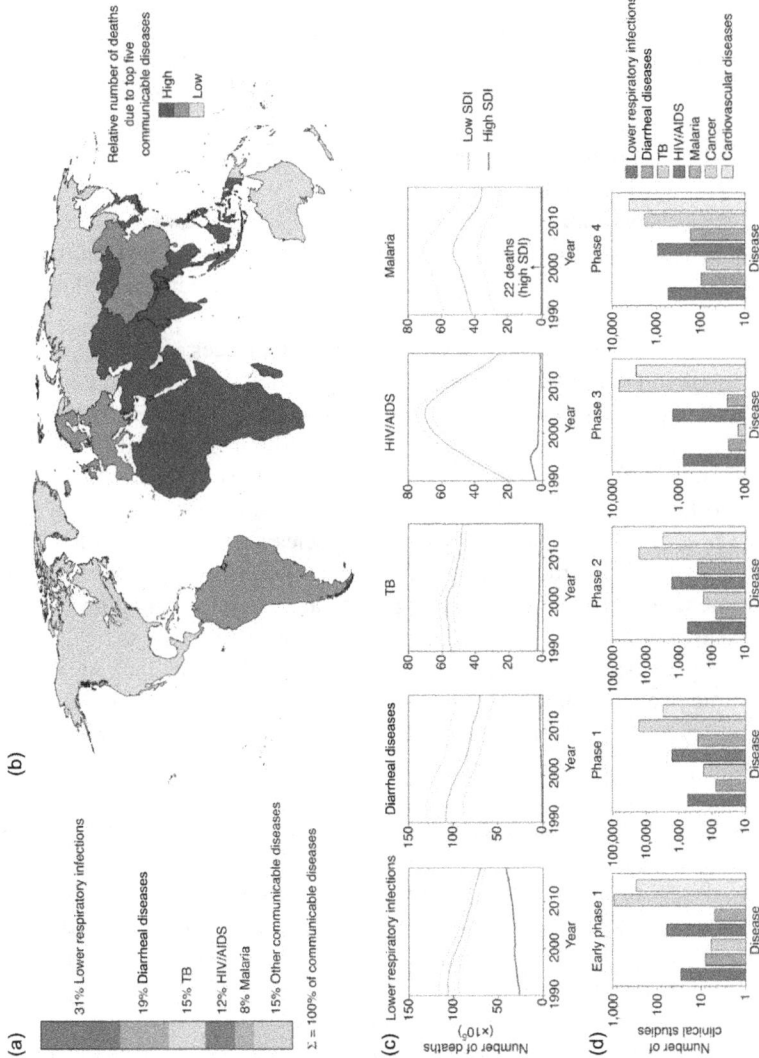

FIGURE 13.1 Infectious diseases represent a chronic healthcare burden around the world and as such are high-priority targets for investigational drugs. (a) The communicable diseases with the five highest mortality rates are lower respiratory infections, diarrheal diseases, TB, HIV infection, and malaria. (b) Low SDI countries are disproportionately affected by these top five communicable diseases. (c) Temporal trends in mortality rate for the five diseases. Although mortality rates from these communicable diseases is declining, there is considerable disparity between low and high SDI countries. The solid lines represent the mean values and the dotted lines show the uncertainty interval. (d) The number of clinical studies listed in clinicaltrials.gov for various diseases.

Source: Reproduced with permission from Kirtane et al., 2021.

and reduce adverse effects during the management of infectious diseases (Xiong et al., 2014). Abed and Couvreur (2014), Forier et al. (2014), Han et al. (2017), and other studies have shown that nanoparticle-based approaches have an important opportunity to decrease the progression of resistance or completely shift acquired resistance (Kumar, Curtis and Hoskins, 2018), through encouraging intracellular uptake, altering the route of drug distribution in subcellular organelles, influencing drug–pathogen communications, and/or imposing an anti-biofilm effect.

Furthermore, multiple studies have demonstrated that nanoparticles are excellent at boosting cellular and humoral immunity, which in turn can increase the effectiveness of adjuvants and antigens (Stewart and Keselowsky, 2017). Nanoparticles are capable of delivering antigens to specific lymphoid tissues, cell types that present antigens, along with subcellular compartments that are intriguing while shielding them from proteolytic degradation (Al-Halifa et al., 2019). Based on these characteristics, nanoparticles enable subunit vaccines to be administered at lower dosages while continuing to deliver desired immunological responses. They also significantly reduce nonspecific immune activation carried on by systemic administration of soluble antigens (Lybaert et al., 2018).

Additionally, antigens are capable of being given to mucosal surfaces with pinpoint accuracy, producing the anticipated mucosal immunity for defense against infections that spread through the mucosa (Narasimhan, Goodman and Vela Ramirez, 2016). Additionally, cross-presentation can be significantly increased through nanoparticle-mediated intracellular administration of exogenous antigens, making it highly favored for both preventative and therapeutic vaccines (Smith, Simon and Baker, 2013). In recent times, bioinspired nanoparticles alongside optimized surface bio-physicochemical characteristics have been produced using nanotechnology and biomimetic techniques for delivering medications and vaccine development (Parodi et al., 2017). In order to create these biomimetic nanoparticles, which have a variety of benefits, the performance, complexity, and biological compatibility of biological substances are merged with the variation, tailorability, and repeatability of synthetic nanomaterials (Meyer, Sunshine and Green, 2015). Nature-inspired nanoparticles alone can serve as potent nanotherapies or nanovaccines toward infectious diseases because of their inherent activity. They may also perform as sophisticated nanocarriers that allow targeted delivery of medicines or vaccinations.

Additionally, to deal with the molecular and cellular occurrences that predominate *in vivo* biopharmaceutical and pharmacokinetic properties of biomimetic nanotherapies that are being developed, mechanistic investigations should be carried out. In context with recent developments in the medical and life sciences as well as the advancements in nanotechnology, it is imperative to keep expanding the kinds and uses of biomimetic nanoplatforms. Additional cutting-edge innovations can be incorporated, such as computational drug design, materials genome, and sophisticated artificial intelligence, for the development of more effective and useful nanoparticles that use bioengineering methodologies. Given the noteworthy clinical effectiveness of bioinspired nanovaccines and nanomedicines, it is hoped that the biomimetic tactic-based nanotherapeutic area will soon offer innovative therapies over infectious diseases (Dong et al., 2019).

13.2   RESOLUTION FOR ANTIBIOTIC RESISTANCE

Despite notable effectiveness of antibiotics, there continue to be several obstacles that treatments for microbial infections must overcome, most notably propensity of bacteria to acquire antibiotic resistance. Due to the dwindling supply of potent medications, multidrug-resistant (MDR) germs appear to be a persistent worry. Bacterial infections are a severe global healthcare concern with dire repercussions. There is currently a battle between the development of therapies and the emergence of antibiotic resistance in microorganisms as a consequence of the swift growth of antibiotic resistance in microorganisms and the sluggish and decreasing development of novel antibiotics (Courtney et al., 2016).

Figure 13.2 shows the mechanisms for antibacterial activity of nanoparticles. Pathogens gain resistance against antibiotics by different mechanisms like alterations in membrane permeability, multidrug efflux pumps development, deoxyribonucleic acid (DNA) alterations, drug-degrading activity of enzymes, as well as longer intracellular residence durations, where therapeutic level of drugs cannot be easily achieved (Alekshun and Levy, 2007), consequently requiring higher doses and repeated administrations of drugs and eventually leading to toxicity or adverse side effects. This complicates compliance and therefore increases the chances to acquire drug resistance. Focus of current research is to solve these problems as well as to enhance the antimicrobial efficacy of available drugs by employing medication delivery systems that might be targeted in an accurate manner (Briones, Colino and Lanao, 2008).

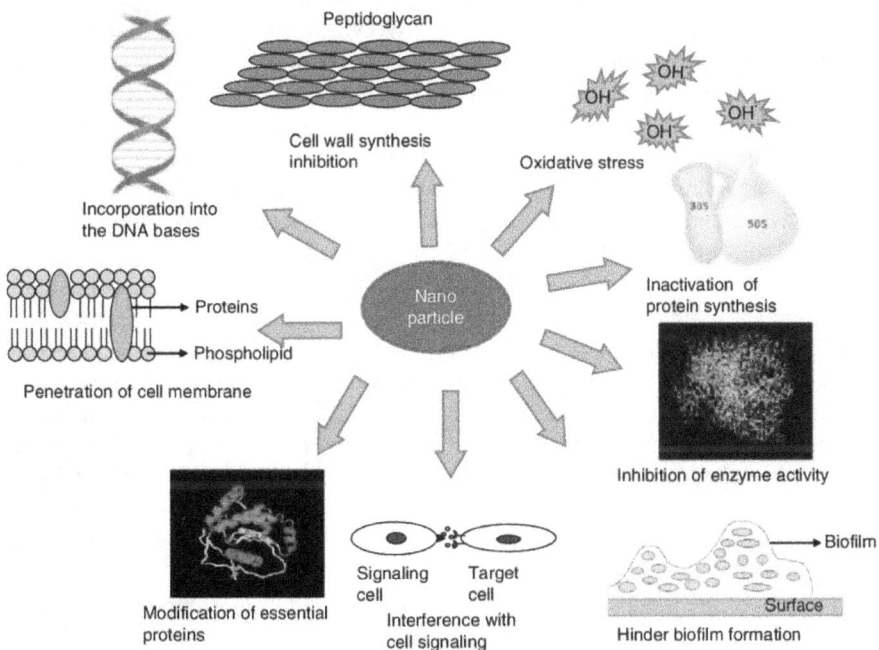

FIGURE 13.2   Mechanisms for antibacterial activity of nanoparticles.

Source: Reproduced with permission from Singh, Smitha and Singh, 2014.

Nanotechnology has advanced significantly over the last ten decades. It is expected that nanomaterials, especially as antibacterial substances, would eventually bridge the gaps left by repeated failures of conventional antibiotics. These materials seem to be extremely promising as they have received quite a lot of attention. The utilization of nanoparticles (NPs) has risen by over fourfold, and recent studies emphasizes the antibacterial potential of NPs, particularly against bacteria that are resistant to antibiotics (Qayyum and Khan, 2016). Additionally, using NPs as a medication carrier might promote and enhance the usage of conventional antibiotics. Regardless of the kind of drug and pathogen, metallic and organic NPs are being demonstrated to synergize the eradication effectiveness of antimicrobial drugs in combination with other treatments (Aditya et al., 2013).

Additionally, the antibacterial potential of NPs is being thoroughly investigated, and it has been discovered that nanoscale components including inorganic ions and polymers have strong antibiotic action on their own. According to some concepts, the ability of NPs to function as antibacterial agents is triggered through three main mechanisms: oxidative stress, metal ion discharge, and nonoxidative stress. These three mechanisms must occur simultaneously in order for bacteria to acquire antibacterial resistance. As a result, bacterial cells discover it more challenging to develop resistance toward NP-mediated antibacterial therapy (Sirelkhatim et al., 2015).

Drugs can be delivered specifically using NPs as delivery mechanisms, and their prolonged, regulated release allows them to make it to the therapeutic intracellular depth. It is possible to prevent drug degradation before it reaches the target and unfavorable drug interactions while also optimizing the physicochemical properties of the associated drug. Other benefits of NP delivery platforms include improved drug solubility, simultaneous administration of various medications, and longer systemic circulation, all of which have been supported by numerous studies (Davis, Chen and Shin, 2009). This has led to the endorsement of numerous NP-based therapies, including the use of NPs as vaccines for methods of administration to treat a wide range of infections that exhibit resistance for conventional therapies. Additionally, numerous therapies are presently going toward the preclinical and clinical testing phases (Chetoni et al., 2016).

A variety of MDR clinical strains of bacteria, including *MRSA*, extended-spectrum-lactamase-generating *Klebsiella pneumoniae*, carbapenem-resistant *Escherichia coli*, and *Salmonella typhimurium*, were reported to be destroyed by recently discovered photoexcited QDs. The redox potentials produced by photogenerated charge transporters, which inhibit MDR bacteria via particular reactions that engage the cellular redox environment quantum dots, are completely in control of the lethal impact (Courtney et al., 2016). AgNPs appear to exhibit antibacterial activity without distinguishing between susceptible and resistant strains, according to research involving these particles (Qayyum and Khan, 2016). These NPs adhere to the cell membrane, impair it, and consequently render it more porous. Once within the cell, silver ions also produce free radicals and raise the quantity of ROS that impede respiratory enzymes and trigger inflammatory reactions, finally leading to apoptosis. In this method, it has been discovered that AgNPs have greater antibacterial action than drugs like gentamicin or vancomycin toward *MRSA* and *Pseudomonas aeruginosa* (Saeb et al., 2014).

Additional metallic NPs that were originally synthesized to combat antimicrobial resistance include Mn, Cu, Zn, Pt, Al, or Ti. These can be used as transporters or as naked NPs due to their antibacterial and magnetic properties, which enhance the therapeutic effect. ZnO-NPs, which have strong antibacterial action, were utilized against a variety of microorganisms. However, the restriction on aggregation renders them hazardous for mammalian cells (Kulshrestha et al., 2014). Although excessive accumulation of copper is harmful, like various other metals, copper nanoparticles are gaining popularity because of their antibacterial and antifungal capabilities. Contrary to silver or gold, the human body has copper-transporters responsible for regulating copper homeostasis (Usman et al., 2013). Others, such as calcium fluoride nanoparticles (CaF_2-NPs), are discovered to have anticariogenic property against *S. mutans*. This is because CaF_2-NPs stick to the surface of teeth and continuously discharge fluoride ions that not only reduces virulence activities of *S. mutans* but also encourages remineralization (Kulshrestha et al., 2016).

It is also vital to take into account the numerous processes involved in antibacterial action. Pathogenic bacteria possess surfaces that are negatively charged beneath physiological conditions, which is capable of being used for effective bacterial targeting with cationic NPs (Sambhy, Peterson and Sen, 2008). Anionic NPs offer better targeting because HIV infection causes infected cells to express positively charged proteins (Gunaseelan et al., 2010). Active targeting is a different approach to combating resistant strains of microorganisms. Active targeting relies on recognizing particular chemicals or ligands on infected cells. The following can be accomplished through altering the surface of NPs, which enables NP-based medicine delivery systems to target only the pathogenic areas. Receptors, temperatures, or magnetic characteristics all can be targeted with active targeting. A variety of NPs and bactericidal polymeric compounds and peptides have been used to target various bacterial species (Byrne, Betancourt and Brannon-Peppas, 2008). Additionally, antimicrobial peptides (AMPs) are brief (10–40 amino acid) cationic peptides which are frequently utilized for efficient cell targeting (Bahnsen et al., 2013).

Integrating nanoporous silica nanoparticles (NPSNPs) containing poly(4-vinylpyridine) utilizing a bismaleimide as a bonding agent and loading chlorhexidine within allowed for controlled release of drugs through pH-sensitive platforms for delivery. Under physiological pH, the polymer acts as a gatekeeper by blocking pore openings to stop the liberation of cargo molecules. When the pH shifts to an acidic level, which typically happens during a bacterial infection, the polymeric strains protonate, the polymers straighten out owing to electrostatic repulsion, which opens the pores and then eventually the cargo is freed (Fullriede et al., 2016). By using these techniques, antibiotic-resistant microorganisms might be eliminated. Traditional antibiotics are unable to carry out such smart tasks. As a result, nanomaterials have a higher probability of overcoming the challenges caused by antimicrobial resistance (Zaidi, Misba and Khan, 2017).

13.3   SMART APPROACHES FOR NONCOMMUNICABLE DISEASES

Noncommunicable diseases (NCDs), which include cardiovascular diseases, obesity, dyslipidemia, cancer, chronic respiratory conditions, kidney diseases, and diabetes, are among the biggest fatalities worldwide and a growing threat to global health. Currently, NCDs cause more deaths than all other communicable diseases combined. On an annual basis, 41 million individuals globally die from NCDs, or more than 7 out of 10 fatalities (*About global NCDs*, 2022). The NCD kills annually 15 million individuals prematurely, before they reach the age of 70. This has been exacerbated by changing economic, social, and structural conditions, including more people relocating to cities, and the widespread adoption of lifestyle choices that are unhealthy (*About global NCDs*, 2022).

A series of metabolic diseases known as diabetes mellitus are characterized by elevated blood glucose levels (hyperglycemia). Diabetes is becoming more prevalent nowadays. It is predicted that there will be more than 400 million adults globally who will be suffering from the disease by 2030 (Shaw, Sicree and Zimmet, 2010). The annual global expenses of treating diabetes and its consequences come to US$500 billion without factoring in indirect expenses like lost productivity (Zhang et al., 2010). One intriguing instance concern superparamagnetic iron oxide nanoparticles (SPION)-containing bioengineered cells which have been discovered to release insulin when hyperthermia is induced externally using alternating magnetic currents. The capacity of the cells to produce insulin required *in vivo* for controlling the amount of glucose in the blood has been demonstrated in this investigation. Nanoparticles have been synthesized to protect and distribute nucleic acids to specific cells (Li and Mahato, 2011). For instance, in animal models for early diabetes, DNA encoding the cytokines interleukin-10 (IL 10) and interleukin-4 has been delivered to white blood cells to block the T cell response to residual innate islet cells, avoiding the occurrence of diabetes in 75% of utilized laboratory animals (Ko et al., 2001).

In contrast, to increase the release of insulin and islet viability (Oh et al., 2003), a gene that produces glucagon-like peptide 1 is being given using nanoparticles. Magnetic nanoparticles covered with the proper peptide-major histocompatibility complexes (pMHC-NPs) have been demonstrated to develop a population of I minimal-avidity autoreactive CD8+ T cells toward memory-like autoregulatory cells, preventing and reversing type 1 diabetes in 75% of laboratory mice (Tsai et al., 2010). This was done by employing a nonobese diabetic induced laboratory mouse model. Figure 13.3 shows the application of nanotechnology in the management of diabetes.

The widespread type of dementia is Alzheimer's disease (AD), a neurodegenerative disease that first manifests as memory loss and cognitive decline before causing harm to the physiological systems (Sonawane, Ahmad and Chinnathambi, 2019). Numerous studies have shown a correlation between the number of soluble masses of the amyloid beta (Aβ) peptide and the level of dementia among Alzheimer's disease (AD) patients (Fan et al., 2018). They aggregate together resulting in insoluble fibrils, and they eventually combine to generate recognizable plaques (Yang et al., 2005). As a result, the majority of current investigations are focused on preventing their aggregation.

Nanomaterials have been employed for this because of their extraordinary small dimensions and ability to traverse the blood–brain barrier (BBB). An aggregation can be prevented by OX26 mAB-conjugated solid lipid nanoparticles (SLNs) and the phytochemical agent-grape resveratrol that acts as a neuroprotective, anti-inflammatory substance (Cartiera et al., 2010). The hydrophobic lipid nucleus of SLNs enables the

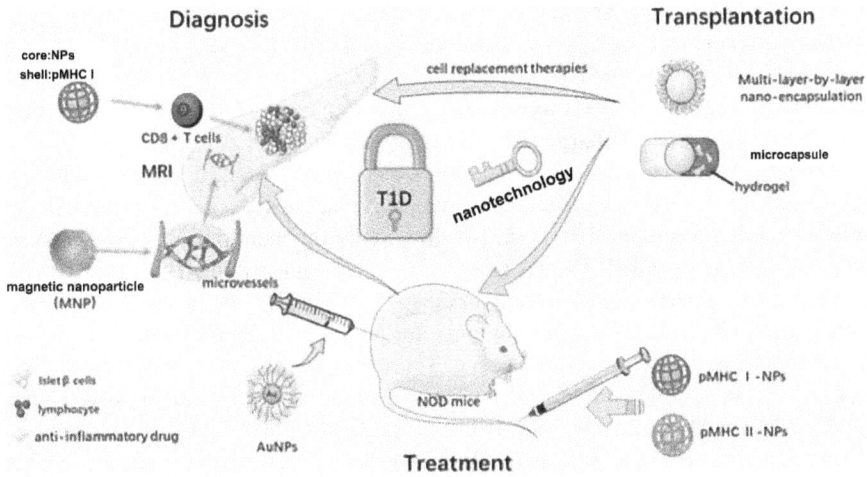

FIGURE 13.3 The application of nanotechnology combining with immunology in the diagnosis, treatment, and islet cells translation of T1D in diabetes.

Source: Reproduced with permission from Pan et al., 2020.

dispersion of the drug, enhancing bioavailability (Mathew et al., 2012). Additionally, they are quickly opsonized and cleared from the circulatory system, providing compelling evidence that these SLN do not concentrate within the bloodstream inappropriately, reducing the risks that are associated with them (Misra et al., 2012). Similar to this, a mouse arteriole aggregate had been successfully identified by a monoclonal antibody targeting fibrillary human amyloid 42, which was coupled with iron oxide NPs (Kundu et al., 2016).

The second most frequently occurring neurodegenerative disorder is Parkinson's disease (PD) (Esteves et al., 2015). The dopaminergic (DA) neurons within the substantia nigra pars compacta, which is located in the midbrain selectively perish and α-syn Lewy bodies begin growing in this pathological condition (Niu et al., 2017). It is discovered that six mutations, including SNCA, PINK 1, DJ-1, ATP13A2, parkin, and LRKK2, are responsible for familial PD (Vekrellis, Rideout and Stefanis, 2004). In the meantime, the relationship between α-syn and the onset of PD has been confirmed, researchers are looking for novel approaches to block its expression (Desplats et al., 2012). In a current investigation, short hairpin RNA (shRNA) as well as an *N*-isopropylacrylamide derivative were immobilized on oleic acid and incorporated into magnetic iron oxide nanoparticles (NPs). *N*-Isopropylacrylamide also received nerve growth factor addition. ShRNA is a potential treatment for PD since it successfully disrupted α-syn production (Ozansoy and Başak, 2013).

Another neurodegenerative condition, amyotrophic lateral sclerosis (ALS), is characterized by damage to the motor neurons, motor cortex region, and the spinal cord. Patients with ALS have abnormal levels of mutated superoxide dismutase (SOD). Misfolded SOD 1 has been proposed as the explanation for the orderly course of diseases. As a result, SOD level reduction is a major focus of research (Debnath et al., 2017). Although antisense oligonucleotides (ASOs) can successfully quiet the proteins, they are ineffective since they cannot cross the BBB. ASOs have been embedded onto lipid-covered calcium phosphate NPs to get over this issue. These are successfully introduced ASO toward a cell line that resembled neurons when they had a negative electrical charge (Bhatt et al., 2015).

Anxiety, restless movements, and chorea are symptoms of Huntington's disease (HD), that can be described as an autosomal-dominant neurodegenerative condition. It has been demonstrated that oxidative stress and mitochondrial abnormalities can be identified in biological samples taken from individuals who have neurodegenerative illnesses like HD. Electron transport chains within HD brains are also dysfunctional (Lin and Beal, 2006). Investigators are on the hunt for novel substances that might be able to suppress the formation of 3-nitroproponoic acid (3-NP), a neurotoxin that causes the development of ROS. Additionally, positive outcomes appeared when 3-NO-induced mice were supplied with SLNs that were laden with rosmarinic acid (Robinson et al., 2018). It has also been shown that siRNA, that can silence or alter the expression of mutated HTT, is carried by β-cyclodextrin (CD) NPs. Although CDNPs partially exhibited toxicity and significantly reduced the total amount of mutated gene mRNA, the entire toxicity profile was satisfactory (Vij et al., 2010).

The gene of cystic fibrosis transmembrane conductance (CFTR) has mutations in the life-threatening genetic condition known as cystic fibrosis. A variety of endothelium cells of tissues exhibit aberrant transit patterns, which are its defining features. As a result, the mucus becomes abnormally sticky and thickened, obstructing the organs. The lung is the main organ that is obstructed. This results in the development of recurring bacterial infections that gradually erode the lung tissues. As a consequence, the pulmonary disease broadens to the point where it causes mortality (Chen et al., 2006). The CFTR gene repair appears to be an appealing approach for treating this condition. Another intriguing method used to treat CFTR infections involved ciprofloxacin complex-loaded biodegradable nanoparticles (NPs). This strategy was chosen to combat the infections that have become inherent to the illness itself. *Pseudomonas aeruginosa* was the organism that these antibiotic-incorporated NPs were designed to eradicate. Following therapy, mucus was examined for results. The mucus reportedly became substantially less turbid, demonstrating a decrease in pathogenic bacteria, and the stability of colloidal particles was demonstrated (Sato et al., 2012).

Acute kidney injury (AKI) represents a serious kidney condition characterized by a rapid reduction in renal function as well as significant morbidity, mortality, and medical expenses. Moreover, it additionally poses a high risk of developing chronic kidney disease (CKD) (Coca, Singanamala and Parikh, 2012). AKI represents one of the most dangerous and frequent consequences among hospitalized patients, causing around 2 million fatalities annually throughout the world (Luo et al., 2017). The most effective pharmacological therapy available at the moment is costly generalized supportive care (Kellum et al., 2021). In addition to traditional medicines, flavonoids—a phytochemical agent—has a significance in AKI. However, the use of flavonoids for the management of AKI is very constrained due to their low solubility in water and permeation capabilities. The accessibility and effectiveness of flavonoids can be enhanced by nanocarriers (Córdoba-David et al., 2020). Employing polyvinyl alcohol (PVA) and Eudragit E100, Zhang and colleagues developed water-soluble eupafolin nanoparticles that can overcome the physicochemical issues with the initial form eupafolin. It increases the water solubility through lowering the particle size and all without harming healthy renal cells. Eupafolin NPs have improved antioxidant and anti-inflammatory actions, which can reduce LPS-induced kidney injury (Zhang et al., 2017).

Obesity is a chronic and complicated condition, as defined by the International Classification of Diseases, that affects people all over the world and has a negative impact on quality of life (Sandoval-Vargas et al., 2021). Overweight and obesity are both defined by the World Health Organization (WHO) as the abnormal accumulation of body fat that has adverse health implications. Dyslipidemia has been recognized as an indicator of obesity and poses significant health concerns to those who are affected. Due to the existence of adipose tissue malfunction, obesity and dyslipidemia are regarded as the primary contributors to the metabolic syndrome. Zhang et al. (2018) examined two perspectives on recent developments in nanotherapeutics as a new technique for treating obesity. One perspective focused on the inhibition of ability to digest, and the other concentrated on the improvement of energy expenditure. Even though administered nanocarriers are an effective way to control body weight, researchers noted that a number of issues still need to be resolved. These include the understanding of the pathways involved in the maintenance of energy homeostasis, the reduction of adverse effects, the assessment of the biocompatibility in administration for a long time, and, obviously, the completion of effective clinical studies and further commercialization (Trandafir et al., 2022).

Using a total of three distinct strategies, including (i) the repression of angiogenesis within the white adipose tissues of the body (WATs), (ii) the conversion of WATs to brown adipose tissues (BATs), and (iii) the photothermal lipid breakdown of WATs, Sibuyi et al. explained nanotechnology-based therapies to be a possible alternative which can be utilized to address obesity and overwhelmed the drawbacks associated with standard therapies. The combined nanocarriers demonstrated high tolerability, decreased adverse reactions, and improved efficacy in a repeatable manner, thereby demonstrating the viability of the theory that focused on nanotherapy can be used to treat obesity while minimizing its comorbidities (Sibuyi et al., 2019).

On a global scale, cardiovascular disease remains the most prevalent cause of death. The difficulties encountered in cardiovascular medicine are a result of poor target precision, low distribution efficiency, and off-target action of current medicines. Cardiovascular disease is another area where nanotechnology is expanding. Individuals with hypertriglyceridemia may benefit from fenofibrate nanoformulations that are currently available on the market for assistance with solubility and absorption issues. The anti-inflammatory cytokine IL (interleukin)-10 was incorporated into nanoparticles in a different investigation employing a related type IV collagen-targeting method. IL-10 nanotherapy improved macrophage-mediated elimination of apoptotic debris and demonstrated comparable protective impacts on severe atherosclerosis in Ldlr-/- animals. This suggests that reducing local inflammation may also have proefferocytic effects (Flores et al., 2019).

13.4   APPROACHES IN GLOBAL SANITARY ISSUES

Menstrual hygiene, geriatric hygiene, pediatric hygiene, and personal hygiene are all important aspects of global sanitation. Sanitary napkins, adult diapers, baby diapers, undergarments, etc. are important in this case. Every woman should be concerned about menstrual hygiene since it lowers her susceptibility to infections of the reproductive tract (RTIs). Commercially accessible feminine hygiene items include sanitary napkins, tampons, underpants shields, towels, wipes, and pads for removing cosmetics. The feminine sanitary pad or serviette is a crucial disposable absorbent hygiene item among these. Its purposes include absorbing and holding onto menstrual fluid flow, isolating it from the skin, and ensuring comfort, avoiding odor, and remaining firmly anchored (Yadav et al., 2016).

Adult diapers and underpant shields are among the items offered in the geriatric personal care marketplace's absorbent category of products that are relevant to adult incontinence. The present product selection is wide-ranging and made to accommodate requirements of both sexes along with individuals of all ages (Ajmeri and Ajmeri, 2010). A common consumer item, disposable baby diapers, produce about 77 million tons of solid waste that goes to landfills each year and degrade at least over 500 years. Additionally, their use is expanding globally (Febo and Gagliardini, 2019).

Superabsorbent polymers (SAPs) along with various compounds have been used for a few decades to boost the ability of disposable diapers, sanitary napkins, and other easily available sanitary items to absorb moisture. Unfortunately, it is typical that those sanitary napkins and diapers do not react well against moist circumstances due to the several chemical compounds present within them, particularly when used as feminine pads during menstruation, superabsorbent polymers, commonly known as regular pads, can produce rashes and even inflammation. The average nappy materials can hold 30 times its own weight in human fluids, demonstrating how effective these supplies are at soaking multiple times their own individual weight in fluids However, the substance is not biodegradable; under ideal circumstances, a nappy may take 500 years to disintegrate (Yadav et al., 2016).

Compared to superabsorbent polymers (ordinary pads), the nanofiber product is more pleasant to use and leaves less residues after use. The structure of the nanofiber material is additionally much smoother, leading to a thinner and softer item that does not require to be transformed as frequently as the conventional pads, thereby providing a more affordable choice, having a smaller environmental impact, and being safer for humans compared with the current superabsorbent polymer materials. Experiments with saline and synthetic urine supported this finding, showing that the electrospun nanofiber material was significantly more absorbent compared with commercially available items. Since the invention of nanotechnology, which promises to have a positive impact on both the environment and global health, hygiene products are now safer to ingest and dispose of (Yadav et al., 2016).

Electrospinning is a simple and inexpensive method for producing fibers with diameters ranging from 10 nm to 10 m. Electrospun fibers can be used in a variety of applications due to their significant surface-to-volume proportion, tunable porosity, and adaptable shape with controlled diameter. As previously stated, the main goal of this study is to maximize the high absorption potential of electrospun nanofibers by making use of their huge surface area (Yadav et al., 2016).

Engaging superabsorbent polymer (SAP) encapsulating strategies, S. Yadav et al. developed cellulose acetate electrospun cellulose acetate (CA) nanofibers that were characterized by their surface shape, comfort, and mechanical attributes. Different assessments, including free absorbency, equilibria absorbency, absorbency during high loadings, and percentage debris, were carried out in various mediums, including distilled water, a solution of saline, and artificial urine, in order to prove their applicability in female hygiene applications. The outcomes were then contrasted to certain well-known commercial feminine hygiene products. It is discovered that adding SAP as encapsulating agents of CA nanofibers reduced the porosity and area of the surface of (CA) nanofibers. Moreover, in addition to their ability to swell, it reduced their ability to absorb more fluids than using just CA nanofibers alone. This clearly indicates that in the event CA nanofibers are employed to produce the absorbent center in feminine sanitary towels without affecting the absorption effectiveness, the consumption of superabsorbent polymers SAP (or in general SAPs) can be avoided. The potential to use these nanofibrous membranes in adult diapers and baby diapers is demonstrated by the previously mentioned electrospun membranes (Yadav et al., 2016).

Moreover, a Japanese textile business, Seiren, claims that its Deoest® odor-eliminating underpants fabricated with the aid of nanotechnology can miraculously absorb unpleasant scents (Onoghwarite and Ikechukwu, 2018). This inventive product leads to higher demands in personal hygiene products. Furthermore, the company named Goldwin, which sells Speedo® swimsuits in Japan, emphasizes that its upgraded MXP® pants with nanotechnology can absorb the odor from 4 L of perspiration. The pants are made of a lightweight, odor-removing, sweat-absorbing, antibacterial, antistatic, and eucalyptus and nanotechnology packed fabric from Toray. Due to their minimal washing requirements, these odor-eliminating pants also conserves water (Onoghwarite and Ikechukwu, 2018). These innovations lead to merits in personal hygiene problems globally.

REFERENCES

Abed, N. and Couvreur, P. (2014) "Nanocarriers for antibiotics: A promising solution to treat intracellular bacterial infections," *Int. J. Antimicrob. Agents*, 43(6), pp. 485–496. doi: 10.1016/j.ijantimicag.2014.02.009.

About global NCDs (2022) *Cdc.gov*. Available at: www.cdc.gov/globalhealth/healthprotection/ncd/global-ncd-overview.html (Accessed: April 22, 2023).

Aditya, N. P. et al. (2013) "Advances in nanomedicines for malaria treatment," *Advances in Colloid and Interface Science*, 201–202, pp. 1–17. doi: 10.1016/j.cis.2013.10.014.

Ajmeri, J. R. and Ajmeri, C. J. (2010) "Nonwoven personal hygiene materials and products," In R.A. Chapman (Ed.), *Applications of nonwovens in technical textiles*. Boca Raton Boston, Washington, and Oxford, UK: Elsevier, pp. 85–102.

Alekshun, M. N. and Levy, S. B. (2007) "Molecular mechanisms of antibacterial multidrug resistance," *Cell*, 128(6), pp. 1037–1050. doi: 10.1016/j.cell.2007.03.004.

Al-Halifa, S., Gauthier, L., Arpin, D., Bourgault, S. and Archambault, D. (2019) "Nanoparticle-based vaccines against respiratory viruses," *Front. Immunol.*, 10, p. 11. doi: 10.3389/fimmu.2019.00022.

Bahnsen, J. S. et al. (2013) "Antimicrobial and cell-penetrating properties of penetrating analogs: Effect of sequence and secondary structure," *Biochimica et biophysica acta*, 1828(2), pp. 223–232. doi: 10.1016/j.bbamem.2012.10.010.

Beaglehole, R. and Bonita, R. (2010) "What is global health?," *Global Health Action*, 3(1), p. 5142. doi: 10.3402/gha.v3i0.5142.

Bhatt, R. et al. (2015) "Development, characterization and nasal delivery of rosmarinic acid-loaded solid lipid nanoparticles for the effective management of Huntington's disease," *Drug Delivery*, 22(7), pp. 931–939. doi: 10.3109/10717544.2014.880860.

Briones, E., Colino, C. I. and Lanao, J. M. (2008) "Delivery systems to increase the selectivity of antibiotics in phagocytic cells," *Journal of Controlled Release: Official Journal of the Controlled Release Society*, 125(3), pp. 210–227. doi: 10.1016/j.jconrel.2007.10.027.

Byrne, J. D., Betancourt, T. and Brannon-Peppas, L. (2008) "Active targeting schemes for nanoparticle systems in cancer therapeutics," *Advanced Drug Delivery Reviews*, 60(15), pp. 1615–1626. doi: 10.1016/j.addr.2008.08.005.

Cartiera, M. S. et al. (2010) "Partial correction of cystic fibrosis defects with PLGA nanoparticles encapsulating curcumin," *Molecular Pharmaceutics*, 7(1), pp. 86–93. doi: 10.1021/mp900138a.

Charrois, G. J. R. and Allen, T. M. (2004) "Drug release rate influences the pharmacokinetics, biodistribution, therapeutic activity, and toxicity of pegylated liposomal doxorubicin formulations in murine breast cancer," *Biochimica et biophysica acta*, 1663(1–2), pp. 167–177. doi: 10.1016/j.bbamem.2004.03.006.

Chen, J. et al. (2006) "Rare earth nanoparticles prevent retinal degeneration induced by intracellular peroxides," *Nature Nanotechnology*, 1(2), pp. 142–150. doi: 10.1038/nnano.2006.91.

Chen, X. et al. (2020) "What is global health? Key concepts and clarification of misperceptions: Report of the 2019 GHRP editorial meeting: Report of the 2019 GHRP editorial meeting," *Global Health Research and Policy*, 5(1), p. 14. doi: 10.1186/s41256-020-00142-7.

Chetoni, P. et al. (2016) "Solid lipid nanoparticles as promising tool for intraocular tobramycin delivery: Pharmacokinetic studies on rabbits," *European Journal of Pharmaceutics and Biopharmaceutics: Official Journal of Arbeitsgemeinschaft für Pharmazeutische Verfahrenstechnik e.V*, 109, pp. 214–223. doi: 10.1016/j.ejpb.2016.10.006.

Coca, S. G., Singanamala, S. and Parikh, C. R. (2012) "Chronic kidney disease after acute kidney injury: A systematic review and meta-analysis," *Kidney International*, 81(5), pp. 442–448. doi: 10.1038/ki.2011.379.

Córdoba-David, G. et al. (2020) "Effective nephroprotection against acute kidney injury with a star-shaped polyglutamate-curcuminoid conjugate," *Scientific Reports*, 10(1), p. 2056. doi: 10.1038/s41598-020-58974-9.

Courtney, C. M. et al. (2016) "Photoexcited quantum dots for killing multidrug-resistant bacteria," *Nature Materials*, 15(5), pp. 529–534. doi: 10.1038/nmat4542.

Davis, M. E., Chen, Z. (georgia) and Shin, D. M. (2009) "Nanoparticle therapeutics: An emerging treatment modality for cancer," In Peter Rodgers (Ed.), *Nanoscience and technology*. New Jersey, USA and London, UK: Co-Published with Macmillan Publishers Ltd, pp. 239–250.

Debnath, K. et al. (2017) "Poly (trehalose) nanoparticles prevent amyloid aggregation and suppress polyglutamine aggregation in a Huntington's disease model mouse," *ACS Applied Materials and Interfaces*, 9, pp. 24126–24139.

Desplats, P. et al. (2012) "Combined exposure to Maneb and Paraquat alters transcriptional regulation of neurogenesis-related genes in mice models of Parkinson's disease," *Molecular Neurodegeneration*, 7(1), p. 49. doi: 10.1186/1750-1326-7-49.

Dickey, S. W., Cheung, G. Y. C. and Otto, M. (2017) "Different drugs for bad bugs: Antivirulence strategies in the age of antibiotic resistance," *Nat. Rev. Drug. Discov.* 16(7), pp. 457–471. doi: 10.1038/nrd.2017.23.

Dong, X. et al. (2019) "Targeting of nanotherapeutics to infection sites for antimicrobial therapy," *Advanced Therapeutics*, 2(11), p. 1900095. doi: 10.1002/adtp.201900095.

Dunham, G. C. (1945) "Today's global frontiers in public health: I. a pattern for cooperative public health," *American Journal of Public Health and the Nation's Health*, 35(2), pp. 89–95. doi: 10.2105/ajph.35.2.89.

Esteves, M. et al. (2015) "Retinoic acid-loaded polymeric nanoparticles induce neuroprotection in a mouse model for Parkinson's disease. Front," *Aging Neurosci*, 7.

Fan, S. et al. (2018) "Curcumin-loaded PLGA-PEG nanoparticles conjugated with B6 peptide for potential use in Alzheimer's disease," *Drug Delivery*, 25(1), pp. 1091–1102. doi: 10.1080/10717544.2018.1461955.

Febo, P. and Gagliardini, A. (2019) "Baby diapers past and present: A critical review." Available at: https://api.semanticscholar.org/CorpusID:235328297.

Flores, A. M. et al. (2019) "Nanoparticle therapy for vascular diseases," *Arteriosclerosis, Thrombosis, and Vascular Biology*, 39(4), pp. 635–646. doi: 10.1161/ATVBAHA.118. 311569.

Forier, K., Raemdonck, K., De Smedt, S. C., Demeester, J., Coenye, T. and Braeckmans, K. (2014) "Lipid and polymer nanoparticles for drug delivery to bacterial biofilms," *J. Control. Release*, 190, 607–623. doi: 10.1016/j.jconrel.2014.03.055.

Fullriede, H. et al. (2016) "pH-responsive release of chlorhexidine from modified nanoporous silica nanoparticles for dental applications," *BioNanoMaterials*, 17(1–2), pp. 59–72. doi: 10.1515/bnm-2016-0003.

Gunaseelan, S. et al. (2010) "Surface modifications of nanocarriers for effective intracellular delivery of anti-HIV drugs," *Advanced Drug Delivery Reviews*, 62(4–5), pp. 518–531. doi: 10.1016/j.addr.2009.11.021.

Han, C., Romero, N., Fischer, S., Dookran, J., Berger, A. and Doiron Amber, L. (2017) "Recent developments in the use of nanoparticles for treatment of biofilms," *Nanotechnol. Rev.* 6(5), pp. 383–404. doi: 10.1515/ntrev-2016-0054.

Hrkach, J. et al. (2012) "Preclinical development and clinical translation of a PSMA-targeted docetaxel nanoparticle with a differentiated pharmacological profile," *Science Translational Medicine*, 4(128), pp. 128ra39–128ra39. doi: 10.1126/scitranslmed.3003651.

Kaufmann, S. H. E., Dorhoi, A., Hotchkiss, R. S. and Bartenschlager, R. (2018) "Host-directed therapies for bacterial and viral infections," *Nat. Rev. Drug. Discov.*, 17(1), 35–56. doi: 10.1038/nrd.2017.162.

Kellum, J. A. et al. (2021) "Acute kidney injury," *Nature Reviews. Disease Primers*, 7(1), p. 52. doi: 10.1038/s41572-021-00284-z.

Kickbusch, I. (1986) "Health promotion: A global perspective," *Canadian Journal of Public Health. Revue canadienne de sante publique*, 77(5), pp. 321–326.

Kickbusch, I. (1999) "Global + local = glocal public health," *Journal of Epidemiology and Community Health*, 53(8), pp. 451–452. doi: 10.1136/jech.53.8.451.

Kirtane, A. R. et al. (2021) "Nanotechnology approaches for global infectious diseases," *Nature Nanotechnology*, 16(4), pp. 369–384. doi: 10.1038/s41565-021-00866-8.

Ko, K. S. et al. (2001) "Combined administration of plasmids encoding IL-4 and IL-10 prevents the development of autoimmune diabetes in nonobese diabetic mice," *Molecular TherI The Journal of the American Society of Gene Therapy*, 4(4), pp. 313–316. doi: 10.1006/mthe.2001.0459.

Kulshrestha, S. et al. (2014) "A graphene/zinc oxide nanocomposite film protects dental implant surfaces against cariogenic Streptococcus mutans," *Biofouling*, 30(10), pp. 1281–1294.

Kulshrestha, S. et al. (2016) "Calcium fluoride nanoparticles induced suppression of Streptococcus mutans biofilm: An *in vitro* and *in vivo* approach," *Applied Microbiology and Biotechnology*, 100(4), pp. 1901–1914. doi: 10.1007/s00253-015-7154-4.

Kumar, M., Curtis, A. and Hoskins, C. (2018) "Application of nanoparticle technologies in the combat against anti-microbial resistance," *Pharmaceutics*, 10(1), p. E11. doi: 10.3390/pharmaceutics10010011.

Kundu, P. et al. (2016) "Delivery of dual drug loaded lipid based nanoparticles across the blood-brain barrier impart enhanced neuroprotection in a rotenone induced mouse model of Parkinson's disease," *ACS Chemical Neuroscience*, 7(12), pp. 1658–1670. doi: 10.1021/acschemneuro.6b00207.

Li, F. and Mahato, R. I. (2011) "RNA interference for improving the outcome of islet transplantation," *Advanced Drug Delivery Reviews*, 63(1–2), pp. 47–68. doi: 10.1016/j.addr.2010.11.003.

Lin, M. T. and Beal, M. F. (2006) "Mitochondrial dysfunction and oxidative stress in neurodegenerative diseases," *Nature*, 443(7113), pp. 787–795. doi: 10.1038/nature05292.

Luo, M. et al. (2017) "A new scoring model for the prediction of mortality in patients with acute kidney injury," *Scientific Reports*, 7(1), P. 7862. doi: 10.1038/s41598-017-08440-w.

Lybaert, L., Vermaelen, K., De Geest, B. G. and Nuhn, L. (2018) "Immunoengineering through cancer vaccines—a personalized and multi-step vaccine approach towards precise cancer immunity," *J. Control. Release*, 289, 125–145. doi: 10.1016/j. jconrel.2018.09.009.

Mathew, A. et al. (2012) "Curcumin loaded-PLGA nanoparticles conjugated with Tet-1 peptide for potential use in Alzheimer's disease," *PLoS One*, 7(3), p. e32616. doi: 10.1371/journal.pone.0032616.

Meyer, R. A., Sunshine, J. C. and Green, J. J. (2015) "Biomimetic particles as therapeutics," *Trends Immunol.*, 33(9), 514–524. doi: 10.1016/j.tibtech.2015. 07.001.

Miele, E., Spinelli, G. P. and Miele, E. (2009) "Albumin-bound formulation of Paclitaxel (Abraxane® ABI-007) in the treatment of breast cancer," *International Journal of Nanomedicine*, 4, pp. 99–105.

Misra, S. et al. (2012) "P1-264: Neuroprotective potential of solid lipid nanoparticles of sesamol: Possible brain targeting strategy," *Alzheimer's & Dementia: The Journal of the Alzheimer's Association*, 8(4S_Part_5), pp. P199–P199. doi: 10.1016/j.jalz.2012.05.544.

Monno, R. et al. (2001) "*Chlamydia trachomatis* and *Mycobacterium tuberculosis* lung infection in an HIV-positive homosexual man," *AIDS Patient Care and STDs*, 15(12), pp. 607–610. doi: 10.1089/108729101753354590.

Narasimhan, B., Goodman, J. T. and Vela Ramirez, J. E. (2016) "Rational design of targeted next-generation carriers for drug and vaccine delivery," *Annu. Rev. Biomed. Eng.*, 18, pp. 25–49. doi: 10.1146/annurev-bioeng-082615-030519.

Niu, S. et al. (2017) "Inhibition by multifunctional magnetic nanoparticles loaded with alpha-synuclein RNAi Plasmid in a Parkinson's disease model," *Theranostics*, 7(2), pp. 344–356. doi: 10.7150/thno.16562.

Oh, S. et al. (2003) "GLP-1 gene delivery for the treatment of type 2 diabetes," *Molecular Therapy: The Journal of the American Society of Gene Therapy*, 7(4), pp. 478–483. doi: 10.1016/s1525-0016(03)00036-4.

Onoghwarite, O. E. and Ikechukwu, O. P. (2018) "Emerging trends in nanoabsorbents absorption applications," *International Journal of Advances in Scientific Research and Engineering*, 4(11), pp. 201–206. doi: 10.31695/ijasre.2018.32963.

Ozansoy, M. and Başak, A. N. (2013) "The central theme of Parkinson's disease: α-synuclein," *Molecular Neurobiology*, 47(2), pp. 460–465. doi: 10.1007/s12035-012-8369-3.

Pan, W. et al. (2020) "Nanotechnology's application in Type 1 diabetes," *Wiley Interdiscip linary Reviews. Nanomedicine and Nanobiotechnology*, 12(6), p. e1645. doi: 10.1002/wnan.1645.

Pardi, N., Hogan, M. J., Porter, F. W. and Weissman, D. (2018) "Mrna vaccines—a new era in vaccinology," *Nat. Rev. Drug. Discov.*, 17(4), 261–279. doi: 10.1038/nrd.2017.243.

Parodi, A., Molinaro, R., Sushnitha, M., Evangelopoulos, M., Martinez, J. O., Arrighetti, N. et al. (2017) "Bio-inspired engineering of cell- and virus-like nanoparticles for drug delivery," *Biomaterials*, 147, pp. 155–168. doi: 10.1016/j. biomaterials.2017.09.020.

Partridge, A. H., Burstein, H. J. and Winer, E. P. (2001) "Side effects of chemotherapy and combined chemohormonal therapy in women with early-stage breast cancer," *Journal of the National Cancer Institute. Monographs*, 2001(30), pp. 135–142. doi: 10.1093/oxfordjournals.jncimonographs.a003451.

Qayyum, S. and Khan, A. U. (2016) "Nanoparticles vs. biofilms: A battle against another paradigm of antibiotic resistance," *Med. Chem. Comm.*, 7(8), pp. 1479–1498. doi: 10.1039/c6md00124f.

Robinson, E. et al. (2018) "Lipid nanoparticle-delivered chemically modified mRNA restores chloride secretion in cystic fibrosis," *Molecular Therapy: The Journal of the American Society of Gene Therapy*, 26(8), pp. 2034–2046. doi: 10.1016/j.ymthe.2018.05.014.

Saeb, A. T. M. et al. (2014) "Production of silver nanoparticles with strong and stable antimicrobial activity against highly pathogenic and multidrug resistant bacteria," *The Scientific World Journal*, 2014, p. 704708. doi: 10.1155/2014/704708.

Sambhy, V., Peterson, B. R. and Sen, A. (2008) "Antibacterial and hemolytic activities of pyridinium polymers as a function of the spatial relationship between the positive charge and the pendant alkyl tail," *Angewandte Chemie (Weinheim an der Bergstrasse, Germany)*, 120(7), pp. 1270–1274. doi: 10.1002/ange.200702287.

Sandoval-Vargas, D. et al. (2021) "Short communication: Obesity intervention resulting in significant changes in the human gut viral composition," *Applied sciences (Basel, Switzerland)*, 11(21), p. 10039. doi: 10.3390/app112110039.

Sato, S. et al. (2012) "Excess potassium and microstructure control for producing dense KNbO₃ ceramics," *Transactions of the Materials Research Society of Japan*, 37, pp. 65–68.

Shaw, J. E., Sicree, R. A. and Zimmet, P. Z. (2010) "Global estimates of the prevalence of diabetes for 2010 and 2030," *Diabetes Research and Clinical Practice*, 87(1), pp. 4–14. doi: 10.1016/j.diabres.2009.10.007.

Sibuyi, N. R. S. et al. (2019) "Nanotechnology advances towards development of targeted-treatment for obesity," *Journal of Nanobiotechnology*, 17(1), p. 122. doi: 10.1186/s12951-019-0554-3.

Siepmann, J. et al. (2004) "Effect of the size of biodegradable microparticles on drug release: Experiment and theory," *Journal of Controlled Release: Official Journal of the Controlled Release Society*, 96(1), pp. 123–134. doi: 10.1016/j.jconrel.2004.01.011.

Singer, P. A. et al. (2007) "Grand challenges in global health: The ethical, social and cultural program," *PLoS Medicine*, 4(9), p. e265. doi: 10.1371/journal.pmed.0040265.

Singh, L., Kruger, H. G., Maguire, G. E. M., Govender, T. and Parboosing, R. (2017) "The role of nanotechnology in the treatment of viral infections," *Ther. Adv. Infect. Dis.*, 4(4), pp. 105–131. doi: 10.1177/2049936117713593.

Singh, R., Smitha, M. S. and Singh, S. P. (2014) "The role of nanotechnology in combating multi-drug resistant bacteria," *Journal of Nanoscience and Nanotechnology*, 14(7), pp. 4745–4756. doi: 10.1166/jnn.2014.9527.

Sirelkhatim, A. et al. (2015) "Review on zinc oxide nanoparticles: Antibacterial activity and toxicity mechanism," *Nano-Micro Letters*, 7(3), pp. 219–242. doi: 10.1007/s40820-015-0040-x.

Smith, D. M., Simon, J. K. and Baker, J. R., Jr. (2013) "Applications of nanotechnology for immunology," *Nat. Rev. Immunol.*, 13(8), pp. 592–605. doi: 10.1038/nri3488.

Sonawane, S. K., Ahmad, A. and Chinnathambi, S. (2019) "Protein-capped metal nanoparticles inhibit Tau aggregation in Alzheimer's disease," *ACS Omega*, 4(7), pp. 12833–12840. doi: 10.1021/acsomega.9b01411.

Stewart, J. M. and Keselowsky, B. G. (2017) "Combinatorial drug delivery approaches for immunomodulation," *Adv. Drug Deliv. Rev.*, 114, pp. 161–174. doi: 10.1016/j.addr.2017.05.013.

Trandafir, L. M. et al. (2022) "Tackling dyslipidemia in obesity from a nanotechnology perspective," *Nutrients*, 14(18), p. 3774. doi: 10.3390/nu14183774.

Tsai, S. et al. (2010) "Reversal of autoimmunity by boosting memory-like autoregulatory T cells," *Immunity*, 32(4), pp. 568–580. doi: 10.1016/j.immuni.2010.03.015.

Usman, M. S. et al. (2013) "Synthesis, characterization, and antimicrobial properties of copper nanoparticles," *International Journal of Nanomedicine*, 8, pp. 4467–4479. doi: 10.2147/IJN.S50837.

Vekrellis, K., Rideout, H. J. and Stefanis, L. (2004) "Neurobiology of alpha-synuclein," *Molecular Neurobiology*, 30(1), pp. 1–21. doi: 10.1385/MN:30:1:001.

Vij, N. et al. (2010) "Development of PEGylated PLGA nanoparticle for controlled and sustained drug delivery in cystic fibrosis," *Journal of Nanobiotechnology*, 8(1), p. 22. doi: 10.1186/1477-3155-8-22.

Xiong, M. H., Bao, Y., Yang, X. Z., Zhu, Y. H. and Wang, J. (2014) "Delivery of antibiotics with polymeric particles," *Adv. Drug. Deliv. Rev.*, 78, pp. 63–76. doi: 10.1016/j.addr.2014.02.002.

Yadav, S. et al. (2016) "High absorbency cellulose acetate electrospun nanofibers for feminine hygiene application," *Applied Materials Today*, 4, pp. 62–70. doi: 10.1016/j.apmt.2016.07.002.

Yang, F. et al. (2005) "Curcumin inhibits formation of amyloid beta oligomers and fibrils, binds plaques, and reduces amyloid *in vivo*," *The Journal of Biological Chemistry*, 280(7), pp. 5892–5901. doi: 10.1074/jbc.M404751200.

Zaidi, S., Misba, L. and Khan, A. U. (2017) "Nano-therapeutics: A revolution in infection control in post antibiotic era," *Nanomedicine: Nanotechnology, Biology, and Medicine*, 13(7), pp. 2281–2301. doi: 10.1016/j.nano.2017.06.015.

Zhang, H. et al. (2017) "Eupafolin nanoparticle improves acute renal injury induced by LPS through inhibiting ROS and inflammation," *Biomedecine & Pharmacotherapie [Biomedicine & Pharmacotherapy]*, 85, pp. 704–711. doi: 10.1016/j.biopha.2016.11.083.

Zhang, P. et al. (2010) "Global healthcare expenditure on diabetes for 2010 and 2030," *Diabetes Research and Clinical Practice*, 87(3), pp. 293–301. doi: 10.1016/j.diabres.2010.01.026.

Zhang, Y. et al. (2018) "Nanomedicine for obesity treatment," *Science China: Life Sciences*, 61(4), pp. 373–379. doi: 10.1007/s11427-017-9257-1.

14 Opportunities and Challenges of Nanotherapeutics

INTRODUCTION

Nanotherapeutics, a branch of nanotechnology used in medicine, is still developing. It is projected to have a revolutionary impact in the field of healthcare (Poirot-Mazères, 2011). The development of nanotherapeutics-based research has tremendously benefited from public investment and legislation (Bawa, 2011). The continuous advancement of nanotherapeutics offers the promise to offer a number of advantages over conventional drugs, including increased efficacy, bioavailability, adjustments in dose and response, targeting capability, personalization of medicines, and safety (Sajja et al., 2009). The design and manufacturing of multifunctional nanoparticle (NP) composites that are capable of simultaneously transporting diagnostic and therapeutic substances to specified areas might represent the most captivating idea in nanotherapeutics-based investigations (Seigneuric et al., 2010). These features are completely revolutionary and highlight significant advancements in patient diagnosis, care, and follow-up. Nevertheless, critical data about the pharmacokinetics profiles, pharmacodynamics profiles, and toxicological data of several nanomaterials remains unavailable when considering these potential advantages (Seigneuric et al., 2010).

Although recent research suggests that certain portions of these substances may reach the body of individuals and turn harmful at the level of cells in different body fluids, structures, and organs, the scientific knowledge of the possibility of toxicity of nanomaterials remains inadequate at the moment. Due to communication and cultural barriers between the nanotechnology research community and the pharmaceutical industry, collaborations have been hindered and the development of nanotherapeutics-based treatments in drug discovery has slowed. Other challenges include technical issues, a lack of standardization, unpredictability, public awareness, and assets. Nanotechnology has become extremely multidisciplinary due of the wide range of fields involved. This broad range of disciplines could even make it difficult to have meaningful talks and to find a shared language. The manufacturing sector must raise its level of awareness and its capacity to promote interactions among nanotechnology alongside other communities for the purpose to get beyond these obstacles. Nanotechnology combines the expertise of chemists, biologists, genetic engineers, microbiologists, biotechnologists, and many more researchers in various disciplines. The complexity of merging specialties in nanotechnology is likely to result in a development of new firms through substantial collaboration (Metselaar and Lammers, 2020).

A number of medications that make use of nanotechnology have been developed and authorized and commercialized, and many more are currently being researched, despite the fact that nanotherapeutics continues to be in its early stages of development. Potential benefits of nanotherapeutics include earlier diagnosis, better, safer, and increasingly individualized therapies, as well as lowered expenditures on healthcare. According to several experts, nanotherapeutics will lead to a paradigm shift that will alter the healthcare industry over the course of the next ten years (McGrady et al., 2010). However, considerably more effort is required to implement testing standards, evaluate efficacy, and compile safety data for diverse nanotherapeutic agents if substantial advancement is to be achieved toward this aim (Ventola, 2012).

14.1 ADVANTAGES OF NANOTHERAPEUTICS OVER CONVENTIONAL THERAPIES

The fundamental components of nanotherapeutic agents, nanoparticles (NPs), can change in a variety of ways that can alter function (Godin et al., 2010). NPs, by definition, are small particles having a minimum of one dimension falling between the range of 1 and 100 nm. Several larger molecules or massive solids lack in unique structural, optical, and electronic features that NPs possess (Godin et al., 2010). They also possess increased solubility, making it possible to reexamine equivalents in bulk drugs that have been demonstrated to have low solubility (Seigneuric et al., 2010). This characteristic would make it possible to turn insoluble or barely soluble medications into soluble aqueous solutions. The improved bioavailability along with duration of circulation brought on by the tiny dimensions of NPs is a further important benefit. Regardless of any surface alterations, studies have demonstrated that particles less than 200 nm have prolonged circulation durations than larger particles (Ventola, 2012).

One of the distinguishing physical properties of NPs is the large surface area compared to their size. As the size of the particles gets smaller, the total surface area increases exponentially. Increased surface area indicates that a greater proportion of the atoms of the particles are located on their surface as opposed to their core. This phenomenon causes NPs to be more reactive than their bulk solid or typically larger molecule counterparts. The increased surface area of NPs also contributes to their better water solubility and bioavailability (Bawa, 2011). The substantial surface area of nanomaterials additionally renders it possible to construct them with a variety of surface properties, such as conjugation with proteins or electrostatic charges. Certain surface features are chosen on the basis of their strategic suitability for aiming targets and other objectives (Ventola, 2012).

NPs may be able to transport medications to locations that are typically inaccessible by conventional methods because of their small dimensions (Seigneuric et al., 2010). An enhanced permeability of NPs might enable it to penetrate through neovessel pores smaller than 1 μm in diameter and deliver cancer medications into tumors (Sajja et al., 2009). The enhanced permeation of NPs might allow nanoparticles to pass across the blood–brain barrier (BBB) by utilizing various absorption pathways.

NPs may be delivered locally or proactively targeted with the help of ligands that are cellular-specific. Moreover, it is assisted by the features like magnetic localization, dimensions-based selectivity, and additional methods (Galvin et al., 2012). The exterior placement of a static magnetic field near the exact location of action can improve the prospective biodistribution and pharmacokinetic profiles associated with these NPs. For instance, MRI results from one study showed that magnetic nanoparticles (NPs) had moved toward neodymium magnets (NdFeB) which had been positioned beyond the cavity of the peritoneum, above grafts of a cancer in human ovaries (Galvin et al., 2012). NPs can be developed to integrate a wide range of chemotherapeutic drugs that can be directed precisely and promptly to the tumor location for greater efficacy and safety. NPs can also be loaded with contrast materials for imaging reasons. Multifunctional NP combinations or NPs employed in imaging for diagnosis have an advantage over minuscule–molecule contrast agents due to the fact they have an enormous surface area which enables targeting by surface changes and the capacity to carry therapeutic medicines at the same time (Ventola, 2012).

Various diagnostic or therapeutic substances can be coupled with nanoparticle interfaces. Cell-penetrating peptides (CPPs), which improve intracellular transportation, fluorescent agents for imaging, including genetic treatment agents like minor inhibitory RNA (siRNA), represent a few suitable biomolecules for NP interface conjugation (Bhaskar et al., 2010). The delivery of imaging contrast compounds that offer improved sensitivity and specificity aid in tumor identification. It can also be facilitated by surfaces of NPs attached with a specific molecule which attaches to heavily expressed tumor cell receptors (Sajja et al., 2009). Additionally, pharmacological therapy may be conjugated to the interfaces of NPs. Surface conjugation can improve the efficiency of NP drug-distribution platforms while drastically lowering the toxicity by using ligands which bind to the target area selectively (Ventola, 2012).

An essential and potent principle is tunability underlying NP characteristics. NPs have a wide variety of tunable biological, physical, optical, magnetic, chemical, electric, and mechanical properties that are drastically different from the same compounds in larger forms given the altered quantum mechanics that occur at the nanoscale stage (Vaddiraju et al., 2010). Scientists can adjust a variety of various features of nanoparticles by changing the diameters of NPs. For instance, by changing the size of an NP, it is possible to produce different fluorescence colors, enabling the use of color coding or labeling in diagnostic imaging applications (Ventola, 2012).

Besides the aforementioned merits, nanotherapeutic agents have significant pharmacokinetic features which may enhance their significance over conventional strategies. Opsonins, which can be described as proteins in the immune system that activate the immunological complement pathway and identify the NPs for elimination by macrophages along with phagocytes, are often responsible for clearing NPs from bloodstream. Hydrophobic particles are removed from circulation more quickly than hydrophilic ones, while neutral NPs get minimally opsonized than particles that are charged. NPs might be made to be neutral or combined with hydrophilic polymers like polyethylene glycol (PEG) in order to increase the duration of circulation (Galvin et al., 2012) Modifying liposomal NPs by adding a PEG coating may additionally improve their bioavailability for the purpose of preventing uptake by the reticuloendothelial system (RES). Consequently, functionalized liposomes are referred to as "stealth liposomes." NPs are frequently coated with a PEG layer for the purpose of reducing opsonization, decreasing RES absorption, improving biocompatibility, and lengthening circulation duration (Sajja et al., 2009). The coating of hydrophilic polymers (like PEG or dextran) on superparamagnetic iron oxide nanoparticles (SPIO NPs) may also make the nanoparticles water soluble. Alternatively, if they have been coated with substances that aid in the passage of DNA molecules inside cells, they are able to become either amphophilic or hydrophobic. Investigators are now using single-walled with multiwalled carbon nanotubes for nanoelectrodes due to their nanoscale size, electrocatalytic capabilities, and enormous surface area (Vaddiraju et al., 2010).

Nanotechnologies have already revolutionized genetic and biological assessments through the use of equipment that look at molecular biomarkers. Because of *in vitro* and *in vivo* testing procedures, these investigations can be completed more rapidly, reliably, and inexpensively than traditional approaches. For instance, they might utilize nanochips or QDs (Poirot-Mazères, 2011). Additionally, nanotechnologies can provide diagnostic tools that tend to be more sensitive and capable of spotting early indications of metabolic abnormalities, helping to prevent various noncommunicable diseases. Personalized medicine will become more common practice as long as nanotechnologies are used to provide more efficient and effective ways of recognizing molecular biomarkers (Poirot-Mazères, 2011).

14.2   LIMITATIONS OF NANOTHERAPEUTICS

Although nanotherapeutics has many advantages, much more studies remain necessary to assess the safe profiles and toxicity correlated with various NPs (Galvin et al., 2012). Few studies have focused on the pharmacokinetic profiles or toxicology of NPs, while the majority of nanomedical research has focused on drug delivery (Bhaskar et al., 2010). Assessing the impact of NPs on patient populations requires research into the pharmacokinetic and pharmacodynamic characteristics, as well as the potential chronic toxicity of NPs *in vivo*. Investigators and the FDA have a formidable challenge in evaluating any nanotherapeutic substance for safety and efficacy, regardless of its classification as a medication, device, biological, or combined therapy. The FDA is currently working to develop testing guidelines and compile safety data (Ventola, 2012).

Additionally, research is required to evaluate the immunogenicity of NPs (Vaddiraju et al., 2010). Due to their higher reactivity when compared to their typical equivalents, nanotherapeutics can display unexpected adverse consequences. A hypersensitive reaction, which may be brought about by stimulation of the immune complement framework, is the side effect associated with nanotherapeutic injections that is most frequently documented. Finding the crucial dimensions whereby nanoparticles (NPs) start to significantly concentrate in the body might be aided by research on the dimensions and surface characteristics of NPs. NPs have a tendency to concentrate in tissues and cellular environment as a result of their improved capacity to penetrate biological barriers due to the small dimensions. Organs including the liver and spleen can turn into the primary sites of oxidative stress due to the apparent tissue accumulation, retention, and sluggish clearance of such conceivably free radical generating particles, in addition to the presence of many phagocytes within the reticuloendothelial system (RES) Ventola, 2012; Ahadian and Radisic, 2017).

Polymer NPs, where data on safety and effectiveness are already known, constitute the mainstay of nanomedical research for a variety of reasons, including a lack of information on potential toxicity issues. As a matter of fact, the FDA has already given its approval to a number of nanotherapeutic agents that comprise polymer NPs. Lipid NPs are additionally believed to be biocompatible and acceptable, unlike other compounds that might turn detrimental in NP form (Galvin et al., 2012). Therefore, it is much more preferable to use nanotherapeutic agents that are biodegradable, readily soluble, free of toxic effects than it is to employ bio-persistent compounds, including polymer compounds, liposomes, and iron oxide (IO) particles. It may be more difficult to use NPs such as metallic nanocarriers, QDs, and carbon nanotubes which are not biodegradable. The attempts to find further biodegradable forms, materials, and surface modifications should be strengthened by this trait rather than serving to hinder nanomedical research using these NPs (Ventola, 2012).

Furthermore, cytotoxicity, genotoxicity, apoptosis, and oxidative stress are the four branches of nanotoxicity that can be further broken down. A change in the structure of biological organs caused by nanoparticles is referred to as cytotoxicity. When nanotherapeutic compounds alter, modify, or cause abnormalities at the chromosomal level, this is referred to as genotoxicity. Oxidative stress results in the production of reactive oxygen species (ROS) and the disruption of cellular functions, while apoptosis results in programmed cell death. Nanotherapeutics may exert harmful effects on host cells that are already alive (Djurišić et al., 2015; Sengul and Asmatulu, 2020).

Figure 14.1 shows the most significant toxicity varieties of nanomaterials in the body (Aillon et al., 2009). These toxicity manifestations are brought on by various chemical pathways (Lanone and Boczkowski, 2006). It is believed that the generation of oxidative stress via the generation of free radicals is the primary molecular explanation for *in vivo* NP toxic effects. Usually present in high concentrations, free

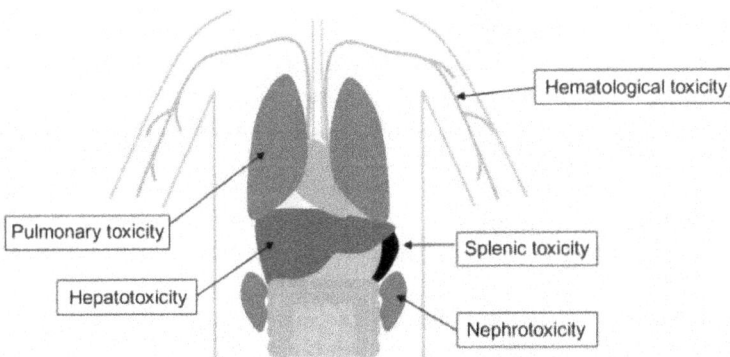

FIGURE 14.1 Major toxicity forms of nanomaterials in the body.

Source: Reproduced with permission from Aillon et al., 2009.

radicals can oxidize lipids, proteins, DNA, and various other biological substances. Certain researchers believe that the aspect ratio and surface area of NPs, like their intrinsic features, can be pro-inflammatory and pro-oxidant. However, in addition to NPs, other variables, which include the reactions of phagocytic cells to external material, a lack of antioxidants, the existence of transition metals, variables in the environment, along with other innate chemical or physical features, can also contribute to the generation of free radicals upon exposure to NPs (Ventola, 2012).

Through the overexpression of reduction-sensitive transcription factors (such NF-B), kinases, as well as activator protein-1, oxidative stress can increase the inflammatory response of the body (Rahman et al., 2005). Large quantities of these free radicals can oxidize and harm biological elements. Due to the poor clearance and accumulation of radicals that are free, as well as the predominance of high quantities of phagocytes, particular organs, especially the spleen and liver, become the primary targets of oxidative stress. Nanotherapeutic agents can also have an impact on organs with a great deal of blood flow, especially the kidney and lung (Arora, Rajwade and Paknikar, 2012). Nanotoxicity can originate from interactions between nanomaterials and the mitochondria and also with the cell nucleus. Fullerenes, gold nanoparticles, carbon nanotubes (CNTs), and block copolymer micelles are a few examples of nanomaterials that may locate to the mitochondria and cause the production of reactive oxygen species (ROS) causing apoptosis (Unfried et al., 2007). Nanoparticles may potentially display additional toxicity pathways as a result of their extensive environmental exposure. Thrombosis and hemolysis can arise from the absorption of nanostructures into the bloodstream. Additionally, interactions between nanomaterials and the immune system raise the danger of immunotoxicity (Dobrovolskaia and McNeil, 2016).

For instance, the resultant particles may be detrimental to living beings if metals like Se, Pb, or Cd are able to leach from nanoparticles and subsequently wind up in the environment. Additionally, it has been suggested that fullerene molecules that are readily soluble in water may cause damage to the brains of largemouth bass, a species of fish that lives in freshwater (Oberdörster, 2004). Dendrimers have also been demonstrated to destroy cell membranes, stimulate the coagulation and complement mechanisms, and induce osmotic damage. The effects of interacting with nanoparticles upon the human body vary based on their dimensions, chemical composition, architecture of the surface, the ability to dissolve, shape, and the extent to which they aggregate together. Typical exposure sites for nanoparticles comprise the gastrointestinal system, the epidermis, and respiratory organs. Nanoparticles possess the ability to alter the way that cells perform. A strategy of essential components for toxicity assessment should comprise the physical and chemical evaluation of nanotherapeutic agents, tissue and cellular analyses, and laboratory animal investigations in order to ensure maximum safety and minimize exposure (Ahadian and Radisic, 2017).

Environmental consequences are also a cause of concern, while being less researched than human health, although there is currently a lot of focus on ecotoxicology, the chemistry of the environment, actions, and destination (Zhu, Zhu and Li, 2008). The various ways that nanoparticles can reach the environment and humans are depicted in Figure 14.2.

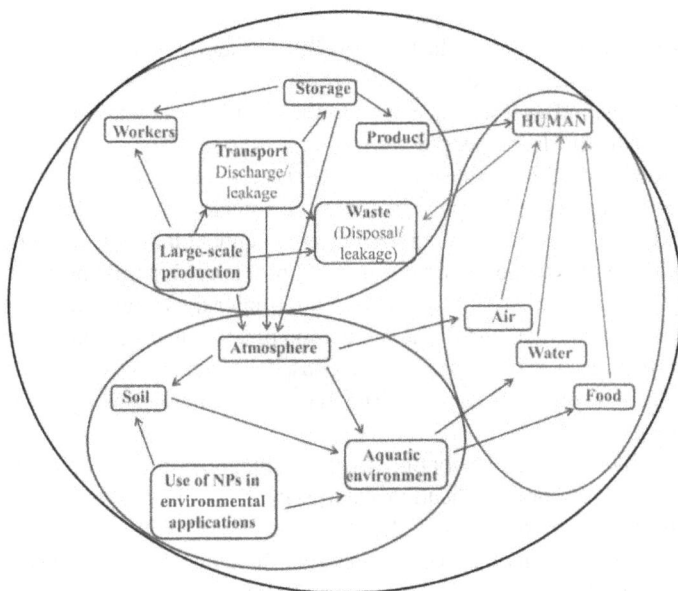

FIGURE 14.2   Multiple scenarios through which nanoparticles enter into the environment and humans.

Source: Reproduced with permission from Viswanath and Kim, 2017.

According to Dhawan and Sharma (2010), there are three possible manners that nanotherapeutic agents may alter the ecology systems. The first factor is direct influence on invertebrates, microbial flora, aquatic creatures, and a variety of other species; the second factor is reaction with additional contaminants that could alter the bioavailability of toxic substances and nutrients; and the third factor is modifications to nonliving ecological structures (Dhawan and Sharma, 2010). It is essential to comprehend the effects of nanomaterials upon the environment along with the well-being of humans for nanomaterials to be developed responsibly and to completely exploit the potential of its utilizations. As nanotechnology develops, concerns are being raised about whether its by-products or materials pose risks to the health of humans or the ecosystem, as well as whether its production generates additional risks or waste products. Regarding the responsible advancement of nanostructures and to completely capitalize on its possible uses, consideration of the effect of nanomaterials upon the ecosystem and human health is a critical stage (Yadav, Mungray and Mungray, 2014).

Although nanotherapeutics exhibit excellent performance in a variety of patients, they may have undesired pharmacokinetic alterations in special groups of people like geriatric and pediatric population. The changes in their physiological condition and anatomical status are the hindered reason for these undesired pharmacokinetic alterations. This may also lead to a challenge for nanotherapeutics. When considering the pharmacokinetic alterations of nanotherapeutic agents in geriatric population, typically elderly people (60 years and older) are the most frequent users of pharmacological therapies (Martin et al., 2019). Elderly patients rarely participate in clinical trials, which is a concern for many medication therapies and is thought to reduce the efficacy after it is transferred to the clinic (Shenoy and Harugeri, 2015). Considering two-thirds of people over 60 consuming four or more medications (Elliott, 2006) and 85% of those over 60 years old consuming at least one medicine, it seems clear that therapies, including nanotherapeutics, will predominantly be delivered to this older age group. In a drug-dependent manner, aging encourages alterations to the pharmacokinetic profiles and pharmacodynamic profiles of almost all drugs (Khan and Roberts, 2018). This could hinder the benefits that a nanotherapeutic agents could provide on the accumulation of a therapeutic drug in the instance of nanotherapeutics. On the other hand, age-associated pharmacokinetic alterations that can reduce the effectiveness of a drug in elderly patients may be overcome using nanotherapeutics.

In terms of absorption, distribution, metabolism, and elimination (ADME), aging is linked to decreased oral medication absorption and modifications to their pharmacokinetic profile (Vinarov et al., 2021). Numerous reasons influence the prolonged absorption of medications and metabolites seen in aged people; however, the main cause is reduced blood flow to the majority of organs, especially the mesenteric system. Importantly, for injectable substances, elderly individuals have comparable pharmacodynamic reactions to them as younger patients (e.g., rapid acting insulin), indicating there are minimal age-related alterations in injectable absorption (Heise et al., 2017). Age is correlated with a reduction in muscle mass, higher fat mass, and increasing bodily water and organ mass. Frailty is frequently connected with a decline in fat mass at extremely advanced ages (>85 years) (Hilmer, Wu and Zhang, 2019). Beyond the age of 50, body fluid levels fall and body fat levels rise by 1% of years (Hilmer, 2008). This results in a reduction in the amount of hydrophilic medication distributed and a spike in the passage of lipophilic medications (Mclean and Le Couteur, 2004). This might have an impact on the transportation of hydrophilic and lipophilic NPs within aging animals, although this has not been studied as yet. According to Payne and Bearden (2006), tissue perfusion declines with age, especially in muscular and splanchnic tissues (Payne and Bearden, 2006). A schematic comparison of the hepatic clearance of nanotherapeutics in a healthy liver and an aging liver is shown in Figure 14.3.

According to Mclean and Le Couteur (2004), aging is related with a 20–50% decline in hepatic blood flow, which affects the ability of the liver to eliminate flow-dependent substrates from the body and perform first pass metabolism. Defenestration of scavenger endothelial system in the liver (LSECs), thickening of the endothelial tissues, and accumulation of collagen are collectively known as pseudocapillarization which affects the passive transport from the bloodstream to hepatocytes (Le Couteur et al., 2008). The hepatic clearance of stream-limited substrates is similarly decreased by these aging changes. Aging has an impact on the mononuclear phagocyte system (MPS), LSECs, immunoglobin G (IgG), and complement systems' phagocytic cells. The generation of cytokines, particularly IL-6, is rising in KCs and macrophages; however, phagocytosis capacity has decreased (Hunt et al., 2019). The metabolism of nanotherapeutic agents in aging animal models and older individuals

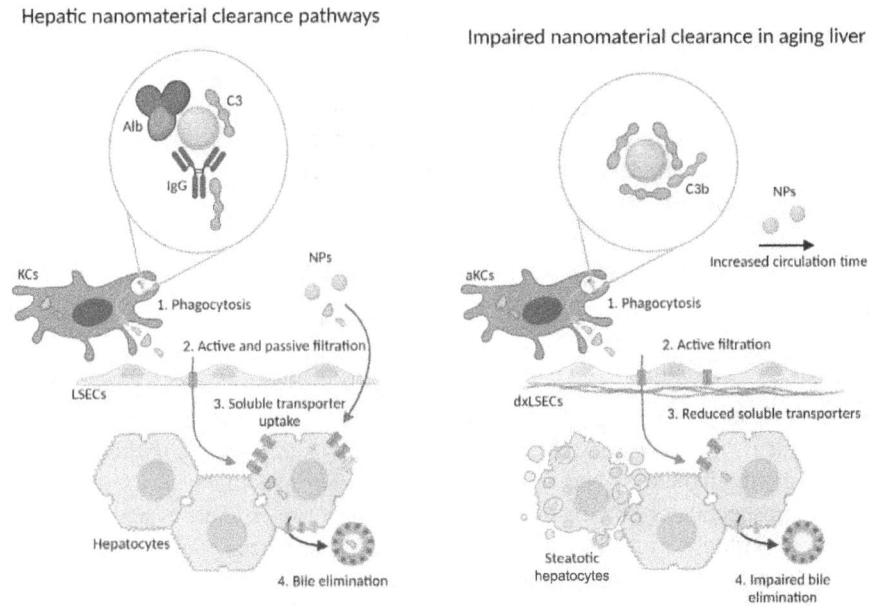

FIGURE 14.3 Hepatic nanomaterial clearance pathways (*left*) are impaired in the aging liver (*right*). Aging decreases circulating albumin and IgG with increased complement activation. Increased activated immune cells promote phagocytosis of nanomaterials by modified complement pathways. Degraded nanomaterials are actively cleared across the liver endothelium with passive transport inhibited by loss of fenestrations and collagen deposits. Hepatic and bile uptake of nanomaterials are limited due to reduced soluble transporters and impaired hepatic metabolism.

Source: Reproduced with permission from Hunt et al., 2022.

may be impacted by a variety of circumstances. Given the decline in phagocytosis by phagocytic cells as well as the passive and active clearance via LSECs, it is possible that aging will result in extended duration in circulation of nanotherapeutics. According to Mclean and Le Couteur (2004), the glomerular filtration rate (GFR) (passive filtration of ultra-particles from the plasma) declines by 15–40% with age. Due to rising renal vascular resistance, the flow of plasma through the kidneys also declines with aging more quickly than GFR (Fliser et al., 2005). When determining the medication dosage given to elderly patients, age-related alterations to renal function constitute a crucial factor to take into account.

The absence of accurate PK data in pediatrics continues to be a serious issue advances in nanotechnology for better drug delivery. It is challenging to design nanoparticle formulations for the pediatric population due to the diversity and distinctions between the patient community and adults. Neonatal, babies, toddlers, as well as children are some of the subgroups among the population that can be distinguished based on age. Pediatric patients differ from adults in terms of their preferred methods of administration, the toxicity of medications, and the bioactivity of both the active substance and formulation excipients. The difficulties with dosing are made worse by rapid growth of children and development, when the doses of some formulations might change by 100 times. Due to the dearth of formulations that are age-appropriate, medical practitioners are forced to utilize medications outside of the recommended dosage range, which increases the risk of toxic effects or subtherapeutic dose. This problem is exacerbated by the paucity of pharmacokinetics (PK) data in pediatrics (Yellepeddi, Joseph and Nance, 2019).

14.3   IMPLEMENTATION OF NANOTHERAPEUTICS

Nanotherapeutic compounds modify the efficacy and toxicity of pharmaceuticals in a manner similar to linkers, antibodies, peptides, and viral vectors. This is important because nanomaterial may be able to compensate for the efficacy and toxicity issues with novel pharmaceutical formulations that were unsuccessful in phase 2 or 3 clinical studies (Harrison, 2016). The difficulties of completing this endeavor is further highlighted by the restricted translation of nanotherapeutics (He et al., 2019). Irrespective of how nanotechnology is thought to be inert or active in their functions within the human body, nanotherapeutics have been categorized as drugs to handle regulatory difficulties with nanotechnology. According to Food and Drug Administration (FDA) recommendations, early phase *in vivo* investigations for all formulations of drugs should include hematology, clinical chemistry, gross pathology, immune response, tissue measurements, and histological analysis. The practical application of nanotherapeutics that are intended to have an extended circulation and become resistant toward metabolism and clearance could prove challenging given the current regulations. Decreased biodegradability and probable accumulation in organs other than the intended target may be major obstacles to approval from regulators. Additionally, using nanomaterials with extremely reactive surface chemistry could encourage the production of ROS, especially when combined with heavy metals (Malaviya, Shukal and Vasavada, 2019). Due to the fact that nanoparticles are essentially medications in and of themselves featuring a wide spectrum of adverse reactions, regulatory assessments of these materials are extremely challenging. Therefore, it is crucial that nanomaterial qualities be taken into account in different regulatory mechanisms that are particularly created with nanomaterial absorption, distribution, cellular uptake, metabolism, therapeutic action, and elimination in mind.

With the aforementioned considerations, nanotechnology should be seen as an enabling technological framework with a variety of possible applications in biotechnology, healthcare, information technology, and cognitive technology. In the past, regulatory systems were dispersed, decentralized, and prone to gaps and problems (Allan et al., 2021; Devasahayam, 2019). However, according to Devasahayam's analysis from 2019, the global legislative metronomy currently in effect at the time is sufficient for adapting to the measurements needed for nanotechnology (nanometrometry).

The legal structure and technical methodologies necessary for the safety and quality monitoring of nanotherapeutics were discussed by Halamoda-Kenzaoui et al. (2021) in a recent study. The International Council for Harmonisation of Technical Requirements for Registration of Pharmaceuticals for Human Use (ICH) guidelines for medical products and CEN—European Committee for Standardization/ISO—International Organization for Standardization—are just a couple of the guidelines that have been published by the European Medicine Agency (EMA) and the FDA, respectively. Additional evaluations are needed due to the complexity and tendency to interact with biological networks. Humanized biodistribution and ADME issues for *in silico* remain crucial topics to overcome. There will be further changes in ADME in older individuals as well as pediatric patients that are not foretold by young laboratory animal models. Finally, to support current physiologically based pharmacokinetic modelling (PBPK) models for the implementation of nanotherapeutics, novel investigations must to be carried out in young and aging animal models. Patients with weak immune systems and other comorbidities must be taken into account as well. Therefore, consideration should be given to each of these crucial areas in order to use nanotherapeutics as a promising perspective to usher in an era of innovation in healthcare (Hunt et al., 2022).

REFERENCES

Ahadian, S. and Radisic, M. (2017) "Nanotoxicity," In Mehdi Razavi and Avnesh Thakor (Eds.), *Nanobiomaterials science, development and evaluation*. Duxford, UK and Cambridge, US: Elsevier, pp. 233–248.

Aillon, K. L. et al. (2009) "Effects of nanomaterial physicochemical properties on *in vivo* toxicity," *Advanced Drug Delivery Reviews*, 61(6), pp. 457–466. doi: 10.1016/j.addr.2009.03.010.

Allan, J., Belz, S., Hoeveler, A., Hugas, M., Okuda, H., Patri, A. et al. (2021) "Regulatory landscape of nanotechnology and nanoplastics from a global perspective," *Regulatory Toxicology and Pharmacology*, 122, p. 104885. doi: 10.1016/j.yrtph.2021.104885.

Arora, S., Rajwade, J. M. and Paknikar, K. M. (2012) "Nanotoxicology and *in vitro* studies: The need of the hour," *Toxicology and Applied Pharmacology*, 258(2), pp. 151–165. doi: 10.1016/j.taap.2011.11.010.

Bawa, R. (2011) "Regulating nanomedicine-can the FDA handle it?," *Current Drug Delivery*, 8(3), pp. 227–234.

Bhaskar, S. et al. (2010) "Multifunctional Nanocarriers for diagnostics, drug delivery and targeted treatment across blood-brain barrier: Perspectives on tracking and neuroimaging," *Particle and Fibre Toxicology*, 7(1), p. 3. doi: 10.1186/1743-8977-7-3.

Devasahayam, S. (2019) "Nanotechnology and nanomedicine in market," *Characterization and Biology of Nanomaterials for Drug Delivery (Elsevier)*, 477–522. doi: 10.1016/b978-0-12-814031-4.00017-9.

Dhawan, A. and Sharma, V. (2010) "Toxicity assessment of nanomaterials: Methods and challenges," *Anal Bioanal Chem*, 398, pp. 589–605.

Djurišić, A. B. et al. (2015) "Toxicity of metal oxide nanoparticles: Mechanisms, characterization, and avoiding experimental artefacts," *Small*, 11(1), pp. 26–44. doi: 10.1002/smll.201303947.

Dobrovolskaia, M. A. and McNeil, S. E. (2016) "Immunological properties of engineered nanomaterials: An introduction," In Marina A Dobrovolskaia, Scott E McNeil (Eds.), *Handbook of immunological properties of engineered nanomaterials*. Tuck Link, Singapore: World Scientific, pp. 1–24.

Elliott, R. A. (2006) "Problems with medication use in the elderly: An Australian perspective," *J. Pharm. Pract. Res.*, 36, pp. 58–66. doi: 10.1002/j.2055-2335.2006.tb00889.

Fliser, D., Wagner, K.-K., Loos, A., Tsikas, D. and Haller, H. (2005) "Chronic Angiotensin II receptor blockade reduces (intra)renal vascular resistance in patients with type 2 diabetes," *Jasn*, 16, pp. 1135–1140. doi: 10.1681/asn.2004100852.

Galvin, P. et al. (2012) "Nanoparticle-based drug delivery: Case studies for cancer and cardiovascular applications," *Cellular and Molecular Life Sciences: CMLS*, 69(3), pp. 389–404. doi: 10.1007/s00018-011-0856-6.

Godin, B. et al. (2010) "Emerging applications of nanomedicine for the diagnosis and treatment of cardiovascular diseases," *Trends in Pharmacological Sciences*, 31(5), pp. 199–205. doi: 10.1016/j.tips.2010.01.003.

Halamoda-Kenzaoui, B., Vandebriel, R., Howarth, A., Siccardi, M., David, C., Liptrott, N. et al. (2021) "Methodological needs in the quality and safety characterisation of nanotechnology-based health products: Priorities for method development and standardisation," *J. Control. Release*, 336, pp. 192–206. doi: 10.1016/j.jconrel.2021.06.016.

Harrison, R. K. (2016) "Phase II and phase III failures: 2013–2015," *Nat. Rev. Drug Discov.*, 15, pp. 817–818. doi: 10.1038/nrd.2016.184.

He, H., Liu, L., Morin, E. E., Liu, M. and Schwendeman, A. (2019) "Survey of clinical translation of cancer nanomedicines-lessons learned from successes and failures," *Acc. Chem. Res.*, 52, pp. 2445–2461. doi: 10.1021/acs.accounts.9b00228.

Heise, T., Hövelmann, U., Zijlstra, E., Stender-Petersen, K., Jacobsen, J. B. and Haahr, H. (2017) "A comparison of pharmacokinetic and pharmacodynamic properties between faster-acting insulin aspart and insulin aspart in elderly subjects with type 1 diabetes mellitus," *Drugs Aging*, 34, pp. 29–38. doi: 10.1007/s40266-016-0418-6.

Hilmer, S. N. (2008) "ADME-tox issues for the elderly. *Expert Opin. Drug Metab. Toxicol.*, 4, pp. 1321–1331. doi: 10.1517/17425255.4.10.1321.

Hilmer, S. N., Wu, H. and Zhang, M. (2019) "Biology of frailty: Implications for clinical pharmacology and drug therapy in frail older people," *Mech. Ageing Dev.*, 181, pp. 22–28. doi: 10.1016/j.mad.2019.111119.

Hunt, N. J. et al. (2022) "Opportunities and challenges for nanotherapeutics for the aging population," *Frontiers in Nanotechnology*, 4. doi: 10.3389/fnano.2022.832524.

Hunt, N. J., Kang, S. W., Lockwood, G. P., Le Couteur, D. G. and Cogger, V. C. (2019) "Hallmarks of aging in the liver," *Comput. Struct. Biotechnol. J.*, 17, pp. 1151–1161. doi: 10.1016/j.csbj.2019.07.021.

Khan, M. S. and Roberts, M. S. (2018) "Challenges and innovations of drug delivery in older age," *Adv. Drug Deliv. Rev.*, 135, pp. 3–38. doi: 10.1016/j.addr.2018.09.003.

Lanone, S. and Boczkowski, J. (2006) "Biomedical applications and potential health risks of nanomaterials: Molecular mechanisms," *Current Molecular Medicine*, 6(6), pp. 651–663. doi: 10.2174/156652406778195026.

Le Couteur, D. G., Warren, A., Cogger, V. C., Smedsrød, B., Sørensen, K. K., De Cabo, R. et al. (2008) "Old age and the hepatic sinusoid," *Anat. Rec.*, 291, pp. 672–683. doi: 10.1002/ar.20661.

Malaviya, P., Shukal, D. and Vasavada, A. R. (2019) "Nanotechnology-based drug delivery, metabolism and toxicity," *Curr. Drug Metab.*, 20, pp. 1167–1190. doi: 10.2174/138920 0221666200103091753.

Martin, C. B., Hales, C. M., Gu, Q. and Ogden, C. L. (2019) "Prescription drug use in the United States, 2015–2016," *NCHS Data Brief*, pp. 1–8.

McGrady, E. et al. (2010) "Emerging technologies in healthcare: Navigating risks, evaluating rewards," *Journal of Healthcare Management*, 55(5), pp. 353–364; discussion 364–5. doi: 10.1097/00115514-201009000-00011.

Mclean, A. J. and Le Couteur, D. G. (2004) "Aging biology and geriatric clinical pharmacology," *Pharmacol. Rev.*, 56, pp. 163–184. doi: 10.1124/pr.56.2.4.

Metselaar, J. M. and Lammers, T. (2020) "Challenges in nanomedicine clinical translation," *Drug Delivery and Translational Research*, 10(3), pp. 721–725. doi: 10.1007/s13346-020-00740-5.

Oberdörster, E. (2004) "Manufactured nanomaterials (fullerenes, C60) induce oxidative stress in the brain of juvenile Largemouth bass," *Environmental Health Perspectives*, 112(10), pp. 1058–1062. doi: 10.1289/ehp.7021.

Payne, G. W. and Bearden, S. E. (2006) "The microcirculation of skeletal muscle in aging," *Microcirculation*, 13, pp. 275–277. doi: 10.1080/10739680600618710.

Poirot-Mazères, I. (2011) "Chapter 6. Legal aspects of the risks raised by nanotechnologies in the field of medicine," *Journal international de bioethique [International Journal of Bioethics]*, 22(1), p. 99. doi: 10.3917/jib.221.0099.

Rahman, I. et al. (2005) "Glutathione, stress responses, and redox signaling in lung inflammation," *Antioxidants & Redox Signaling*, 7(1–2), pp. 42–59. doi: 10.1089/ars.2005.7.42.

Sajja, H. K. et al. (2009) "Development of multifunctional nanoparticles for targeted drug delivery and noninvasive imaging of therapeutic effect," *Current Drug Discovery Technologies*, 6(1), pp. 43–51. doi: 10.2174/157016309787581066.

Seigneuric, R. et al. (2010) "From nanotechnology to nanomedicine: Applications to cancer research," *Current Molecular Medicine*, 10(7), pp. 640–652. doi: 10.2174/156652410792630634.

Sengul, A. B. and Asmatulu, E. (2020) "Toxicity of metal and metal oxide nanoparticles: A review," *Environmental Chemistry Letters*, 18(5), pp. 1659–1683. doi: 10.1007/s10311-020-01033-6.

Shenoy, P. and Harugeri, A. (2015) "Elderly patients' participation in clinical trials," *Perspect. Clin. Res.*, 6, p. 184. doi: 10.4103/2229-3485.167099.

Unfried, K. et al. (2007) "Cellular responses to nanoparticles: Target structures and mechanisms," *Nanotoxicology*, 1(1), pp. 52–71. doi: 10.1080/00222930701314932.

Vaddiraju, S. et al. (2010) "Emerging synergy between nanotechnology and implantable biosensors: A review," *Biosensors & Bioelectronics*, 25(7), pp. 1553–1565. doi: 10.1016/j.bios.2009.12.001.

Ventola, C. L. (2012) "The nanomedicine revolution: Part 1: Emerging concepts," *P & T: A Peer-Reviewed Journal for Formulary Management*, 37(9), pp. 512–525.

Vinarov, Z., Abrahamsson, B., Artursson, P., Batchelor, H., Berben, P., BernkopSchnürch, A. et al. (2021) "Current challenges and future perspectives in oral absorption research: An opinion of the UNGAP network," *Adv. Drug Deliv. Rev.*, 171, pp. 289–331. doi: 10.1016/j.addr.2021.02.001.

Viswanath, B. and Kim, S. (2017) "Influence of nanotoxicity on human health and environment: The alternative strategies," *Reviews of Environmental Contamination and Toxicology*, 242, pp. 61–104. doi: 10.1007/398_2016_12.

Yadav, T., Mungray, A. A. and Mungray, A. K. (2014) "Fabricated nanoparticles: Current status and potential phytotoxic threats," *Rev Environ Contam Toxicol*, 230, pp. 83–110.

Yellepeddi, V. K., Joseph, A. and Nance, E. (2019) "Pharmacokinetics of nanotechnology-based formulations in pediatric populations," *Advanced Drug Delivery Reviews*, pp. 151–152, pp. 44–55. doi: 10.1016/j.addr.2019.08.008.

Zhu, X., Zhu, L. and Li, Y. (2008) "Comparative toxicity of several metal oxide nano-particle aqueous suspensions to zebrafish (Danio rerio) early developmental stage," *J Environ Sci Health A Tox Hazard Subst Environ Eng*, 43, pp. 278–284.

15 Future Prospects of Nanotherapeutics

INTRODUCTION

Despite gaining traction in the clinical setting, nanotherapeutics continue to focus on novel drugs and their disease implications. Aside from observing from a relatively safe academic vantage point, the nanotherapeutics research community should make a concerted effort to envision clinical practice application in each research project it undertakes (Bregoli et al., 2016). It is anticipated that by raising end-user awareness, beginning with the formulation design and bench trial stages, a more precise understanding of the entire effort and investments required will emerge. It is possible to make wise decisions regarding the preclinical testing setup, manufacturing requirements, and even production methods after carefully considering the market opportunity, therapeutic positioning, and the clinical study design, like its therapeutic endpoints. Investigative nanotherapeutics have to adhere to this method of rigorous strategy development and navigation via clinical translation in order to eventually fulfill their promise of greater beneficial effects for patients (Moghimi, Hunter and Murray, 2005).

In the last three decades, nanotechnology has contributed to great strides in the medical sector. The development of a significant amount of nanotherapeutics has proven their promise in the identification and management of diseases (Choi and Han, 2018). Furthermore, it is predicted that they will eventually replace current diagnostic and therapeutic methods. The current status of nanotherapeutics in preclinical and clinical trials is vital to examine further, as is how it will develop in the future to treat life-threatening diseases, enhance quality of life, and collaborate with the most recent technological breakthroughs. According to Shi et al. (2022), future nanotherapeutics should have three crucial characteristics. They are multifunctionality (by combining features like diagnosis, visualization, and therapy), intelligence (by using artificial intelligence to guide the design of nanostructures and the utilization of nanorobots), and precision and personalization (by including patient classification and specifically chosen regimen selection) (Shi et al., 2022).

Significant contributions have been particularly successful at encouraging scientists to engage in biomedical research and fostering relationships with biological researchers. However, there has been noticeably inefficient use of these assets frequently as a result of inadequate conceptualization and communication, which resulted in misplaced programs (Bawa and Johnson, 2007). Accelerated "translation" of nanotechnologies, or the transfer of scientific discoveries from the lab bench to the clinical setting, has been emphasized from the beginning. While this is an admirable objective, it minimizes the fact that considerable basic study is still required to understand how nanomaterials interact with biological things.

DOI: 10.1201/9781003442202-16

The protracted debate regarding whether carbon nanotubes are harmful or not (Aschberger et al., 2010) is just one illustration of the extent to which important fundamental knowledge exists.

It could be dangerous to attempt to translate concepts to the clinic before fully understanding the basic ways that nanomaterials connect to biological systems. A significant portion of the employees produced by these massive initiatives involves the development of new technology (Armarego, 2022). This is undoubtedly crucial; as already mentioned, a lack of communication among nanotechnologists and bio-medical scientists frequently leads to "seeking the solution of a problem" as opposed to technologies that effectively deal with clinical issues. As a result, the literature on nanotherapeutics is replete with articles that detail ingenious, elegant advancements in nanotechnology along with predictions of its potential clinical or diagnostic application (Sakamoto et al., 2010). However, many of these technologies stagnate instead of developing into useful applications. It is a reason to wonder if massive and well-managed programs are the best approach to advance nanotherapeutics at a time when the National Institutes of Health are facing severe financial constraints. A more productive solution might be giving smaller funds to individual researchers who are connected to a system of multi-institutional core centers in order to gain the maximum performance of nanotherapeutic research (Nordmann and Rip, 2009).

15.1 SUSTAINABLE INNOVATIONS OF NANOTHERAPEUTICS

Comparing nanotherapeutics to traditional small-molecule medications, these latter show distinct advantages regarding clinical performance. In-depth research in the field of nanotherapeutics over the last three decades has resulted in a substantial amount of nanotherapeutic agents being commercialized globally along with a pipeline of candidates becoming translated. According to a recent study by Zhang et al. (2020), a bibliometric study of the Web of Science Core Collection reveals that nano-medical studies have surged in recent years and that, from 2000 to 2019, the total amount of annual publications increased by over tenfold (Figure 15.1 (a)) (Zhang et al., 2020). The study of the delivery of medications and drugs or therapies comprises up to 76% of all nanomedical investigations, and it represents one of the main study fields in nanotherapeutics, contributing to 49% of publications throughout the last two decades (Figure 15.1 (b)) (Zhang et al., 2020). With 26% of all published studies in this area during the last two decades, the United States continues to be the dominant nation in nanotherapeutic research, closely followed by China with 22% (Figure 15.1 (c)). More than 16% of articles come from Europe; Japan and India each contributes 5% and 6%, respectively (Zhang et al., 2020).

According to shifts in the geographical location of nanotherapeutic investigations, Asia is an area for nanotherapeutic research that is developing more quickly than the United States or Europe. It may eventually become the most powerful business marketplace for nanotherapeutics. Nevertheless, the West continues to lead the way in clinical nanotherapeutics translation; other nations and regions should prioritize clinical nanotherapeutics translation as well as fundamental nanotherapeutic research. The global commercialization of nanotherapeutics is expanding (Malviya et al., 2021).

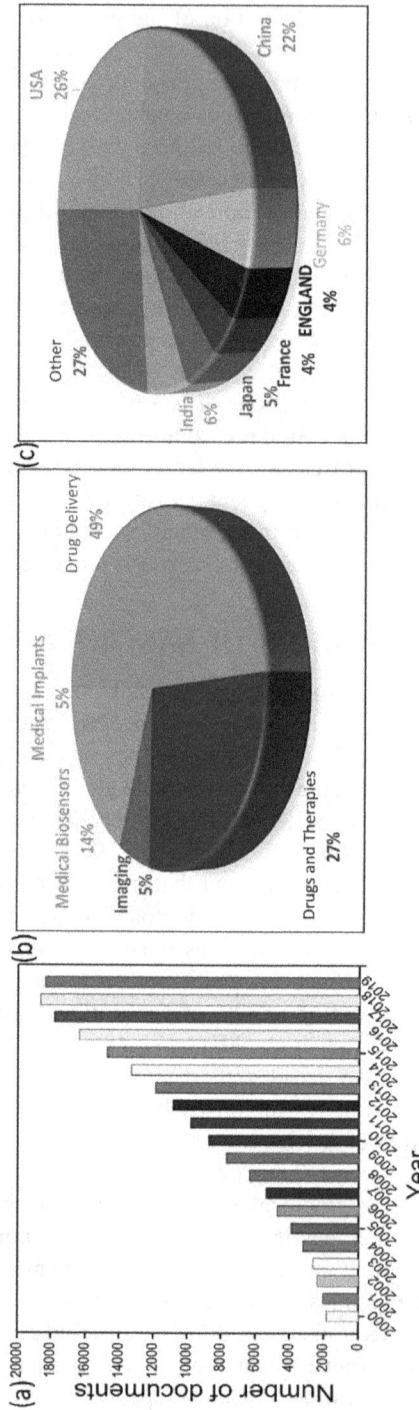

FIGURE 15.1 Bibliometric analysis of research in nanomedicine, from the Web of Science Core Collection. (a) Annual number of nanomedical publications globally. (b) Distribution of publications among fields within nanomedicine. (c) Geographical distribution of nanomedical publications.

Source: Reproduced with permission from Zhang et al., 2020.

North America and Europe presently hold a majority of the global market for nanotherapeutics because of the benefits involved in the sheer number of patented nanotherapeutics as well as their advantageous regulatory systems. Nevertheless, nanotechnology-based healthcare industry in Asia is expanding quickly due to a recent surge in funds for nanotherapeutic research and a boom in demand for better disease remedies. Numerous nanotherapeutics have been given the receive-ahead for entering into commercial production or are now undergoing clinical testing (Zhang et al., 2020).

The total number of journal publications on the topic of nanotherapeutics is continuously increasing, and the fields of "Drug Carriers" along with "Drug Delivery Platforms" are growing especially quickly, in accordance with an analysis performed by Shi et al. (2022). In their research, they have made some significant discoveries. Those conclusions include that the Department of Health and Human Services (NIH and others) has provided more financing for indications besides cancer than it has for cancer, there has been a lot of funding for HIV/AIDS-related applications, and the majority of cancers are being affected, although there are many clinical studies for non-cancer symptoms like pain and infections, the majority of them are concentrated on breast, cutaneous, metastatic, and ovarian cancers. Since the majority of the clinical trials of nanotherapeutics are currently in phases I and II, it may take some time before they have a significant impact on patients. Moreover, Shi et al. (2022) revealed that the bulk of current trials are testing nab-paclitaxel/Abraxane and liposomes, which are two well-known nanotherapeutic formulations, along with other treatments. However, since 2009, there have been more clinical trials using various nanotherapeutic formulations. Only a small percentage of the experiments involve dendrimers or micelles. Taken as a whole, the report presents an impression of nanotherapeutics that continue to receive significant funding and study, however with few recent advances. It remains uncertain whether nanotherapeutics will ever offer the "silver bullet" for the treatment of cancer or other disorders (Zhang et al., 2020).

Furthermore, nanoparticles or nanostructures have been detected in many medicines or diagnostic tools under development or already available. Technologies for tissue engineering, systems for delivering drugs for diagnosis or therapy, tests for sensing, drug evaluation, and different kinds of assays are among them. Some products, like sunscreen, skincare items, and dietary additives, are OTC (over-the-counter). Doxil and Abraxane are two examples of nano-based medications that have been approved by governments (such as the Food and Drug Administration in the United States), while many others are through various levels of clinical and preclinical testing (Juliano, 2012; Zhang et al., 2020).

15.2   FUTURE OF NANOTHERAPEUTICS

The therapeutic efficacy of conventional medications may be increased by integrating nanotechnology. Nevertheless, since several nanotherapeutics do not particularly target lesions, techniques cannot prevent their toxic effects toward healthy tissues. The development of precise, highly effective medications that concentrate in lesions instead of accumulating in healthy nontargeted regions is one of the top priorities for the upcoming generation of nanotherapeutics.

The development of intelligent medication delivery devices with active targeted delivery and stimulus responsiveness has been a crucial requirement in the advancement of nanotherapeutics. These intelligent systems for delivering drugs offer both an excellent chance and an important hurdle for the forthcoming development of nanotherapeutics in terms of their potential to destroy pathological tissues while safeguarding normal tissues. A number of excellent research papers have just been released that list the nanotherapeutic formulations that have been granted approval by the Food and Drug Administration (FDA) or additional regulatory agencies worldwide, or at least those that are undergoing clinical trials (McGoron, 2020).

Figure 15.2 illustrates the challenges that must be solved for clinical translation of nanotherapeutic medicines beyond the laboratory benchtop (Metselaar and Lammers, 2020). Most of the evaluations focus on cancer specifically, while others provide more general assessments of nanotherapeutics. It was anticipated that novel formulations of doxorubicin (Doxil) would appear soon after the introduction of the liposomal dosage form formulation in 1995 (Barenholz, 2012). A year later, daunorubicin liposomal drug (DaunoXome) received approval. A perspective posed by Venkatraman mentioned that "has nanomedicine lived up to its potential?" (Venkatraman, 2014). Five novel nanomedicine formulations have been authorized since that article was published. Nanomedicines will increasingly fulfill their

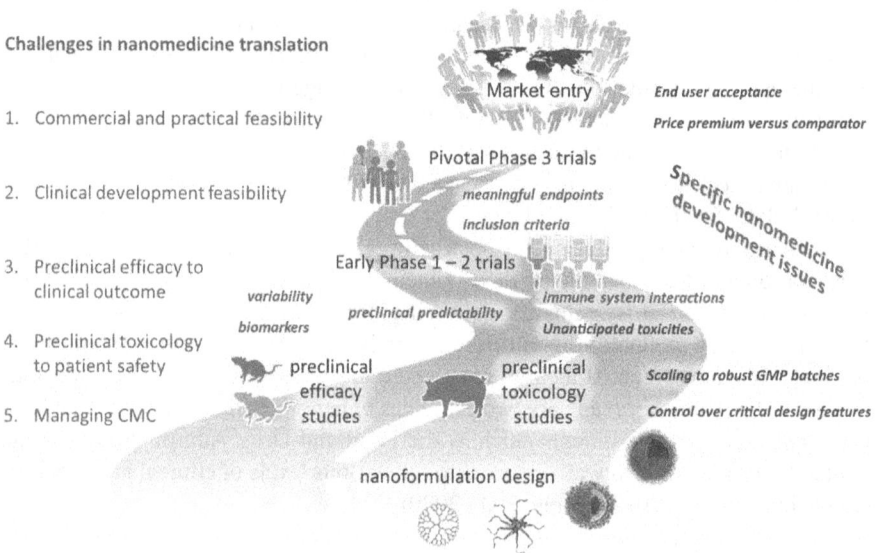

FIGURE 15.2 Challenges in nanomedicine translation. Five key challenges of nanomedicinal product development are depicted top-down, from the vantage point of the end user. Practical and clinical development feasibilities come first, followed by preclinical and pharmaceutical aspects of nanomedicine research and development. This way of route planning allows one to identify—right from the start—where and which specific issues can be encountered along the way.

Source: Reproduced with permission from Metselaar and Lammers, 2020.

promises to patients over the next two decades, according to van der Meel, who wrote "Cancer Nanomedicine: Oversold or Underappreciated?" (Van Der Meel, Lammers and Hennink, 2017). Sarmento has raised the question, "Has medication research and development using nanomedicines advanced as much as we'd hoped?" and responds, "Nanomedicines have not yet had a significant impact on clinical practice" (Sarmento, 2019).

The term "advanced impact" is significant because nanotherapeutics has had an effect, even if it may not have yet delivered the "silver bullet" that Richard Feynman (who was a Nobel Laureate in Physics in 1965) anticipated in his well-known 1959 American Physical Society speech, "There is plenty of room at the bottom." The results seem uneven, particularly when it comes to cancer. The majority of licensed nanotherapeutics do not exist for combating cancer, despite the enormous number of papers in journals and studies that receive funding in the field that are related to nanomedicine (McGoron, 2020).

The investigation of human clinical studies intended to assess nanotherapeutic formulations provides another glimpse at the intriguing possibilities of the field. In a recent investigation, Shi et al. (2022) searched the ClinicalTrials.gov database with the help of keywords. For the purpose of this evaluation, the research type "investigational (clinical trials)" was used to filter the search. Using the initial keyword search, the user can locate criteria connected to the outcomes of the search by analyzing the "topics" of the findings and identifying those that appear frequently to further narrow down the search. According to the results, the "Search Details" page shows how many times specific keywords and synonyms have been searched. The data was processed using additional keywords alongside the base keywords. Although liposomes and nab-paclitaxel (Abraxane) are the subjects of the largest number of clinical trials investigating nanotherapeutics, many other nanoparticle medication formulations have recently come under study. Many of the studies are focused on, and the majority of them are for, oncology indications. The majority are in phase I or phase II. Considering liposome technological advances and nab-paclitaxel are widely established, leaving them out offers insight into additional novel nanotherapeutic uses (Zhang et al., 2020).

Prior to starting clinical investigations, researchers must submit an investigational new drug (IND) application to the FDA taking into account the clinical trials. A study by D'Mello et al. was done on FDA-internal data from 1974 to 2015. It demonstrates that between 1994 and 2015, submissions to the Centre for Drug Evaluation and Research (CDER) regarding nanomaterial substances fluctuated between 10 and 25 per year, growing sporadically throughout the 1980s and peaking in 2006 (D'Mello et al., 2017). Throughout the same time period, the number of new products utilizing nanomaterials that were approved annually ranged from 1 to 7. Liposomes comprised the vast majority of the nanomaterials employed in pharmaceuticals between 2010 and 2015, the bulk of cancer-related indications (40%), and the bulk of intravenous delivery techniques (63%) (D'Mello et al., 2017). The findings of the researchers state that more medication products with nanomaterials are anticipated to be submitted in the near future. The form and complexity of nanotherapeutic formulations are also expected to rise, according to the scientists. It is obvious that the revolutionary nanotherapeutic formulations are still in the early stages of evaluation, and it is anticipated that very few of them will progress to phase III clinical trials and access marketplaces. This, however, is not unique to nanotherapeutics because it is a widespread issue in the development of drugs in general. However, the evidence suggests that there is still interest in using nanotechnology in medicine, and in particular, in developing medications based on nanotherapeutics (McGoron, 2020).

15.3 CONCLUSIONS

Nanotechnology offers extraordinary advantages when used in medicines, medical devices, and innovative drug discovery. Additionally, the patent cliff and expirations have made it possible for pharmaceutical corporations to implement fresh venture plans. Although many popular medications are losing their patent protection, the development of nanotherapeutics has completely changed the pharmaceutical sector. The total number of patent applications has risen considerably as nanopharmaceutical enterprises have developed. Pharmaceutical corporations have created innovative approaches and strategies to modify medications that are close to losing their patent protection using nanotechnology. The potential for revenue growth for nanotherapeutics is very promising. The information provided above offers a thorough analysis of the market for nanotherapeutic medicines, taking into account a variety of influencing factors such as current trends, regulatory laws, and technological advancements in the sector (Foulkes et al., 2020).

The "drug transport type," "uses," "distribution channel," and "specific areas" are the market segments that nanotherapeutics have been established. The facts that have been discussed before provide a way to gain thorough understanding of the market and aid in the development of strategic judgments that are well-informed. Some important factors that need to be considered before combining the industries are revealed by the current investigation. In 2017, the market for nanotherapeutic drugs was estimated at $40.37 billion, and by 2026, it is anticipated to grow to $79.29 billion (*Global Nanopharmaceutical Drugs Market: Focus on nanodrugs and its application in therapeutics, competitive landscape, and country—analysis and forecast (2018–2026)*). Government and corporate funding to promote the advancement of regenerative medicines, an upsurge in the frequency of chronic illnesses and genetic abnormalities, an expansion in the cost of healthcare globally, and the growing aging of people worldwide are the main factors propelling the expansion of this industry. The market for nanotherapeutic pharmaceuticals is also being driven by the expanding coverage of insurance and compensation laws in developed markets, including the United States, Germany, Japan, and the United Kingdom.

Additionally, the anticancer therapeutic field dominated the worldwide nanotherapeutic marketplace in 2017 among the other therapeutic fields. The use of nanoparticles presents a chance to change cancer research in general. Numerous medication candidates are undergoing clinical testing and could soon enter the market. The most promising nanotherapeutics should adhere to the regulatory approval process, have an adaptable structure that is simple to scale up for cGMP production, and be able to keep for a long time before being administered to individuals. The FDA as well as the Nanotechnology Characterization Laboratory collaborate to develop and evaluate the nanotherapeutics platform (Bansal et al., 2020).

The worldwide nanotherapeutics marketplace is divided into four geographical segments based on geography: North America, Asia-Pacific, Europe, and Rest of the World (RoW). The market for nanotherapeutic medicines is the largest in the world, with North America accounting for 51.78% of the sales in the market in 2017. However, during the time frame expected, revenue in Europe and Asia-Pacific is anticipated to expand at a considerable CAGR of 5% and 7%, respectively (*Global Nanopharmaceutical Drugs Market: Focus on nanodrugs and its application in therapeutics, competitive landscape, and country—analysis and forecast (2018–2026)*). Although there are many prospects, nanotherapeutics confront more difficulties than conventional medicines. Although traditional medications continue to rule the market, they are increasingly using nanotechnologies to lessen adverse effects and boost effectiveness. An essential route for modernizing conventional medications is represented by nanotherapeutics. The investment has grown exponentially on its own, and the majority of its consequences are likely not yet fully felt. However, entrepreneurs must take the initiative to shepherd the discoveries to clinical settings if nanotherapeutics are expected to make an actual impression (Thapa and Kim, 2023).

REFERENCES

Armarego, W. L. F. (2022) "Nanomaterials," in *Purification of laboratory chemicals.* Burlington, USA and Oxford, UK Elsevier, pp. 586–630.

Aschberger, K., Johnston, H. J., Stone, V., Aitken, R. J. et al. (2010) "Review of carbon nanotubes toxicity and exposure: Appraisal of human health risk assessment based on open literature," *Critical Reviews in Toxicology*, 40, pp. 759–790.

Bansal, M. et al. (2020) "Nanomedicine: Diagnosis, treatment, and potential prospects," in *Environmental chemistry for a sustainable world.* Cham: Springer International Publishing, pp. 297–331.

Barenholz, Y. (2012) "Doxil(R)-the first FDA-approved nanodrug: Lessons learned," *J. Controlled Release*, 160(1), pp. 117–134.

Bawa, R. and Johnson, S. (2007) "The ethical dimensions of nanomedicine," *The Medical Clinics of North America*, 91(5), pp. 881–887. doi: 10.1016/j.mcna.2007.05.007.

Bregoli, L. et al. (2016) "Nanomedicine applied to translational oncology: A future perspective on cancer treatment," *Nanomedicine: Nanotechnology, Biology, and Medicine*, 12(1), pp. 81–103. doi: 10.1016/j.nano.2015.08.006.

Choi, Y. H. and Han, H.-K. (2018) "Nanomedicines: Current status and future perspectives in aspect of drug delivery and pharmacokinetics," *Journal of Pharmaceutical Investigation*, 48(1), pp. 43–60. doi: 10.1007/s40005-017-0370-4.

D'Mello, S. R. et al. (2017) "The evolving landscape of drug products containing nanomaterials in the United States," *Nature Nanotechnology*, 12(6), pp. 523–529. doi: 10.1038/nnano.2017.67.

Foulkes, R. et al. (2020) "The regulation of nanomaterials and nanomedicines for clinical application: Current and future perspectives," *Biomaterials Science*, 8(17), pp. 4653–4664. doi: 10.1039/d0bm00558d.

Global Nanopharmaceutical Drugs Market: Focus on nanodrugs and its application in therapeutics, competitive landscape, and country—analysis and forecast (2018–2026) (no date) *ReportLinker.* Available at: www.reportlinker.com/p05644015 (Accessed: April 28, 2023).

Juliano, R. L. (2012) "The future of nanomedicine: Promises and limitations," *Science & Public Policy*, 39(1), pp. 99–104. doi: 10.3152/030234212x13214603531969.

Malviya, R. et al. (2021) "Commercial utilities and future perspective of nanomedicines," *PeerJ*, 9(e12392), p. e12392. doi: 10.7717/peerj.12392.

McGoron, A. J. (2020) "Perspectives on the future of nanomedicine to impact patients: An analysis of US federal funding and interventional clinical trials," *Bioconjugate Chemistry*, 31(3), pp. 436–447. doi: 10.1021/acs.bioconjchem.9b00818.

Metselaar, J. M. and Lammers, T. (2020) "Challenges in nanomedicine clinical translation," *Drug Delivery and Translational Research*, 10(3), pp. 721–725. doi: 10.1007/s13346-020-00740-5.

Moghimi, S. M., Hunter, A. C. and Murray, J. C. (2005) "Nanomedicine: Current status and future prospects," *FASEB Journal: Official Publication of the Federation of American Societies for Experimental Biology*, 19(3), pp. 311–330. doi: 10.1096/fj.04-2747rev.

Nordmann, A. and Rip, A. (2009) "Mind the gap revisited," *Nature Nanotechnology*, 4(5), pp. 273–274. doi: 10.1038/nnano.2009.26.

Sakamoto, J. H. et al. (2010) "Enabling individualized therapy through nanotechnology," *Pharmacological Research: The Official Journal of the Italian Pharmacological Society*, 62(2), pp. 57–89. doi: 10.1016/j.phrs.2009.12.011.

Sarmento, B. (2019) "Have nanomedicines progressed as much as we'd hoped for in drug discovery and development? *Expert Opin. Drug Discovery*, 14(8), pp. 723–725.

Shi, Y. et al. (2022) "The future of nanomedicine," in *Nanomedicine*. Singapore: Springer Nature Singapore, pp. 1–28.

Thapa, R. K. and Kim, J. O. (2023) "Nanomedicine-based commercial formulations: Current developments and future prospects," *Journal of Pharmaceutical Investigation*, 53(1), pp. 19–33. doi: 10.1007/s40005-022-00607-6.

Van Der Meel, R., Lammers, T. and Hennink, W. E. (2017) "Cancer nanomedicines: Oversold or underappreciated? *Expert Opin. Drug Delivery*, 14(1), pp. 1–5.

Venkatraman, S. (2014) "Has nanomedicine lived up to its promise?," *Nanotechnology*, 25(37), p. 372501. doi: 10.1088/0957-4484/25/37/372501.

Zhang, C. et al. (2020) "Progress, challenges, and future of nanomedicine," *Nano Today*, 35(101008), p. 101008. doi: 10.1016/j.nantod.2020.101008.

Index

For Product Safety Concerns and Information please contact our EU
representative GPSR@taylorandfrancis.com
Taylor & Francis Verlag GmbH, Kaufingerstraße 24, 80331 München, Germany

www.ingramcontent.com/pod-product-compliance
Lightning Source LLC
Chambersburg PA
CBHW070715220326
41598CB00024BA/3171